The Pericardium

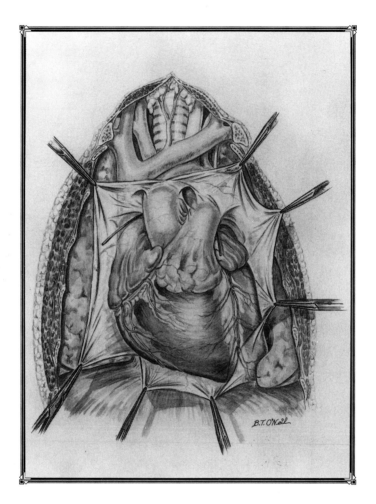

The opened normal pericardium and heart in situ. The epicardial mesothelium is transparent; the parietal pericardium–mesothelium and fibrosa– is translucent. A curved probe is in the pericardial tranverse sinus (see also Figures 2.1 and 2.3). (From Spodick, Acute Pericarditis, 1959; author's copyright.)

The Pericardium
A Comprehensive Textbook

David H. Spodick, M.D., D.Sc.,
F.A.C.C., F.C.C.P., F.A.C.P.

Professor of Medicine
University of Massachusetts Medical School;
Director of Clinical Cardiology
and Cardiovascular Fellowship Training
Saint Vincent Hospital
Worcester, Massachusetts

Marcel Dekker, Inc.
New York•Basel•Hong Kong

Library of Congress Cataloging-in-Publication Data

Spodick, David H.
  The pericardium : a comprehensive textbook / David H. Spodick.
    p. cm. — (Fundamental and clinical cardiology ; v. 27)
  Includes index.
  ISBN: 0-8247-9316-1 (hardcover : alk. paper)
  1. Pericardium—Diseases. I. Title. II. Series.
[DNLM: 1. Pericardium. 2. Pericarditis. W1 FU538TD v.27 1997 /
WG 275 S762p 1997]
RC685.P5S725 1997
616.1'1—dc20
DNLM/DLC
for Library of Congress   96-43173
                                                        CIP

The publisher offers discounts on this book when ordered in bulk quantities. For more information, write to Special Sales/Professional Marketing at the address below.

This book is printed on acid-free paper.

Marcel Dekker, Inc.
270 Madison Avenue, New York, New York 10016

Current printing (last digit):
10 9 8 7 6 5 4 3 2 1

PRINTED IN THE UNITED STATES OF AMERICA

To Carolyn,
for her love and care and her support and forbearance
while this book was being written.

Preface

"Pericardiology" is a term that might express concisely the comprehensive scope of this book. I used it to name a course at Heart House, headquarters of the American College of Cardiology in Bethesda. Indeed, this book attempts to express the fruit of an exceptional personal exposure to pericardial disease in the context of recent advances in medical and surgical diagnosis and therapy and in physiology, immunology and oncology and infectious, metabolic and traumatic diseases. It relies extensively on the work of others as well as personal clinical and laboratory observations, formal investigations and publications.

AUTOBIOGRAPHICAL EXCURSUS AS PREFACE

I am often asked: "How did you get so interested in pericardial disease?" The answer is that it was inevitable, given extraordinary opportunities to diagnose, manage and investigate pericardial disorders, coupled with a deep personal interest in physiology and bedside medicine. I hope readers will forgive me for expanding on this answer in highly personal, indeed autobiographical, terms.

As a junior house officer, I saw sporadic cases of pericardial disease and a few weeks of what must have been a small enterovirus epidemic in England while I was with the U.S. Air Force Medical Service. As a senior resident at New England Medical Center, I had two patients with severe tuberculous pericarditis, one with cardiac tamponade that resolved after pericardiocentesis and another with tamponade followed by accelerated effusive-constrictive pericarditis. Inspired by a consummate teacher, Louis Selverstone, I became fascinated with tamponade physiology and plotted these patients' venous pressures and roentgenographic responses to the disease and its treatment. In both cases, increasing venous pressure fell dramatically after pericardial drainage, along with shrinking of the cardiopericardial silhouette. However, though the less fortunate second patient maintained his newly reduced heart shadow, within days the venous pressure reascended, an abnormal third heart sound appeared and he required pericardiectomy. After a search at the Boston Medical Library, I published these cases with an exhaustive literature review. This also stimulated two publications in the Bulletin of Tufts–New England Medical Center: "Observations in Cardiac Tamponade: Physiological Considerations" and "Pain Mechanisms in Pericardial Disease." Later, first as a cardiology resident and then as a Special Postdoctoral Fellow of the National Heart Institute under David Littmann, my treatment of a succession of tamponaded patients led to publication of a small series on electrical alternation. Thereafter, during my 19 years at the Lemuel Shattuck Hospital, the original patient population provided a veritable pericardial pandemic. Cases were varied, frequently complicated, and numerous owing to very large specialized units including chest disease, rheumatology, oncology, radiation therapy and renal dialysis, in addition to the other in- and outpatient services of a large hospital. My private affiliation at neighboring Faulkner Hospital extended these opportunities to observe, manage and consult on additional patients.

Pericardial disease on the rheumatology service varied from subclinical to severe; our Chief Resident, Edward Cathcart, and I published, in the *New England Journal of Medicine*, a case-control study demonstrating rheumatoid heart disease in 254 cases and 254 matched control subjects; among the cases, 6 had clinical pericarditis while 6 of 15 autopsies revealed rheumatoid pericarditis— a proportion comparable to other series and consistent with this common but usually clinically silent lesion. Pericardial disease was nearly always dramatic on the oncology service, with typically large to massive effusions and frequent electrical alternation (duly published). Along with radiation therapy, some malignancies also produced classic and occasionally elastic constriction, as well as effusive-constrictive pericarditis (also reported). Nephrology provided frequent acute uremic and infectious pericarditis in all their clinical and hemodynamic phases and later the new, recalcitrant "dialysis pericarditis," while improved survival now permitted the emergence of occasional uremic constriction. Urgent pericardiocentesis was required when new patients' first dialyses rapidly decreased blood volume, precipitating previously compensated or occult cardiac tamponade.

This pericardial pandemic inspired my first book, *Acute Pericarditis*, followed by *Chronic and Constrictive Pericarditis*. It also permitted large, prospectively acquired series describing and codifying the variety of electrocardiographic and acoustic phenomena in uncomplicated acute pericarditis and documenting the apparent absence of significant arrhythmias. During a College of Physicians scholarship as visiting colleague at St. George's Hospital, I repeatedly visited several London hospitals and clinics to see ordinary and unusual cases of pericardial disease.

A meeting on pericardial disease at the University of Kentucky, directed by Ralph Shabetai, gave me an opportunity to organize my large accumulation of historical material on the pericardium and its diseases, with idiomatic translations from ancient Greek and Latin graciously provided by the professors of the classics at Harvard and Boston universities. This was published in the *American Journal of Cardiology* (then the College's official publication) as "The Hairy Hearts of Hoary Heroes" and later amplified in a chapter contributed to Noble Fowler's superb book *The Pericardium in Health and Disease*. Meanwhile, advances in the microanatomy and macro- and microphysiology and chemistry of the pericardium, accompanied by expanding clinical experience, warranted a new book. In dread of the effort required to do another single-author work, I co-opted 27 other authors and edited *Pericardial Diseases*, which was selected by the American College of Physicians as one of 70 recommended books.

At the Saint Vincent and other core hospitals affiliated with the University of Massachusetts, I have opportunities to continue to observe, manage and consult on many patients with a variety of acute, subacute, chronic and recurrent pericardial diseases. This resulted in publications that include the following topics: procainamide-induced lupus with rapid pericardial constriction; measurement of atrial natriuretic factor (ANF) before and immediately after pericardiectomy for constriction; frequency of atypical ECG changes in acute pericarditis; and 24-hour ECG (Holter) monitoring in 50 consecutive patients with acute pericarditis, the results of which—no significant arrhythmias in the absence of heart disease—confirmed both consistent clinical experience and a 100-patient series from a monitored unit at the Lemuel Shattuck Hospital.

Finally, as a "born again" echocardiographer, my daily task of directly observing cardiac anatomy and physiology "in action" amplified my experiences in pericardiology and made further investigations inevitable. One investigation showed that even small effusions that never cause clinical tamponade could significantly exaggerate respiratory effects on the heart, as demonstrated by the precise and sensitive, though relatively nonspecific, systolic time intervals; this was later confirmed by hemodynamicists and became incorporated in P. S. Reddy's concept of tamponade as "not all or none."

A new, comprehensive book seems warranted not only by my progressive personal experience, but also by particular advances in our understanding of normal and abnormal pericardial physiology, immunology, effusion and tamponade and improved imaging methods for effusion and constriction. These advances include notable contributions by Fowler, Shabetai, Reddy, Klopfenstein,

Friedman, Sarnoff, LeWinter, Tyberg, Hancock, Maisch, and Maruyama as well as the astute clinical observations of Soler, Permanyer, Bayes, Millaire and my friend and colleague Abdul Hakim Khan. In striving for comprehensiveness, I have sought to incorporate the vast clinical, hemodynamic, investigative and experimental work on the normal and diseased pericardium by cardiac and medical clinicians, surgeons, anatomists, physiologists, nephrologists, anesthesiologists, intensivists and traumatologists in the light of a lifetime's clinical and investigative activity, published and unpublished. An extensive experience with the most difficult current problem, recurrent and incessant pericarditis, continues among patients (some of them physicians) referred from the United States and other countries by physicians trying to cope with the most stubborn and frustrating forms of pericardial disease.

ACKNOWLEDGMENTS

This work relied heavily on silent and active collaborators at Saint Vincent Hospital—Maureen Smith, Linda Duffy and their director, Joan Yanicke of the Dumphy Medical Library, and on illustrations supplied over the years by Jane Griesbach, medical artist-photographer (who must work a 25-hour day) and her assistant, Charlene Baron. Pathologist Henry Soto graciously analyzed organs and tissue specimens. The collaboration of numerous house officers, medical students and cardiac fellows at the Lemuel Shattuck and Saint Vincent Hospitals (many of whom are my coauthors and often first authors of journal articles) was indispensable for numerous personal investigations and publications, including several very large prospective series, characterizing certain aspects of pericardial disease like electrocardiography and auscultatory phenomena, epistenocardiac pericarditis, and the unexplained high incidence of left-sided pleural effusion in acute pericarditis. All such collaborators were equally essential to advising me of cases at our own and other hospitals and in publishing smaller series and reports of cases of clinical and physiologic significance. To all the foregoing, I am endlessly grateful.

Contents

PART III.   ETIOLOGIC AND PATHOGENETIC FORMS OF
         PERICARDIAL DISEASE

The Pericardium

1

Perspectives: The Pericardium in Health and Disease

ORGANIZATION AND OBJECTIVES OF THIS BOOK

This work is the outgrowth of a professional lifetime's commitment to the pericardium in health and disease. It attempts to present the gamut of pericardial conditions by pathogenesis, diagnosis and treatment, introduced by basic descriptions of normal and abnormal pericardial anatomy, physiology and response patterns to virtually every kind of disease. Indeed, it would be only faintly facetious to assert: "Everything causes pericardial disease." That variety is only one of its many attractive and instructive aspects.

The text proper is designed to cover the spectrum of pericardial disease in appropriate depth for comprehensive understanding and clinical usefulness, with special emphasis on the most frequent forms and complications. Some less common conditions, like cholesterol pericarditis, are covered in disproportionate detail because of extensive clinical and laboratory investigations which shed light on other conditions. Tables and diagrams are designed to reinforce the essential points, while inclusively covering each important area. Rarely, details deliberately omitted from the text appear in tables. Some schemata better outlined by tabulation are mentioned in the text but detailed in tables. For example, every verified echo-Doppler sign of cardiac tamponade and constriction is tabulated, while the text covers nearly all of them. On the other hand, current understanding of the macrophysiology of tamponade is schematized and that of pulsus paradoxus diagrammed comprehensively. At the end of each chapter is a list, entitled "Key Points," recapitulating the chapter's highlights and selected "pearls."

To avoid literary excess baggage, phrases like "It has been shown" are usually omitted (any demonstrably valid result has indeed "been shown"). Only the results of experimental work are included, with only selective mention of methodology, despite its importance. Examples include Fowler's and Shabetai's brilliantly conceived classic investigations showing pulsus paradoxus to depend on right heart filling in inspiration; when changes in right ventricular volume during breathing are prevented, pulsus paradoxus cannot occur. Another example is the characterization of pericardial rubs in detail by phase structure, location, breathing behavior and palpability, without giving the details of simultaneous phonocardiography and auscultation by three mutually blinded observers in a 100-patient prospective study. Normal and tamponade physiology are presented intensively without discussing the relative merits of pericardial pressure measurement by catheter versus flat balloon. Finally, the text omits the rich history of pericardial investigation from Richard Lower in the 17th century and Cohnheim in the 19th century through the consistently brilliant work of 20th-century clinicians and physiologists.

LOGIC OF ORGANIZATION: CHAPTER SEQUENCE

Most chapters are self-contained monographs that can be read by themselves. Indeed, only novels, biographies, histories and detective stories are best read "linearly" from cover to cover because of inescapable time sequences. Textbooks are only so read by conscientious reviewers who can then detect "overlap" and "repetitiveness"; here, both are deliberately included because comprehensive presentation of some conditions makes overlap and repetition unavoidable—although only to an extent that seems absolutely necessary to keep chapters independent as well as interdependent. Frequent references to other chapters, tables, figures and particular pages emphasize interdependence.

The text is designed to deal with the concerns of cardiologists, internists, surgeons, rheumatologists, intensivists, anesthesiologists, traumatologists and, of course, anyone else who wishes to seek breadth and depth in its subjects. The first seven chapters present the fundamentals, including clinical fundamentals, of the pericardium and its disorders in the widest sense. Chapter 14, "Noneffusive Sequelae of Pericardial Inflammation," was moved from this section to juxtapose it to Chapter 15, "Constrictive Pericarditis," because the noneffusive sequelae are mostly cicatricial and adhesive. It is therefore within the group from Chapters 8 through 15, which is designed "Clinical Pericardial Disease." Chapters 16 through 25, "Etiologic and Pathogenetic Forms of Pericardial Disease," omit congenital disease, which is discussed in Chapter 6. The final two chapters, "Recurrent and Incessant Pericarditis" and "Chronic Pericardial Effusion and Chronic Tamponade," present some of the less common but diagnostically and especially therapeutically more troublesome conditions. Although most treatises on pericarditis place "idiopathic pericarditis" early, here it will be found near the end. Ultimately, nothing is idiopathic, and while a great many cases never have clear etiologic proof, diagnostic advances are continually reducing this category. Therapeutic advances should increase the need for specific diagnoses by providing more specific treatment, as in viral diseases.

DELIBERATE ASYMMETRY

Although I hope all subjects are covered comprehensively and in sufficient depth, one role of this book is as a clinical guide and vade mecum. Since every physician uses a stethoscope, auscultation is concentrated in Chapter 4, as well as being included as appropriate to each form of pericardial disease. Independent, detailed exposition is also give to electrocardiography (ECG) (Chapter 5) because it is a test that is widely familiar and often at least basically understood among physicians of all kinds. Furthermore, on a practical level, certain major as well as finer points of ECG that are important in pericardial diseases tend to get missed by most current computer programs. Because thrombolysis has provoked hemopericardium in patients misdiagnosed as having acute infarction, there is heavy emphasis on "diagnostic" EGCs as well as typical and atypical variants with many illustrations.

There is also strong emphasis on echo-Doppler diagnosis (distributed among appropriate chapters), because it is usually the most readily available efficient and cost-effective imaging method and it dynamically illustrates both pathophysiology and anatomy in cardiac tamponade and constriction. Indeed, echocardiography has revolutionized diagnosis. Its details are more familiar to the nonradiologist than those of magnetic resonance imaging (MRI) and computed tomography (CT)—although these are included here. Thus, MRI and CT are less emphasized but detailed in the compressive pericardial disorders because detection of fluid and recognition of tissue and fluid textures by CT and MRI are more certain than for many pericardial "thickenings" demonstrated by transthoracic and even transesophageal echocardiography. Yet, MRI and CT present considerable logistical problems, especially during emergencies. Spectral and color Doppler, moreover, are well suited to pathphysiologic analysis. Thus, for example, echo-Doppler study can be critically time- (read "life-") saving for patients with aortic dissection or intramural hematoma. Chest x-ray evidence is described but, except for pericardial calcifications, is mainly nonspecific, even when chest films—as they frequently do—give initial clues to pericardial disease. Finally, traumatic (including surgical) pericardial disease has been relatively neglected in the nonsurgical literature, although cardiopericardial traumata have become frequent. Consequently, these forms are included in some detail.

Deliberate asymmetry also complements what I trust is the creative redundancy mentioned earlier, because overlapping conditions demand appropriately overlapping presentation, while clinical importance and the extent of significant information compel proportionately broad and deep presentation. Thus, tamponade physiology is integrated with its clinical characteristics, diagnosis and treatment (Chapter 11), while its pathophysiology is detailed in the context of clinical considerations (Chapter 12). Chapter 13 describes and analyzes pulsus paradoxus, which must be understood for itself as well as in connection with the preceding two chapters and to explain its customary absence in pericardial constriction (Chapter 15). Each of these chapters can stand alone because of deliberate overlap. On the other hand, their instructional and practical value deepens by reading them seriatim.

CATEGORIZATION/CLASSIFICATION OF PERICARDIAL DISORDERS

Many clinical conditions might be described with equal accuracy under more than one rubric or pathogenesis. For example, pericarditides in most of the vasculitis–connective tissue disease group (Chapter 19), particularly the recurrent forms, have strong immunopathic features. This is true also of the postcardiac injury syndrome(s). Thus, the post–myocardial infarction (Dressler's) syndrome can be catalogued both with infarct pericarditis and with post-pericardiotomy syndrome or post–cardiac injury syndromes because of common features. Similarly, hepatitis B and polyarteritis each cause pericarditis. However, there is a form of hepatitis B that includes a variant of polyarteritis; pericarditis can be described under either or both. Systemic lupus erythematosus (SLE) is a multisystem autoimmune vasculitic disease frequently causing pericarditis; SLE pericarditis may also be caused by certain drugs, yielding related but pathogenetically and prognostically different categories. Finally, an expanding number of pericardial disorders could come under the specific rubric "iatrogenic," many of them traumatic or drug-related. Since "iatrogenic" must be a catchall, such "diseases of medical progress" are mainly presented where they appear to fit most characteristically.

Pericardial involvements attributed to diseases of rare etiology and unusual pathogenesis are included where the evidence appeared strong enough to consider them verified. However, coincidence of a rare and a common disease, for example, infectious or even neoplastic pericarditis in a patient with rheumatoid arthritis—approximately half of whom have evidence of pericarditis at autopsy and many have asymptomatic pericardial effusions—may account for individual case reports. Consequently, in many cases, it is difficult clinically to rule in or out any apparent etiology. For example, I diagnosed neoplastic effusive-constrictive pericarditis in a patient with breast cancer; at operation, pericardial tissue was free of cancer and typical of rheumatoid scarring. However, even pathologic evidence can be inconclusive. For example, finding a dracuncular worm in constrictive pericardial tissue made this organism a plausible but not absolutely proven cause.

REFERENCES

In this volume, unlike my previous books, specific references have been omitted for individual facts and investigative results, so that the reader must necessarily concede the benefit of the doubt for both knowledge and bona fides. I hope the reader can trust me to have included adequate references to original work in the list completing each chapter, among which some books and extended reviews also appear. Indeed, in this day of ready recourse to computer searches, the literature on any subject can be exhaustively accessed quite rapidly. Even some individual case reports have been included to the extent that the presentation is convincing and seems to make valid points (case reports, after all, are the "salt and pepper" of medicine). On the other hand, an example of a durable anecdotal hand-me-down is the report of a sword swallower who perforated his esophagus and with it his pericardium. Pericardial, not to mention esophageal, wounds must be rare in the small community of sword swallowers or it would go out of business. I have not been able to verify this reference, now over a century old, to check the original publication, which has been cited in many reports.

STATISTICS

Diagnosis and differential diagnosis depend on understanding probabilities. Understanding probabilities will not make a good poker player or diagnostician, but disregarding them makes a bad one. However, in most pericardial disease, the remarkably imprecise statistical base continues to make most exact numbers misleading. Because of this, precise incidences and percentages of certain findings are avoided in favor of qualitative descriptors like "frequent," "occasional" or "rare." This is mainly because there are few reports of adequate-sized series without considerable ascertainment biases. For example, institutions with large oncology services report high percentages of pericardial effusions to be large as well as malignant. Similarly, pericardial effusion in acquired immunodeficiency syndrome (AIDS) is given as from 16 to 63% of patients in seven series, inner-city hospitals being responsible for the high range. Finally, lupus pericarditis is reported in between 7 and 50% of all systemic lupus erythematosus, while various recent series of Coxsackie virus disease report between 4 and 43% of cases to have pericarditis—each much too wide a spread to usefully tabulate, while metaanalyses are impossible. Moreover, contemporary diagnostic methods are much swifter and surer than even those of one or two decades ago, leading to earlier recognition and treatment of many conditions, which invalidates previous case mixes, frequencies of symptoms and signs (contaminated in the past by those due to complications) and exact incidences of vanishing complications like pericardial calcifications. Therefore, the descriptors I used are judgmental, based on personal experience and acquaintance with the literature. Again, I must beg the benefit of the doubt for both experience and judgment.

APPROACHES TO EMPHASIS AND TEACHING POINTS

I have employed various methods to emphasize certain points and also facilitate for readers the location of the information on the same page or elsewhere. These include liberal use of *italics*, which not only stress the fundamental points but should "spring from the page," making it easier to locate and review certain subjects, diseases or processes. There is also liberal parenthetic reference to other pages and chapters that touch or elaborate on comparable subjects. This is also the role of tables and subheads; the latter, along with illustrations and diagrams, not only concentrate the salient points but also, I trust, serve to break up solid blocks of text, making reading easier.

Finally, I hope that readers, while finding this book informative and useful, will derive some of the same pleasure I have had in investigating and practicing amid the remarkable spectrum of normal and abnormal pericardial physiology and anatomy and the clinical, graphic and pathophysiologic expressions of pericardial disease.

2

Pericardial Macro- and Microanatomy: A Synopsis

The pericardium is macro- and microanantomically specialized to serve its relatively complex passive and active normal functions. Grossly, there are two pericardial layers, the *serosa* and the *fibrosa*, with appropriate nerves, blood vessels and lymphatics (Frontispiece; Figure 2.1). The serosa is a complete sac lined by mesothelial cells attached by loose connective tissue to the heart surfaces, the juxtacardiac great vessels and the inner aspect of the fibrosa, lying on these structures like a collapsed plastic bag. It contains 15 to 35 ml of serous pericardial fluid, an ultrafiltrate of the blood plasma. This mesothelial sac is clasped externally by the fibrosa, which continues superiorly an average of 6 cm above the aortic root and over the arch of the aorta, where it blends with the deep cervical fascia. However, the fibrosa itself is not a true sac, although it is closed by firm attachment of its projections, which accompany the serosa over the proximal great vessels. It is loosely anchored by *ligaments* to the manubrium and xiphoid process of the sternum and more firmly attached to the central tendon of the diaphragm. The monocellular serosa directly covering the heart surfaces is the *visceral pericardium*, also called "*the epicardium*" (Figure 2.2). The fibrosa together with the reflections of the serosal sac internally attached to it is the *parietal pericardium*, also referred to simply and confusingly as "*the pericardium.*" The parietal pericardium varies in thickness between 1 and 3.5 mm due to variations in the fibrosa. Ultramicroscopic pores have been discovered between the pericardium and the adjacent pleura in some species.

7

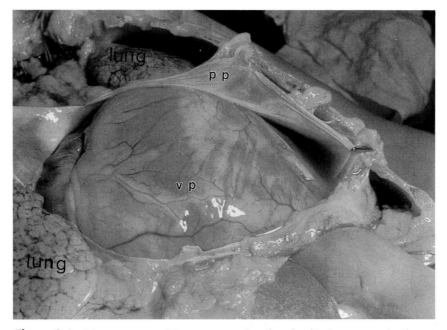

Figure 2.1 Macroanatomy of the normal pericardium in situ (sternum and adjacent ribs removed). PP = parietal pericardium composed of *fibrosa* lined by mesothelial *serosa* continuous with the serosa of the visceral pericardium (VP), thus lining the entire pericardial sac. The serosa is transparent, as seen on the visceral pericardium, which glistens but permits full visualization of all heart surfaces. Because of the tough outer fibrosa, the normal parietal pericardium (PP) is only translucent. (Inflammation and its consequences can render it opaque.) Proximity of the lungs (labeled), pleural cavities and rib cage is evident.

THE PERICARDIAL SINUSES, RECESSES AND RESERVE VOLUME

The pericardial "cavity" is a nonuniform, mainly potential space. During life, most of the normal fluid is undetectable except in the major sinuses (Figure 2.3) and in the atrioventricular grooves. Behind the proximal ascending aorta and pulmonary artery and in front of the atria and superior vena cava is a short, serosa-lined pericardial passage, the *transverse sinus*, where the serosa encloses the terminal portions of the venae cavae and the pulmonary veins with separate recesses surrounding one-third to two-thirds of the circumference of the proximal pulmonary artery. Posteriorly, it forms an inverted U, framing a pericardial projection posteriorly, the *oblique sinus*. At the level of the tracheal bifurcation, the serosal *superior sinus* clasps the ascending aorta. In addition to these major sinuses, computed tomographic scans disclose numerous smaller

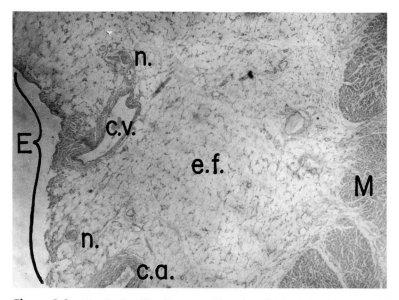

Figure 2.2   The "epicardium": serosa (E), epicardial fat (ef) with nerves (n), a coronary arteriole (ca) and a coronary vein (CV). M = myocardium. (From Spodick, Acute Pericarditis, 1959; author's copyright.)

recesses not easily detected at surgical or postmortem examination. Taken together with the pericardial sinuses, these recesses increase the pericardial capacity to accommodate increased fluid (or other contents) and contribute to the *pericardial reserve volume* (Figure 3.1).

THE MESOTHELIUM

The serosal mesothelial cells tend to interdigitate and overlap, maintaining mechanical stability or permitting changes in surface configuration. Projecting *microvilli* (Figure 2.4) presumably reduce friction and facilitate exchange of fluid and ions; relatively perpendicular in systole, they become oblique during diastole. Proteinaceous *cystoskeletal filaments* include *keratins* for structural support and *actin filaments* that appear to be involved in cellular shape changes. A basal lamina underlies the mesothelium but is not strongly adhesive, so that serosal cells easily fall off with even gentle handling at surgery or necropsy.

THE FIBROSA

The fibrosa is mainly fibrocollagenous tissue that is wavy in youth and progressively straightens during aging (Figure 2.5). *Elastic fibers*, numerous early in

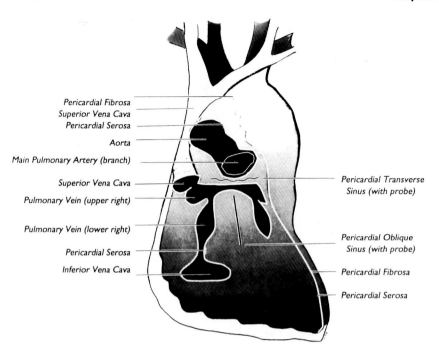

Pericardial Fibrosa
Superior Vena Cava
Pericardial Serosa
Aorta
Main Pulmonary Artery (branch)
Superior Vena Cava
Pulmonary Vein (upper right)
Pulmonary Vein (lower right)
Pericardial Serosa
Inferior Vena Cava

Pericardial Transverse
Sinus (with probe)

Pericardial Oblique
Sinus (with probe)

Pericardial Fibrosa

Pericardial Serosa

Figure 2.3   Schema of the pericardial sinuses. Probe in transverse sinus.

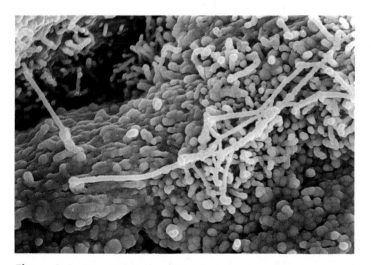

Figure 2.4   Mesothelium: scanning electron micrograph showing microvilli.

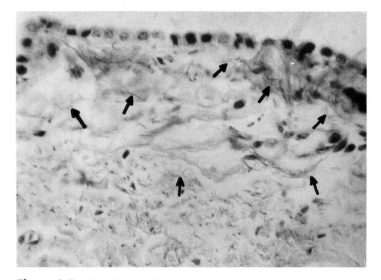

Figure 2.5 The fibrosa. Elastic tissue stain showing the single layer of mesothelial cells (here, cuboidal) and elastic fibers (arrows). (From Spodick, Acute Pericarditis, 1959; author's copyright.)

life, become less densely distributed with aging; they are mainly *elastin*, an extracellular protein with stress-strain characteristics like rubber. The pericardial fibrous tissue (Figure 2.6) is arranged in *fascicular bundles* that are thicker over the thinner parts of the heart (e.g., the right ventricle) except the left atrium, which is tightly clasped by a denser fibrosal mesh. Their seemingly purposeful organization appears to be determined by mechanical factors, particularly external traction forces like respiratory movements and internal pressures from changes in the heart transmitted through the pericardial fluid. As they extend over the aortic arch, the fibers become parallel and virtually ligamentous, seemingly to support the proximal aorta and arch against the thrust of blood ejecting from the left ventricle. However, pericardial collagenous tissue may not be continuous at points of reflection from the great vessels, a weakness that can permit air and fluids to dissect along the perivascular sheaths and enter the pericardial space (see page 87).

NERVES, ARTERIES, LYMPHATICS AND LYMPH NODES

The *phrenic nerves* course downward over the anterior parietal pericardium and supply most of it. (They must be protected during cardiac and pericardial sur-

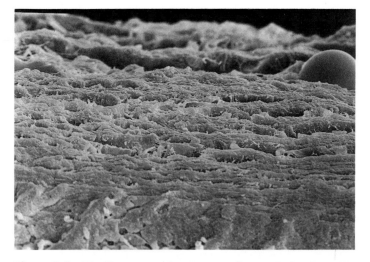

Figure 2.6   The fibrosa: scanning electron micrograph showing collagenous fascicles.

gery.) *Vagal* supply to the posterior pericardium is via the esophageal plexus. Parietal pericardial *lymphatics* drain to corresponding anterior and posterior mediastinal nodes, while the superficial plexus of cardiac lymphatics drains the visceral pericardium to the tracheal and brachial mediastinal lymph nodes. Usually one or two *lymph nodes* lie within the fibrosa near the inferior vena cava orifice. Finally, the pericardial *arterial supply* comes from small aortic twigs posteriorly, with the internal thoracic (internal mammary) arteries perfusing its superior, lateral and inferior portions. Of surgical and echo-doppler importance, in a significant number of people the left superior and inferior pulmonary veins join to form a common trunk in the pericardium.

SUBEPICARDIAL FAT AND CONNECTIVE TISSUE

Between the cardiac surfaces and the mesothelium of the epicardium is a variable amount of connective tissue and a fat layer that increases with increasing body weight. Markedly increased epicardial fat sometimes invades the myocardium. This layer improves the capability of computed tomography and magnetic resonance imaging to delineate the pericardium, but on echocardiography can be confused with pericardial effusion. Increased epicardial fat in obese patients is only loosely related to body fat but is disproportionately increased in coronary disease; the layer undergoes *serious atrophy* in some chronic diseases, but increases with corticosteroid therapy. Whether such changes have

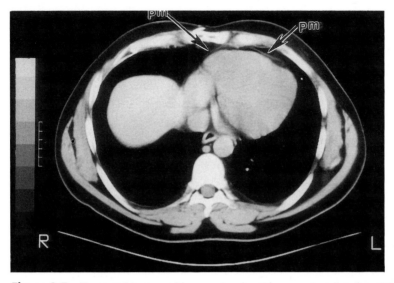

Figure 2.7 Computed tomographic scan showing thin normal pericardium ("Pm"; arrows) rendered visible by underlying epicardial fat (black lucency).

functional effects is unknown, but subepicardial fat contains a prostaglandin-like *angiogenic factor* and important parasympathetic ganglia are in its *sinoatrial fat pad* at the margin of the right atrium, superior vena cava, and right superior pulmonary vein.

OVERVIEW

The dissected normal parietal pericardium ("the pericardium") is relatively thin, (2–4 by CT), as also shown on computed tomography (Figure 2.7), and may be grossly unremarkable, yet the foregoing makes quite clear that its composition along with the visceral pericardium ("the epicardium") and their gross, microscopic and ultramicroscopic structure imply much more for cardiac function in health and disease. Moreover, pericardial susceptibility to virtually every kind of medical and surgical disease often converts it, because of its location and distribution, from a protector and physiologic facilitator of the heart to that organ's bad neighbor.

KEY POINTS

1. Major pericardial components: mesothelial *serosa*, a sac clasped by fibrocollagenous *fibrosa* and projected over proximal great vessels.

2. Collagenous and elastic tissues of fibrosa functionally organized.
3. Pericardial recesses and sinuses contribute to *pericardial reserve volume*, accommo-
    dating modest increases over the normal 15 to 35 mL of pericardial fluid.
4. Both *phrenic nerves* course through anterior pericardium, with clinical and surgical
    consequences.

BIBLIOGRAPHY

Gray H. Anatomy of the Human Body, 24th ed. Lewis, W.H. (ed.). Philadelphia: Lea
    & Febiger, 1946, pp. 522–524.
Spodick, D.H. Macro- and micro-physiology and anatomy of the pericardium. Am. Heart
    J. 1992; 124:1046–1051.
Spodick, D.H. Diseases of the pericardium. In: Parmley, W.W., and Chatterjee, K.
    (eds.). Cardiology. Vol. 2. Philadelphia: Lippincott, 1988, chap. 43.
Spodick, D.H. Acute Pericarditis. New York: Grune & Stratton, 1959, chap. 1.

3

Physiology of the Normal Pericardium: Functions of the Pericardium

Table 3.1 summarizes of the role of the pericardium in health based on clinical and experimental observations.

Physical Effects of the Pericardium

Purely mechanical and physical effects belong mainly to the parietal pericardium, while chemical agents are produced by the serosal mesothelium of both layers. *The normal parietal pericardium retracts when it is incised, indicating that it is under some stress.* Indeed, the pericardium contributes to resting intracavitary diastolic pressure. Moreover, by exerting a stress (magnified by any increase in pericardial fluid pressure), normal pericardium restricts overall heart filling with a much greater effect on thinner parts, especially the right ventricle and atrium, which probably depend on pericardial constraint for much of their normal cavitary pressures and dimensions. (After pericardiectomy, right ventricular size increases.) The pericardium also helps limit acute cavitary overdistension following ruptured papillary muscle, acute pulmonary embolism or acute myocarditis; by this mechanism it also appears to limit the stroke volume response to exercise in patients with cardiomegaly and chronic heart failure.

Pericardial responses to the foregoing are not homogeneous because the pericardium is *anisotropic*, due to interlacing and layering of its fibrosal fibers

Table 3.1 **Functions of the Normal Pericardium**

Mechanical functions: Promotion of cardiac efficiency, especially during hemodynamic overloads.

I. **Relatively inelastic cardiac envelope.**
    A. Maintenance of normal ventricular compliance (volume-elasticity relation).
    B. Defense of the integrity of any Starling curve: Starling mechanism operates uniformly at all intraventricular pressures because presence of pericardium
        1. Maintains ventricular function curves.
        2. Limits effect of increased left ventricular end-diastolic pressure.
        3. Supports output responses to:
            a. Venous inflow loads and atrioventricular valve regurgitation (particularly when acute).
            b. Rate fluctuations.
        4. Hydrostatic system (pericardium plus pericardial fluid) distributes hydrostatic forces over epicardial surfaces.
            a. Favors equality of transmural end-diastolic pressure throughout ventricle, therefore uniform stretch of muscle fibers (preload).
            b. Constantly compensates for changes in gravitational and inertial forces, distributing them evenly around the heart.
    C. Limitation of excessive acute dilation.
    D. Protection against excessive ventriculoatrial regurgitation (atrial support).
    E. Ventricular interaction: relative pericardial stiffness
        1. Provides a mutually restrictive chamber favoring balanced output from right and left ventricles integrated over several cardiac cycles.
        2. Permits either ventricle to generate greater isovolumic pressure from any volume.
        3. Reduces ventricular compliance with increased pressure in the opposite ventricle (e.g., limits right ventricular stroke work during increased impedance to left ventricular outflow).
    F. Maintenance of functionally optimal cardiac shape.
II. **Provision of closed chamber with slightly subatmospheric pressure in which:**
    A. The level of transmural cardiac pressures will be low, relative to even large increases in "filling pressures" referred to atmospheric pressure.
    B. Pressure changes aid atrial filling via more negative pericardial pressure during ventricular ejection.
III. **"Feedback" cardiocirculatory regulation via pericardial servomechanisms**
    A. Neuroreceptors detect lung inflation and (via vagus): alter heart rate and blood pressure.
    B. Mechanoreceptors: Lower blood pressure and contract spleen.
IV. **??Limitation of hypertrophy associated with chronic exercise**

Membranous functions
I. **Reduction of external friction due to heart movements.**
    A. Production of pericardial fluid.
    B. Generation of phospholipid surfactants.

Table 3.1 Continued

II. **Buttressing of thinner portions of the myocardium** (reciprocal variations in parietal pericardial thickness).
    A. Atria.
    B. Right ventricle.
III. **Defensive immunologic constituents in pericardial fluid.**
IV. **Fibrinolytic activity in mesothelial lining.**
  V. **Prostacyclin (PGE2, PGI2 and eicosanoids)** released into pericardial sac in response to stretch, hypoxia and increased myocardial loading/work.
VI. **Synthesis and release of endothelin**, increased by angiotensin III stimulation.
VII. **Barrier to inflammation from contiguous structures.**

Ligamentous function
    A. Limitation of undue cardiac displacement.
    B. Modify pericardial stress/strain by limiting directions of traction of its fibers.

(Figure 2.6), to the proportion of collagen and elastic tissue over particular zones and to dynamic forces from contact with underlying chambers during the cardiac cycle such that *dynamic variations in regional pericardial shape tend to conform to the pressure-volume changes in the subjacent chamber.* For example, cyclic changes in pericardial areas over the right atrium vary reciprocally with those of the right ventricle. However, during tamponade, these become synchronized (although their amplitude is decreased). It should be emphasized that these changes are acute. *Hypervolemia exaggerates all such pericardial effects:* When cardiac volume is acutely increased by rapid fluid infusion, much of the increased ventricular diastolic pressure is borne by the pericardium, which ensures only a minimal change in diastolic ventricular transmural pressures (page 21), while increasing pericardial constraint. This is dramatic during volume loading in patients who have had cardiomyoplasty.

When the heart, chest and pericardium are normal and the patient is *euvolemic*, the parietal pericardium appears to have minimal direct influence on cardiac dimensions, pressures or chamber interactions. There is virtually no such effect during *hypovolemia*, probably because decreased preload and reduced heart size free the heart from restraint by both the pericardium and the cardiac fossa. For the same reason, nitroglycerin and erect posture reduce pericardial effects on the myocardium. Both chronic pericardial effusion and chronic cardiomegaly lead to stretching ("give") and hypertrophy of the parietal pericardium, increasing its compliance and decreasing its constraining effects on the heart compared to acute changes. Another component of pericardial "give" is time-dependent *creep* preceded by *stress relaxation.*

NORMAL PERICARDIAL MACROPHYSIOLOGY

At least under the conditions of operative anesthesia and sternotomy, *pericardiotomy* augments right ventricular filling and stroke volume consistent with improved systolic function, owing to the Frank-Starling relationship. Moreover, this occurs with a decrease in right atrial pressure, suggesting increased diastolic compliance. Both of these indicate "baseline" pericardial constraint of the right heart. Indeed, experimental *pericardiectomy* results in mild acute chamber dilations and chronically sometimes in myocardial hypertrophy—further evidence that *the normal pericardium subtly, but significantly, constrains the normal heart.* However, pericardial constraint accounts for most of the resting diastolic right atrial and ventricular cavity pressures and contributes substantially to those on the left. (This is well documented when a balloon transducer is used to measure epicardial radial stress.) Yet, the parietal pericardium is not needed to sustain life, as shown following its surgical removal or congenital absence (Chapter 6). However, under a variety of pathologic conditions during physiologic challenges, the pericardium has multiple effects on both cardiac function and symptom provocation. As indicated in Table 3.1, *the major functions of the pericardium—mechanical, membranous and ligamentous—*result from its macro- and microstructure (Chapter 2).

The normal parietal pericardium is tough and stiffer than cardiac muscle, although thin enough to be translucent (Figure 2.1). The relative stiffness of the parietal pericardium is also related to regional fiber orientation; i.e., more parallel fibers produce more pericardial stiffness. Its mechanical functions mainly relate to (1) its contribution to *cardiac* stiffness, (2) the effects of a chamber filled with fluid at subatmospheric pressure surrounding the heart and (3) to incompletely understood circulatory "feedback" regulation of pericardial *neuro-* and *mechanoreceptors*. On mechanical stretching, the parietal pericardium shows an initial "give" mainly due to stretching of the elastic fibers and straightening of the wavy collagen fibers of the fibrosa. Thereafter, rapidly increasing resistance to increasing stretch produces characteristic *stress-strain curves*. This response is also a principal determinant of the similar *pressure-volume curves* of intact pericardium (Figure 3.1) : both the excised tissue's curve and the intact sac's curve have a "J" shape with an initial slow rise in pressure as volume increases—and, correspondingly, of strain as stress increases—followed by a "knee" or angle, after which there is a sharp rise. With the pericardium intact, the pressure-volume curve of the ventricles is exactly parallel. Moreover, any acute *increase of pericardial fluid or of intracardiac volume tends to couple the pericardium to the heart more closely,* exaggerating this effect of the normal pericardium. *Pericardial constraint also operates during cardiac pressure loading—*e.g., acutely increased arterial or venous pressure—to limit myocardial stretch (and, hence, reduce cardiac release of

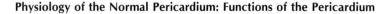

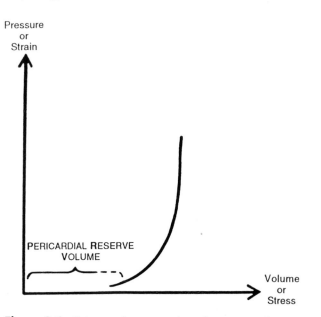

Figure 3.1 Schema of stress-strain and pressure-volume curves of the normal pericardium. After the relatively small *pericardial reserve volume* is exhausted by filling of
the pericardial sinuses and recesses, the curve at first rises gently; with continued filling at some point more acutely, the time scale and exact proportions are variable depending on the *rate of filling* of the intact pericardial sac.

atrial peptides; page 188). Removal or opening of the parietal pericardium
makes the ventricular pressure-volume curve significantly more gentle ("shift
to the right"), permitting ventricular pressure to begin to rise later, at a higher
cardiac volume, and thereafter to increase more gradually. Finally, the pericardium particularly constraints the atria, limiting both their reservoir and booster
pump functions.

Pressure-Volume Relationships (Figure 3.1)

Normal intrapericardial pressure approximates and varies with pleural pressure
during respiration: nearly always negative; extremes: –5 to +5 mm Hg. At the
earliest increase in pericardial fluid, pressure changes tend to be small due to
the *pericardial reserve volume—the volume by which the unstressed pericardium
exceeds the cardiac volume.* The pericardial reserve volume is provided by (1)
the normal slight slackness of the parietal pericardium, (2) the pericardial recesses and (3) its major sinuses: the transverse, the superior and (especially)
the oblique sinuses (Figure 2.3).

At necropsy, 100 to 200 mL of fluid will distend the normal pericardium by exceeding its reserve volume. However, with an intact heart and pericardium, during life, physiologic effects of very small increments are detectable *as long as the change is acute*; even large amounts of fluid chronically accumulated do not produce such marked effects. For example, patients with chronically enlarged hearts maintain normal intrapericardial pressure. Chronic cardiomegaly permits this due to a slow parallel increase in pericardial size. Thus, chronic increase in heart size is paced by gradual pericardial stretch. Subsequently there is *pericardial hypertrophy*; in such chronic responses, both pericardial weight and surface area increase.

The Pericardial Hydrostatic System

The pericardium plus its normal serous fluid distributes hydrostatic forces over the surface of the cardiac chambers. This favors approximation of end-diastolic transmural pressure throughout the ventricles and consequently uniform stretch of muscle fibers, tending to balance preload and permitting the apparent Frank-Starling mechanism to operate uniformly over the range of intraventricular pressures. (Note: In addition to any increased fluid pressure, *pericardial contact pressure*, measured by flat balloons rather than catheters, and not yet fully understood, may better represent the normal pericardial constraint of cardiac volume.) The pericardial hydrostatic system also constantly compensates for changes in gravitational and inertial forces, distributing them around the heart. Finally, such a hydrostatic system favors a net balanced output from both ventricles when output is integrated over several cardiac cycles.

Ventricular Interaction and Pericardial Constraint of the Heart

Ventricular interdependence, expressed as *ventricular interaction*, describes the effects of the movements and physical changes of one ventricle on activities of the other, like filling, contraction and even relaxation. While the normal right ventricle is much more compliant than the left ventricle, the pericardium constrains both similarly and tends to equalize their compliances. Of course, interaction also occurs without the pericardium due to continuity of the circumferential myocardial muscles and especially through the ventricular septum—the common right and left ventricular wall—as long as the septum is compliant.

Diastolic *cardiac chamber interactions are greatly magnified by the presence of the pericardium.* (Systolic interaction is only minimally affected.) For example, acute obstruction of left ventricular outflow dilates the left ventricle, tightening the pericardium and consequently limiting right ventricular filling and output. Comparably, *acutely increased size of the right ventricle* during cardiocirculatory volume overloads or right ventricular infarction raises intrapericardial pressure significantly, imposing a steeper pressure-volume curve (increased stiffness) on the constrained left ventricle. This is also seen continuously through minimally during normal breathing: *inspiration* increases right ventricular filling, which slightly reduces left ventricular filling and consequently output and decreases arterial blood pressure; *expiration* reverses the process. This sequence is exaggerated by even small increases in pericardial fluid (Chapter 10) and markedly so in cardiac tamponade (Chapter 12); it produces pulsus paradoxus (Chapter 13), a physiologic misnomer, since it is a marked exaggeration of this normal state.

The very important pericardial contributions to ventricular interaction help to explain *reduced ventricular compliance when there is increased pressure in the other ventricle*. Moreover, the parietal pericardium also permits either ventricle to generate greater isovolumic pressure from any diastolic volume when the pericardium is intact than when it is opened or removed. Finally, since pericardiectomy tends to result in a more spherical heart, the parietal pericardium may help maintain functionally optimal cardiac shape, e.g., the normal ellipsoidal, "football" shape of the left ventricle.

Transmural Pressures

Pressure curves obtained by catheters in the normal pericardial sac resemble mirror images of the pressure in the subjacent cardiac chamber, especially the right atrium and right ventricle. The *transmural pressure of the pericardium itself* (*PTMP*: pericardial pressure minus pleural pressure) is approximately zero, though usually slightly negative, as long as cardiac cavity pressures are normal, since intrapericardial pressure both approximates and varies with pleural pressure at the same hydrostatic level. *Myocardial transmural pressure* (*TMP*: intracavitary pressure minus adjacent intrapericardial pressure), normally less than 3 mm Hg, in turn depends on intrapericardial pressure. This is an extremely important relationship, because myocardial transmural pressure (TMP) at end-diastole is a measure of preload, which is the actual chamber-distending pressure; TMP is thus a true "filling pressure." Consequently, *the normal mainly negative pericardial pressure ensures distending (transmural) cardiac pressures slightly greater than cavitary pressure*. For example, a normal pericardial pressure of –2 mm Hg, when subtracted from a chamber diastolic pressure of 5 mm Hg, produces a myocardial TMP of 7 mm Hg [i.e., 5–(–2) = 7]. Accordingly, when the ventricles contract during ejection, rapidly reducing their volume, the corresponding sharp fall in pericardial pressure promotes atrial filling by a corresponding sharp increase in atrial transmural pressure (the increased intrapericardial negativity during ventricular systole is then "subtracted," i.e., added, as above, to atrial pressure, thus exaggerating atrial transmural distending pressure). Finally, the closed pericardial chamber, normally at slightly subatmospheric pressure, ensures that the levels of transmural myocardial pressures are low relative to even large increases of cavitary diastolic pressures.

To extend the foregoing example: with an elevated atrial or ventricular pressure, say 15 mm Hg, a pericardial pressure of –2 m Hg produces a diastolic myocardial TMP of only 17 mm Hg [15–(–2) = 17].

Finally, ventricular performance is largely determined by end-diastolic fibre length. End-diastolic volume is determined by end-diastolic transmural pressure due to pericardial constraint, especially during dilating ventricular dysfunction. The pericardium not only limits acute dilation, but in both normal and abnormal left ventricles, increases early diastolic filling at the expense of later filling, with selectively increased subendocardial bloodflow. This should improve oxygen delivery and distribution for the increased requirements of dilated ventricles.

Normal Respiratory Effects

Average intrapericardial pressure not only approximates pleural pressure but also varies with its respiratory changes—about –3 mmHg at end-expiration to –6 mmHg at end-inspiration. The normal inspiratory fall in pleural pressure reduces pericardial, right atrial, right ventricular, pulmonary wedge and systemic arterial pressures slightly. Because in inspiration pericardial pressure decreases somewhat more than atrial pressure, right atrial and other central *transmural* (distending) pressures increase, augmenting systemic venous return and right heart filling and therefore right ventricular preload and output. Consequently, pulmonary artery flow velocity increases. At the same time inspiratory aortic flow decreases as aortic transmural pressure increases (increasing impedance to ejection) while systemic venous return is increasing. Moreover, as it crosses the lungs, any inspiratory "pooling" of the increased right ventricular output tends to reduce the gradient for left heart filling. The corresponding slight inspiratory decrease in the left ventricular transmural pressure and increased left ventricular afterload (impedance to ejection) reduce left ventricular stroke output. Consequently, changes in left heart flow velocities, left ventricular output and systemic arterial blood pressure vary directly, while changes in right heart flow velocities, pressures and output vary inversely with respiratory changes in pleural ($\cong$ pericardial) pressure. *These are directionally identical with the far greater changes in the same measurements during pulsus paradoxus* (Chapter 13).

Passive Pericardial Functions

Membranous functions of the pericardium result from its physical presence and are partly inferential. Thus, the pericardium appears to buttress the thinner parts of the myocardium, particularly the right atrium and ventricle, to be a barrier to inflammation from contiguous structures and to reduce friction due to heart movements. (The latter may be related to normal pericardial fluid but is probably largely due to pericardial phospholipids; page 24). *Ligamentous functions* of the pericardium limit cardiac displacement via superior, inferior, lateral and anterior attachments to adjacent structures (page 17). Moreover, these ligaments probably modify the stress/strain relations of the parietal pericardium while limiting the directions of traction on its fibers.

MICROPHYSIOLOGY OF THE NORMAL PERICARDIUM

Servomechanisms

Cardiocirculatory feedback regulation via *pericardial servomechanisms* contributes to pericardial mechanical function and perhaps membranous function. These include (1) *neuroreceptors* in the epicardium and the fibrosa that detect lung inflation and may operate via the vagus nerves to alter blood pressure and heart rate, (2) *sympathetic efferents* that do the opposite and (3) *mechanoreceptors* sensitive to changes in ventricular stretch, determined by ventricular volume and transmural pressure; pericardial constraint may attenuate their activity by limiting cardiac distension. *Pericardial dysfunction* is sensed by mechanoreceptors with phrenic afferents that appear to monitor beat to beat changes in cardiac volume. Mechanoreceptors with unmyelinated fibers signal myocardial tension and appear to reflexly match contraction strength with peripheral resistance, as with exercise. Some of these receptors' output can contract the spleen and lower blood pressure, and (4) *chemoreceptors* sensitive to substances in the pericardial fluid. The latter actually include "hybrid" mechanoreceptors responding to digitalis glycosides and perhaps contributing to their bradycardic effects.

Normal Pericardial Fluid

Normally, there are 15 to 35 mL of serous fluid in the pericardium, mainly an ultrafiltrate of plasma that may include some overflow of myocardial interstitial fluid as well as myocardial lymph drainage. *Protein concentration* is lower than in plasma, but with a relatively high albumin component, owing to albumin's lower molecular weight and ease of transmembrane transport as compared to a complete protein. *Electrolyte concentrations* are as predicted for a plasma ultrafiltrate, yielding a pericardial fluid osmolarity consistent with such an ultrafiltrate and therefore less than plasma osmolarity.

Mesothelial Metabolic Activity

The mesothelium has cyclooxygenase, prostacyclin synthetase and lipoxygenase activities. *Prostaglandin E2, eicosanoids* and large amounts of *prostacyclin*

(PGI2) are continually released by the entire pericardial mesothelium, especially from the visceral layer, into the pericardial cavity in response to pericardial stretching, to increases in myocardial work and loading conditions, and to hypoxia. They are also stimulated by angiotensin II and bradykinin. These prostanoids are capable of altering pericardial sympathetic neurotransmission and myocardial contractility. They may influence pericardial function but also modulate the caliber and tone of the underlying coronary vessels (i.e., direct vasodilation by prostaglandin and indirectly by opposing coronary spasm). Mesothelial synthesis and release of *endothelin*, increased by angiotensin II stimulation, also may have a contributory role, but as a vasoconstrictor. Since increased pericardial prostaglandins inhibit efferent sympathetic effects, they also act as modulators of sympathetic neurotransmission, with multiple effects on cardiac electrophysiology, possibly including reduction of reperfusion-induced arrhythmias.

In addition to the prostacyclins mentioned, small amounts of *complement* (C3, C4, CH50), other *immune factors, myocardial cellular enzymes* and re-lated compounds are continually released into the pericardial fluid. During transmural cardiac injury and necrosis (as in myocardial infarction) pericardial fluid "washes" the cardiac surfaces, diluting substrates leaked into it that might adversely affect the superficially coursing sympathetic nerve fibers. Moreover, pericardial prostacyclin is generated during hypoxia and work (e.g., exercise) and may potentiate the chronotropic and algesic properties of bradykinin, par-ticularly during angina, and perhaps also the pain of pericardial inflammation.

Prostacyclin is also a very potent inhibitor of platelet aggregates and may inhibit thrombosis in the major coronary vessels as well as clotting when there is blood in the pericardium. This mechanism may operate during intrapericardial bleeding, when *fibrinolytic activity* in the intact mesothelial serosa opposes both intrapericardial clotting and formation of adhesions. However, after any kind of pericardial injury, including physical and chemical trauma, pericardial fibrin-olytic activator activity decreases.

Although pericardial fluid has a grossly "obvious" lubricant function, a variety of surfactant *phospholipids* within it are capable of greatly reducing friction between otherwise hydrophilic surfaces, consistent with the classical theory of "boundary" lubrication.

Interestingly, a peculiar cell-to-cell interaction between pericardial mesothe-lium and ventricular myocytes in tissue culture, demonstrated only in vitro, has not yet found a place in the complex scheme of pericardial microphysiology.

Finally, the effects on the heart, its nerves and the coronaries of intra-pericardially injected substances, like those produced by the pericardial mesothe-lium itself (page 23) suggest that the pericardial sac can be used as a vehicle for local delivery of therapeutic agents and gene products affecting these tissues.

KEY POINTS

1. The normal parietal pericardium is *relatively* inelastic, with structurally determined complex mechanical and membranous functions and apparently simple ligamentous functions.
2. Mechanical pericardial effects on the thin right ventricle are stronger than on the left ventricle.
3. *Pericardial pressure* approximates and varies with pleural pressure and is usually slightly negative, which increases myocardial transmural pressures; its cyclic respiratory changes contribute to corresponding respiratory changes in cardiac function.
4. Hypervolemia and acute cardiac dilatation increase pericardial effects on the heart; hypovolemia, decreased ventricular preload, and acute cardiac shrinkage (e.g., nitroglycerin effect) decrease pericardial effects.
5. The pericardium contributes strongly to *ventricular interdependence (interaction)*, with right ventricular diastolic pressure a major determinant of left ventricular diastolic pressure particularly under *abnormal* conditions. With a *normal* thorax and cardiocirculatory system, the pericardium definitely but only minimally influences cardiac pressures, dimensions and interactions.
6. Pericardial *servomechanisms* include modulation of vagal neuroreceptors, sympathetic efferents and mechanoreceptors with a variety of cardiocirculatory effects.
7. Normal serous pericardial fluid has the characteristics of a plasma ultrafiltrate modified by any myocardial lymph.
8. Pericardial mesothelium produces large amounts of prostacyclin (PGI2) and related substances that may have direct and indirect coronary vasodilatory effects.
9. Mesothelial endothelin may oppose this. Mesothelial fibrinolytic activity opposes thrombosis during intrapericardial bleeding but may be inhibited by various traumas.

BIBLIOGRAPHY

1. Applegate, R.J., Santamoer, W.P., Klopfenstein, H.S., Little, W.C. External pressure of undisturbed left ventricle. Am. J. Physiol. 1990; 158:H1079–H1086.
2. Dauterman, K., Pak, P.H., Maughan, W.L., et al. Contribution of external forces to left ventricular diastolic pressure—Implications for the clinical use of the starling law. Ann. Intern. Med. 1995; 122:737–742.
3. Hills, B.A., Butler, B.D. Phospholipids identified on the pericardium and their ability to impart boundary lubrication. Ann. Biomed. Eng. 1985; 13:573–586.
4. Miyazaki, T., Pride, H.P., Zipes, D.P. Prostaglandins in the pericardial fluid modulate neural regulation of cardiac electrophysiological properties. Circ. Res. 1990; 66:163–175.
5. Nolan, R.D., Dusting, G.J., Jakubowski, J. Martin, T.J. The pericardium as a source of prostacyclin in the dog, ox and rat. Prostaglandins 1982; 24:887–902.
6. Shabetai, R. Function of the Pericardium *In*: Fowler, N.O. (ed.). The Pericardium in Health and Disease. Mount Kisco, New York: 1985, Futura, pp. 22–26.
7. Spodick, D.H. Threshold of pericardial constraint: The pericardial reserve volume and auxiliary pericardial functions. J. Am. Coll. Cardiol. 1985; 6:296–297.

8.   Spodick, D.H. Macro- and microphysiology and anatomy of the pericardium. Am. Heart. J. 1992; 124:1046–1051.
9.   Spodick, D.H. The normal and diseased pericardium: Current concepts of pericardial physiology, diagnosis and treatment. J. Am. Coll. Cardiol. 1983; 240–251.
10. Toyoda Y, Okada M, Kashem MA, Tsukube T. Effects of cardiomyoplasty on right ventricular diastolic filling during volume loading. J Am Coll Cardiol 1996; 27: 327A
11. Traboulsi, M., Scott-Douglas, N.W., Smith, E.R., Tyberg, J.V. The right and left ventribular intracavitary and transmural pressure-strain relationships. Am. Heart J. 1992' 123:1279.
12. Woody M, Mehdi K, Zipes DP, Brantley M, Trapnell BL, March KL. High efficiency adenovirus-mediated pericardial gene transfer in vivo. J Am Coll Cardiol 1996; 27: 31A.

4

Auscultatory Phenomena in
Pericardial Disease

Most pericardial auscultatory phenomena are direct or indirect consequences of the pericardial process itself. Additional sounds may be generated by related or unrelated valve or myocardial disease. Pericardial auscultatory phenomena fall into four categories: pericardial rubs, altered heart sounds, murmurs and the effect of pneumohydropericardium (spontaneous or induced) (Table 4.1)

PERICARDIAL RUBS (TABLE 4.1A)

The pericardial friction sound or rub (redundantly, "friction rub"), the hallmark of acute pericarditis, sometimes is also audible in subacute and even chronic pericardial disease. Pericardial rubs are considered to be due to friction between inflamed, scarred or tumor-invaded visceral pericardial surfaces (*endopericardial rub*; "pericardial friction rub") or, infrequently, between the parietal pericardium and the adjacent pleura or chest wall (*exopericardial rub*) or both (*endo-exopericardial rub*). Endopericardial rubs may also be due to absence of surfactant pericardial phospholipids that lubricate what would otherwise be hydrophilic surfaces (page 24). Rarely, dissecting aortic hematoma may undermine the visceral pericardium or irritate both pericardial layers to produce a rub. Endopericardial rubs occur in "garden variety" acute pericarditis (Chapter 8) with acute and subacute inflammation of the visceral pericardium, often rather monotonal over any short period (Figure 4.1), and nearly always disappear with resolution of acute inflammation. Exopericardial rubs can result from penetrat-

Table 4.1 Auscultatory Phenomena in Pericardial Disease

A. **Pericardial rubs**
1. Endopericardial: all 3; any 2 or 1
     Ventricular systolic
     Atrial
     Ventricular early diastolic
2. Exopericardial
     Pleuropericardial
     Conus rubs: acute pulmonary embolism; thyroid "storm"
     Pericardium-chest wall: pericardial effusion; postsurgical
3. Combined
B. **Abnormal heart sounds**
1. First heart sound: diminution in tamponade and constriction
2. Second heart sound
     Diminution in tamponade and constriction
     Relative/absolute increase of P2
     Splits
       Fixed
       Sudden: A2 early on first beat of inspiration
3. Third heart sound
     Earlier than normal and abnormal S3
     Intense, often palpable (constriction)
     Suppressed (tamponade)
4. Fourth heart sound (sinus rhythm)
     Presence inconstant, except elastic constriction
C. **Murmurs**—epiphenomena due to:
     Cardiac disease, associated or unassociated with pericardial disease
     Local effects of unequal or regional pericardial adhesions, constriction,
     calcification or partial pericardial absence
     Atrial septal defect: ? special/fortuitous relation to constriction.
D. **Clicks:** Nearly always due to abnormal valves or valve apparatus, *esp*. A-V valves
   prolapse when ventricular volume reduced by effusion or constriction
E. **Pneumohydropericardium**
     Splashes
     Mill-wheel sound

ing severe acute pericarditis or pericardial effusion in some patients (see below) but otherwise are due to direct extension, inflammation or tumor implantation from adjacent structures.

Exopericardial as well as endopericardial rubs also occur after cardiac surgery and in association with constrictive and nonconstrictive pericardial scarring; most are due to adjacent pleuritis (*pleuropericardial rub*). Pleuropericardial rubs are due either to primarily pleural or to pericardial inflammation or to si-

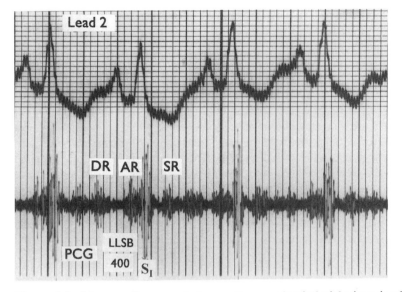

Figure 4.1 Electrocardiogram and phonocardiogram of typical triphasic pericardial rub in atrial systole (AR), ventricular systole (SR) and ventricular diastole (DR). In this example, all three components are distinct but of equal amplitude, giving a monotonal quality on auscultation.

multaneous involvement of both membranes and have respiratory as well as cardiac periodicity. *Conus rubs* accompany (Means-Leman scratches), pulmonary embolism, thyroid "storm" and acute beriberi heart disease; they are ascribed to dilation of the pulmonary conus in a hyperactive heart. When due to subacute or chronic processes, any rub can last indefinitely. Exopericardial rubs are much more likely than endopericardial rubs to change radically with respiration, to have a musical quality and to seem quite superficial. Occasional "*chest wall sounds*" resemble rubs but are usually lower-pitched and sharply localized.

While rubs in acute pericarditis usually cease with accumulation of a significant amount of effusion fluid, they *frequently do not disappear despite even very large effusions* and even during tamponade. Rarely, such rubs "paradoxically" disappear after pericardiocentesis. An audible component of the rubs in such patients is probably exopericardial and requires increased intrapericardial pressure to maintain friction between the parietal pericardium and the pleura or chest wall.

Finally, and especially because intracardiac pacemakers can also cause traumatic pericardial disorders (page 381), the occasional rub associated with a temporary pacemaker normally lying on the endocardium (*endocardial rub*) should not be mistaken for pericardial involvement by pacemaker penetration of the myocardium (page 380).

AUSCULTATORY CHARACTERISTICS

Rubs are composed of mixed- (mainly high-) frequency vibrations (Figure 4.2) and usually are so distinctive on auscultation as not to be confused with most murmurs. Rubs frequently wax, wane and transiently disappear between examinations, unlike most murmurs. Rubs vary from a subtle, distant "scrape" or set of scrapes to grating, scratching or creaking noises, which may become quite loud and even palpable, especially in uremic pericarditis. They may seem to "obliterate" or give the illusion of "going through" the heart sounds while giving a definite impression of "superficiality." Because of their frequency characteristics, pericardial rubs are best heard with the stethoscopic diaphragm and

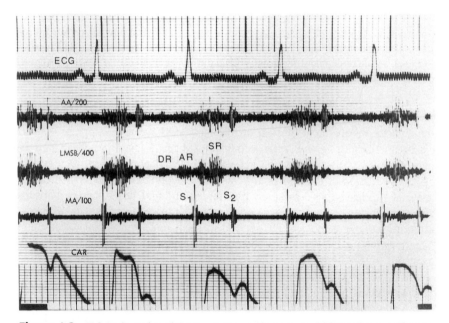

Figure 4.2   Triphasic pericardial rub: electrocardiogram, multifilter phonocardiogram and peaks of carotid pulse. S1 = first heart sound. S2 = second heart sound. Rub components labeled as in Figure 4-1. Rub vibrations are mainly high frequency (top two phonocardiograms) and much reduced at lowest frequency (MA/100). This example shows the most common relative intensity: VR louder than AR, louder than DR; only VR remains at lowest filtration.

may fluctuate with varying pressure of the bell of the stethoscope. Unlike most murmurs, many rubs change quite noticeably with respiration and body position and do not respect the conventional murmur zones of maximum intensity and radiation. However, *the vast majority of rubs are heard best, or only, along the left mid- to lower sternal edge.* There, many rubs may be at their most intense and palpable, resembling the murmur and thrill of a small ventricular septal defect. This localization is probably due to the proximity of the right ventricle to the chest wall and minimal to absent interposition of aerated lung near the left lower sternal edge. The apex is the next likely but much less common location. Occasional rubs may be confined to zones anywhere along the cardiac borders. While pericardial rubs are usually loudest on inspiration, particularly noticeable in the presence of some increase in pericardial fluid (Figure 4.3), they occasionally show no respiratory predilection or even increase in expiration (Figure 4.1). Finally, suspected rubs may be elicited or accentuated by raising all four of the patient's extremities simultaneously, presumably due to right heart distention by the suddenly increased venous return.

RUB COMPONENTS

Rubs have classically been designated as biphasic, "to-and-fro" phenomena. "To and fro" was usually the result of slipshod auscultation. Careful auscultation in patients with heart rates under 120 beats per minute reveals a *triphasic* pattern in well over one-half of patients in sinus rhythm. They occur in atrial sys-

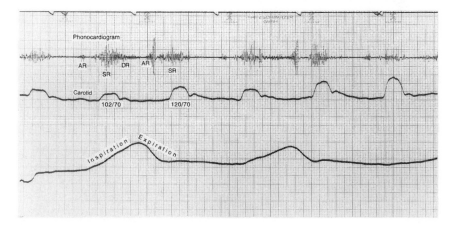

Figure 4.3 Inspiratory amplification of rub. Phonocardiogram, carotid pulse and respiratory thermistor output. Rub components increase during and at peak inspiration and decrease during expiration (the latter best seen at beginning and end of phonocardiogram). Patient with cardiac tamponade. (Pressures: brachial cuff.)

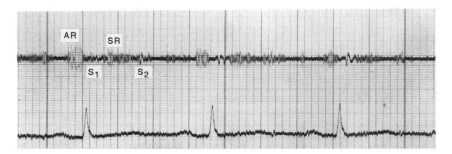

Figure 4.4 Biphasic pericardial rub in atrial and ventricular systole. The atrial rub (AR) is more intense. Patient with pericardial effusion.

tole (*atrial rub*), ventricular systole (*systolic rub*), and early diastole (*early diastolic rub* (Figures 4.1 to 4.3). Only about one-third are biphasic (true to-and-fro; Figure 4.4) rubs and even some of these are due to the absence of atrial systole in cardiac patients with atrial fibrillation or misplaced atrial systole (Figure 4.5). About 10% are monophasic, most often during ventricular systole (Figure 4.6), and it is the ventricular systolic component that nearly always is the loudest in tri- and biphasic rubs. Occasional monophasic rubs are confined to atrial systole (Figure 4.7) or, rarely, early ventricular diastole (Figure 4.8). At rates over 100 beats/minute, the early diastolic and atrial components of triphasic rubs may fuse (*summation rub*; Figure 4.9) but even then can often be distinguished by a change in auscultatory quality beginning with atrial

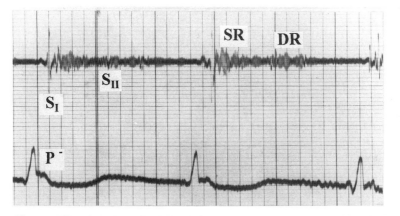

Figure 4.5 Biphasic pericardial rub due to atrioventricular (A-V) dissociation. Atrial systole (P–) occurs during ventricular systole, so that only systolic and diastolic rubs are possible (T wave shows digitalis effect—the cause of the junctional rhythm with A-V dissociation).

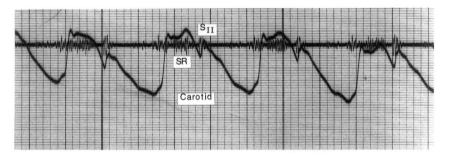

Figure 4.6 Monophasic rub in ventricular systole (SR). The rub begins with the carotid pulse upstroke (which rises well after ventricular systole begins) and ends before the second heart sound (SII).

systole. Finally, some rubs may appear after light exercise; others with less than three components may acquire the remaining one or two components on exercise.

HEART SOUNDS (TABLE 4.1B)

Pericardial rubs often obscure heart sounds by auscultatory masking (Figure 4.9). Pericardial disease itself can alter heart sounds and their auscultatory

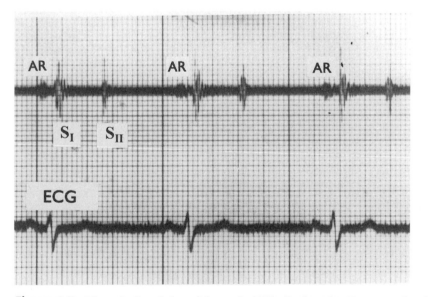

Figure 4.7 Monophasic rub in atrial systole (AR). Begins after P wave and ends before first heart sound (SI).

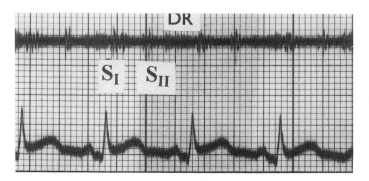

Figure 4.8 Monophasic rub in ventricular diastole (DR). Begins shortly after second heart sound (SII).

appreciation by insulation and particularly by hemodynamic changes. *Insulation of the heart* by fluid should tend to make the heart sounds more remote (Figures 4.3 and 4.4). This could be true also of thick nonconstricting scar, although dense anterior pericardial adhesions and fibrosis might actually improve acoustic coupling of the myocardium to the chest wall and transmit heart sounds better. Thus, fluid is the only more or less definite insulating medium, although it is not rare, even with fairly large nontamponading pericardial effusions, to find clear heart sounds of normal or near normal intensity. *Hemodynamic*

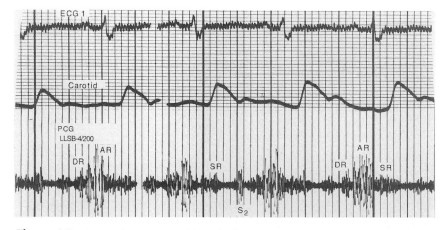

Figure 4.9 Summation rub. Diastolic rub (DR) continues into atrial rub (AR), which in this example is the most intense of all three rub components. DR onset precedes P wave; AR begins toward end of P wave. Auscultation revealed a presystolic change in pitch (frequency) of these rubs. First heart sound is not discernible because of contiguous rub vibrations on each side of it.

changes common to both tamponade and constriction decrease stroke volume and myocardial compliance, tending to decrease the first and second heart sounds, with an accentuated pulmonic component of S2 in some patients with higher pulmonary artery pressures. Constrictive pericarditis produces its hallmark, the abnormal early diastolic sound (EDS), which is a variant of the third heart sound (S3; Figure 4.10), as well as abnormal splitting of the second heart sound (page 36) and a fourth heart sound heard in some cases (page 36). *Note: In pure tamponade, the absence of rapid filling makes an S3 impossible.*

Simultaneous auscultation of A2 and P2 at the left upper sternal edge reveals their splitting characteristics. Although P2 sometimes seems absolutely increased on auscultation, this may be due to confusion with a very early abnormal S3, which can be well transmitted to the left upper sternal edge. During tamponade and subacute—and even chronic—pericardial constriction, any persistent pericardial rubs will tend to alter the perception of contiguous heart sounds. In mixed effusive-constrictive syndromes due to simultaneous scar and fluid, with or without cardiac compression, mixed pictures result, as, for example, many cases of chronic pericardial effusion and some cases of chronic and subacute constriction (pages 438).

The S3 of constriction coincides with the abrupt halt of excessively rapid filling in early diastole, owing to decreased ventricular compliance, small ventricular volumes and diastolic suction with a brief very high filling gradient. The abnormal S3 of constriction occurs earlier than the normal S3 of young people and most other abnormal S3s of myocardial disease and atrioventricular (A-V) valve regurgitation; its relative timing is analogous in behavior to that of opening snaps; i.e., *the greater the hemodynamic impairment and the less the myo-*

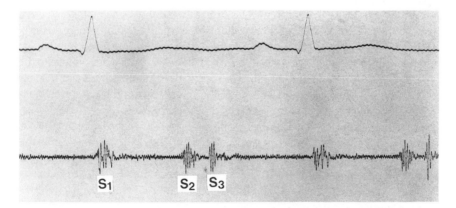

Figure 4.10 Phonocardiogram in constrictive pericarditis with abnormal third heart sound (S3). Rapid paper speed accounts for "wide" Q wave in electrocardiogram.

cardial compliance, the closer the S3 will be to S2. Some very early abnormal sounds are high-pitched and resemble a mitral or tricuspid opening snap. Frequently the abnormal S3 of constriction is the only loud heart sound (sometimes with an intense "knocking" quality) and may be misinterpreted as S1 (Figure 15.27), especially during rapid heart rates and particularly if there is a simultaneous early diastolic thrust of the chest wall, which can be mistaken for the apex beat (Figure 15.26). At the beside the S3 can be timed to follow the crest of the carotid pulse and to coincide with the trough of the *y* descent of the jugular pulse. While patients with heavy calcification can have a particularly loud and sharp abnormal S3, this is probably due to markedly reduced compliance rather than the presence of calcification. Like its timing, S3 intensity varies directly with the abruptness with which ventricular expansion halts, since louder third sounds are correlated with greater diastolic pressures and the steepness of the reascent from the typical early diastolic "dip" of the ventricular pressure and chest wall displacement curves (page 223).

In contrast to ventricles without advanced diastolic restriction, in the tightly constricted ventricle, brief forceful filling in early diastole is *monophasic*, i.e., not followed by a significant slow filling phase so that the abnormal S3 occurs close to the peak of the ventricular volume curve (page 237). In constricted patients with sinus rhythm, a fourth heart sound (S4) is rarely heard and can be ascribed to the high resistance to ventricular filling encountered by effective atrial systolic flow. This suggests lack of impairment of atrial systole by the constrictive process, explaining why S4s are more common in *elastic constriction* (pages 254).

Better appreciated by phonocardiography, constriction produces two patterns of second heart sound (S2) splitting: (1) in the absence of any definite inspiratory fall in systolic blood pressure, there is little change with respiration, producing an almost fixed split of S2. Virtual immobility of the pulmonic component (P2; Figure 15.27) contrasts with the normal situation where inspiratory delay of P2 produces most of the split. This is ascribable to minimal or absent respiration-associated change in right ventricular stroke volume with virtual fixation of the duration of right ventricular systole during the respiratory cycle. (2) In occasional cases with atypically well-marked respiratory changes in the arterial pressure, there is a peculiar form of S2 splitting occurring within one beat after the onset of inspiration (and probably related to the characteristic Doppler flow changes on that beat; page 240). Here, P2 remains virtually fixed but the aortic component of S2 (A2) appears earlier on inspiration. This resembles normal A2 behavior but the maximum fall in arterial pressure and the earliest timing of A2 occur one beat after the onset of inspiration— a more abrupt change—reflecting shortened left ventricular ejection time due to transient underfilling of the left ventricle in these patients.

CLICKS (TABLE 4.1D)

Clicks are high-frequency, fairly discrete vibrations, more common in phono-cardiograms than on auscultation and resembling in timbre opening snaps of stenosed valves and ejection sounds. Classically ascribed to pericardial scarring and calcification, this remains largely speculative (although Fowler demonstrated visually a sound-producing mobile pericardial adhesion).

Most cardiac clicks are due to intracardiac phenomena related to valves or chordae tendineae. Indeed, pseudoprolapse or actual prolapse of mitral and tri-cuspid leaflets due to disproportionate shrinkage of ventricular volume in tam-ponade and constriction has produced clicks.

MURMURS ASSOCIATED WITH PERICARDIAL DISEASE (TABLE 4.1C)

Murmurs are auscultatory phenomena due to turbulent flow across orifices and in tubes. In any kind of pericardial disease they are epiphenomena—either due to coincident heart disease, which may or may not be related to the pericar-dial lesion, or as a result of unusual forms of pericardial scarring. The latter occur when a cicatricial pericardial process involves a valve ring or locally narrows a portion of the heart, the aorta or the pulmonary artery (page 253). Faint systolic murmurs in the absence of valvulopathy may be due to functional impairment of the myocardium or the valves rather than direct encroachment by pericardial scar. Diastolic murmurs, also rare, have been noted under the same circumstances and with normal valves.

Murmurs due to constrictive pericardial scarring, calcification, inflamma-tory cysts or abscesses per se are quite uncommon and result from narrowing of valve orifices by compression or actual physical disruption of the valve. Atrioventricular groove constriction has produced annular mitral and tricuspid stenosis with murmurs indistinguishable in quality and timing from those of A-V valve disease and behaving similarly during respiration and administration of amyl nitrite. Comparable selective scarring has produced systolic murmurs of relative aortic valvular and supravalvular stenosis and pulmonic valvular, supravalvular and infundibular stenosis.

A number of the foregoing appear only postoperatively, the mechanism being apparent at reoperation to remove the selective scarring; others have been due to unexplainable regional scarring or local inequalities within a generalized constricting pericardial scar. Occasional patients have murmurs with gradients demonstrable at catheterization without apparent valve involvement, again, prob-ably due to local variability in the constrictive process, but with an uncertain mechanism.

Murmurs not associated with the pericardial process are most often due to coexisting congenital or acquired heart lesions. For example, there is a repeatedly observed, although uncommon and unexplained, association of atrial septal defect and constrictive pericarditis with the appropriate tricuspid and pulmonic murmurs accompanying otherwise classic constriction.

FORTUITOUS MURMURS

Intrinsic heart lesions and an acute or healed pericarditis may have a common origin. Sometimes this is due to antecedent myopericarditis (Chapter 9) or bacterial endocarditis, particularly of the aortic valve, but also of the mitral valve with the infection spreading to the pericardium. More frequently, rheumatic valvulopathies coexist with a nonconstricting adhesive pericarditis, the residuum of an acute pericarditis that is the hallmark of the most severe rheumatic carditis. Exceptionally, nonconstricting rheumatic mediastinopericarditis has been known to involve the pulmonary arteries sufficiently to cause harsh ejection murmurs and accentuation of P2, typical findings of supravalvular pulmonic stenosis.

EFFECT OF PNEUMOHYDROPERICARDIUM (TABLE 4.1E)

When there is a mixture of air or other gas and fluid in the pericardial sac, either due to gas-producing organisms, a fistula from the respiratory system, esophagus, stomach or colon, or introduced purposely after drainage of fluid (pages 377–378), a metallic tinkle synchronous with systole and occasionally with both systole and early diastole may be heard if the amount of gas is small. Large amounts produce a churning, splashing, *"mill-wheel sound"* due to agitation of the gas-liquid interface by the beating heart.

KEY POINTS

1. Pericardial rubs are usually triphasic, frequently biphasic ("to and fro") and occasionally monophasic.
2. Rubs are relatively frequent during pericardial effusions.
3. Cardiac tamponade and constriction reduce heart sound intensity, usually because of hemodynamic abnormalities. Subsidiary mechanism: insulation due to effusion and possibly by dense scar not coupled to the chest wall.
4. The abnormal diastolic sound of constriction is a very early S3 with the same mode of production. Exceptional earliness and intensity is due to abrupt halting of brief, exceptionally rapid filling by the unyielding scar. It tends to be loud (though frequently without a "knocking" quality) and may be mistaken for S1, especially when palpable.

5. Murmurs are epiphenomena due to valve and heart disease associated or unassociated with the pericardial lesions. Rarely, murmurs are created by pericardial scarring entrapping cardiac or vascular structures.

BIBLIOGRAPHY

1. Hills, B.A., Butler, B.D. Phospholipids identified on the pericardium and their ability to impart boundary lubrication. Ann. Biomed. Eng. 1985; 13:573–586.
2. Spodick, D.H. Pericardial fraction: Characteristics of pericardial rubs in fifty consecutive, prospectively studied patients. N. Engl. J. Med. 1968; 278:1203–1207.
3. Spodick, D.H. Acoustic phenomena in pericardial disease. Am. Heart. J. 1971; 81:114–124.
4. Spodick, D.H. The pericardial rub: A prospective, multiple observer investigation of pericardial friction in 100 patients. Am. J. Cardiol. 1975; 35:357–362.
5. Spodick, D.H., Marriott, H.J.L. Atrial diastolic friction. Chest 1975; 68:122-123.
6. Spodick, D.H. Diseases of the pericardium. In: Chatterjee, et al. (eds.). Cardiology: An Illustrated Text/Reference. Philadelphia: Lippincott, 1991, pp. 10–38, 10–64.

5

Electrocardiographic Abnormalities in Pericardial Disease

Clinical Considerations

Although the pericardium produces no detectable electrical phenomena, pericardial disease can significantly modify the electrocardiogram (ECG). The most striking and specific findings are produced by spread of pericardial inflammation to the superficial, subepicardial layer of the myocardium: a *superficial myocarditis*, nearly always with no apparent myocardial impairment. In the less common circumstance of clinically recognizable *myopericarditis* (Chapter 9), the myocardium is principally involved and dominates the clinical picture, with a variety of ECG changes. In myopericarditis, the only "typical" ECG changes are indistinguishable from Stage III of the ECG progression of acute pericarditis (see below); others are localized changes indistinguishable from those of myocardial ischemia or infarction. In contrast, *to be considered typical, ECG abnormalities in acute pericarditis must be generalized.*

Excess pericardial fluids or dense scar may insulate the heart, tending to decrease voltage, although, during tamponade at least, *hemodynamic impairment is more important than the size of any effusion (unless massive) in reducing ECG voltage.* Pericardial fluids with a potassium concentration exceeding that of the blood, as from hemolyzed red blood cells, can provoke S- and T-wave changes without inflammation. Detectable ECG effects of constrictive scarring also depend more on hemodynamic impairment and fibrosis and calcification of the subjacent myocardium than electrical insulation; any asymmetry of constrictive

40

scarring can mimic disease of a cardiac chamber, valve or great vessel. (See Chapter 15, "Constrictive Pericarditis.)

ACUTE PERICARDITIS (FIGURE 5.1)

Acute pericardial inflammation with a superficial shell of myocarditis provokes ST-T abnormalities, which, when *in typical three- or four-stage sequence* (Table 5.1) are pathognomonic of acute pericarditis; Stage I alone is quasidiagnostic if mimics like "early repolarization" are ruled out. (It is *Stage I* and its *typical variants* (page 50) that computers frequently misinterpret as acute myocardial infarction.) The ST-T changes are primarily due to inflammation on the ventricular surfaces with characteristic evolution involving the ST junction (J) and T waves (Figures 5.2 and 5.3). In the thin-walled atria, this myocarditis cannot be superficial. Moreover, the atria do not have an electrical "gradient" corresponding to the "ventricular gradient," so that the atrial T wave (Ta wave) retains its normal polarity opposite to the P wave (Figures 5.5 and 5.6) but shifts to an early position where it becomes visible in the PR segment, producing *mainly depressed PR segments (with an elevated PR segment, of course, in lead aVR)*. The PR segment deviations have a vector (axis) 180° opposite to the P vector (axis)—usually at –120 to –150° (pointing to the right shoulder), which is normal for the mean atrial T wave (Figures 5.2 through 5.6).

Stage I (Figure 5.7; Table 5.1) is virtually pathognomonic of acute pericarditis when it involves virtually all leads with earliest ST junction elevations that produce an appearance as if the T waves are "jacked up" on the QRS, but otherwise normal; note that there is no morphologic ST "segment" separate from the T wave (Figures 5.1 to 5.3). Minimum lead involvement to be considered typical—i.e., quasipathognomonic—includes I, II, aVL, aVF and V3 through V6. There are no truly reciprocal ST depressions but leads theoretically reflecting "endocardial" events necessarily show depressed J points (Table 5.1) and PR segment elevations. Thus, ST is always depressed in lead aVR, very frequently depressed or isoelectric in V1 and occasionally depressed in V2. Rarely, the Stage I pattern is simulated by a circumcardiac tumor, but usually these J-point elevations are accompanied by terminal T inversions and these changes do not evolve, implying an incessant injury current.

Stage II is evolutionary (Figure 5.1; Table 5.1). In *early* Stage II, all ST junctions return to the baseline more or less "in phase," with little change in the T wave itself; the PR segment may now be depressed if it had not been in Stage I (Figure 5.8). In *late* Stage II, the T waves progressively flatten and invert, mainly in leads that had shown ST elevations (Figure 5.9). *Stage III* (Figure 5.1) shows generalized T-wave inversion in most or all of the leads that had shown J-point elevations (Figure 5.10). If the ECG is first recorded in Stage

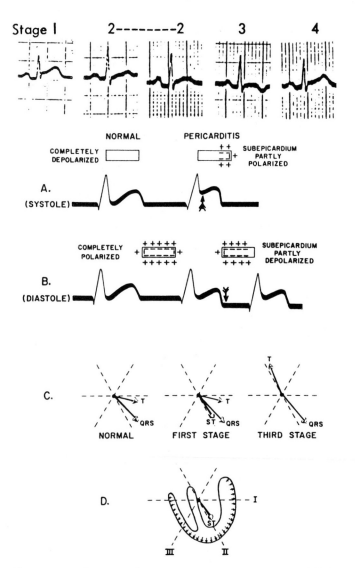

Figure 5.1 Schema and electrogenesis of typical sequential electrocardiographic changes of acute pericarditis. (Adapted from Spodick, *Acute Pericarditis*, 1959; author's copyright.) *Top*: four-stage evolution of J (ST) and T changes (see text). A. *Systolic current of injury* due to polarized subepicardial myocytes. J (ST) directly elevated. B. *Diastolic current of injury* due to partly depolarized subepicardial myocytes. Baseline depressed leaving J (ST) "hung up." (Mechanism not distinguishable because of AC coupling of clinical electrocardiograms). C. *Typical QRS, J (ST) and T vectors* of Stage I and Stage III compared to baseline (normal) ECG (Stages II and IV do not deviate significantly from baseline). D. *J (ST) vector of Stage I* as a function of net direction of injury current due to subepicardial superficial myocarditis (outward arrows around cardiac perimeter).

Table 5.1 Four-Stage ("Typical") ECG Evolution of Acute Pericarditis

Sequence Stage	Leads of "epicardial" derivation: at least I, II, aVL, aVF, V3-6			Leads reflecting "endocardial" potential: aVR, often V1, sometimes V2		
	J-ST	T waves	PR segment	ST segment	T waves	PR segment
I	Elevated	Upright	Depressed or isoelectric	Depressed	Inverted	Elevated or isoelectric
II early	Isoelectric	Upright	Isoelectric or depressed	Isoelectric	Inverted	Isoelectric or elevated
II late	Isoelectric	Low to flat to inverted	Isoelectric or depressed	Isoelectric	Shallow to flat to upright	Isoelectric or elevated
III	Isoelectric	Inverted	Isoelectric	Isoelectric	Upright	Isoelectric
IV	Isoelectric	Upright	Isoelectric	Isoelectric	Inverted	Isoelectric

Abbreviations: ∇J-ST = Junction of S (or T) wave with the end of the QRS complex.
Source: Modified from Spodick, Am J Cardiol 1974; 33:470.

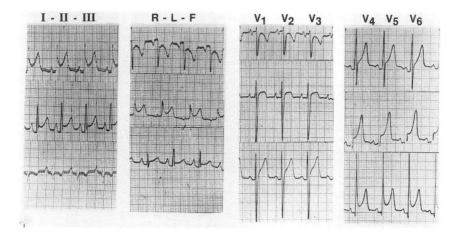

Figure 5.2 Stage I electrocardiogram in a patient with high voltage. J (ST) elevated in all leads except III, where it is isoelectric (common in algebraically "0" QRS, as here): J (ST) typically depressed in leads aVR and V1. PR segments depressed in nearly all leads; typically elevated in aVR and V1 and isoelectric in aVL with an algebraically "0" P wave (PR segment in V2 is transitional between V1 and V3). T waves retain normal concave upslope.

III, pericarditis cannot be diagnosed on ECG grounds, since the tracing is characteristic of diffuse myocardial injury, "biventricular strain" or frank myo-carditis (Chapter 9). Stage III in recent years is seen less frequently, presumably due to effective early anti-inflammatory treatment. In *Stage IV*, the ECG evolves back to the prepericarditis state (Figure 5.1). Occasionally, especially with impending constriction, Stage IV does not occur and there are permanent generalized or focal T-wave inversions and flattening.

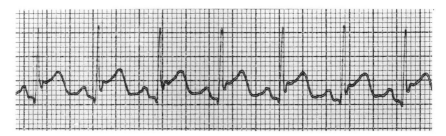

Figure 5.3 Electrocardiographic strip (lead II) showing PR segment depression and J (ST) elevation in relation to the ECG baseline (T-P interval). T waves themselves are "normal" and therefore characteristically have a concave upslope.

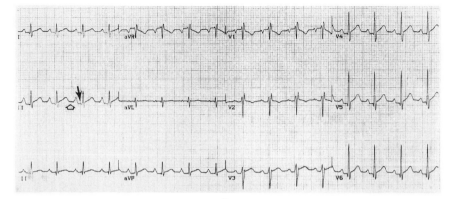

Figure 5.4 Acute pericarditis with PR segment deviations only; no J (ST) deviations. Open arrow: ECG baseline, the T-P interval. Black arrow: PR segment depressed below baseline.

In acute pericarditis, ECG changes may evolve over hours, days, or weeks. The most rapid transition is usually from Stages I to II and the slowest from Stages III to IV.

Electrogenesis of Electrocardiographic Abnormalities (Figure 5.1)

The pericardium is not a contractile tissue. Its inflammation per se cannot affect the events of the cardiac cycle. Electrocardiographic abnormalities during pericarditis seem firmly linked to the accompanying superficial myocarditis but only variable influenced by the presence of effusion.

Superficial myocarditis is virtually always present in cases showing ST-T changes. These may begin to appear even before histologic alterations in the myocardium and may therefore depend in part upon irritative and biochemical factors. Low-voltage complexes in the absence of effusion and edema may result from the insulating action of fibrin.

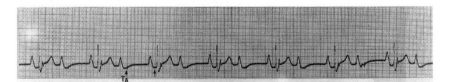

Figure 5.5 Mechansim of PR segment depression. Blocked P waves (every other beat) expose atrial T wave (TA: arrows) which in normal hearts should occur later, hidden in the QRS (see text).

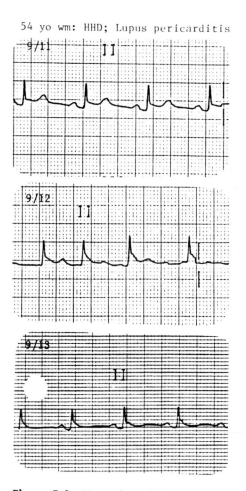

Figure 5.6 Mechanism of PR segment depression: transient disappearance during paroxysmal atrial fibrillation as pericarditis evolves from Stage I to late Stage II, when T waves and PR segments return. (Atrial fibrillation was due to lupus cardiomyopathy.)

ST-T changes in acute pericarditis arise from inflammation (myopericarditis) of a "shell" of superficial myocardium. Unless there is a deeper involvement ("Myopericarditis," Chapter 9), there are no detectable QRS deformities or prolongations, and J (ST) elevation usually does not obliterate preexisting S waves (as is common in acute infarction). The entire subepicardial zone is involved in typical, generalized pericarditis, so that most ECG leads are involved simultaneously and develop "in phase" with each other. The mean (J)

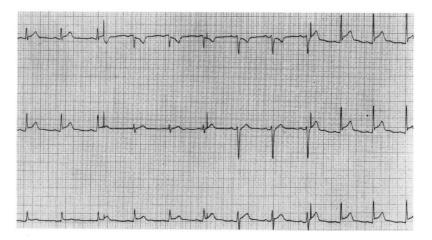

Figure 5.7   Typical, quasidiagnostic Stage I ECG. J (ST) elevated in all leads except aVL (QRS algebraically 0), depressed in aVR and V1. PR segment deviated except aVL where P is small. Quantitative changes less striking than in Figure 5.2 partly because of more normal T and QRS voltages. See also Figures 5.8 and 5.9 (same patient).

ST vector (axis) is usually directed inferiorly and to the left ("southwestward"), i.e., between $+30$ and $+60°$ (Figure 5.10) in normal hearts.

Apparent Stage I J (ST) displacement appears to represent a systolic event (QRST is electrical systole). However, incomplete polarization of the injured

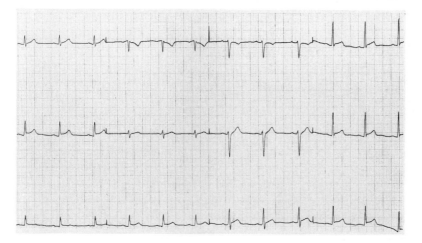

Figure 5.8   Early Stage II (same patient as in Figures 5.7 and 5.9). J (ST) returning to baseline. T waves intact.

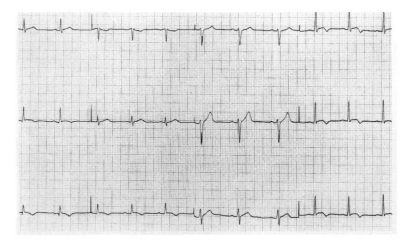

Figure 5.9 Late Stage II–early Stage III (same patient as in Figures 5. and 5.8) J points on baseline, T waves inverting asymmetrically (slightly atypical distribution).

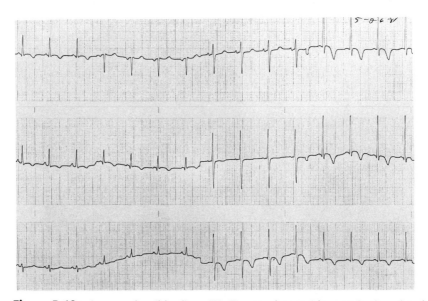

Figure 5.10 Acute pericarditis, Stage III. T waves inverted in most leads and typically upright in aVR and V1. Low, upright T in lead III corresponds to algebraically near-0 QRS voltage.

zone occurs in systole, diastole *or both* (Figure 5.1), as shown by direct current-coupled instruments that are impractical for clinical use. J (ST) displacement results from the partly polarized injured zone (Figure 5.1A,B).

Systolic Injury Current (Figure 5.1A)

During systole, myocardial activation producing the QRS advances normally from the endocardium to the epicardium, where the superficial myocarditis probably alters phase 2 of the transmembrane action potential (TMP) and decreases the duration and intensity of electrical activity in subepicardial muscle, which remains partly polarized. The resultant potential difference between it and the completely depolarized myocardial mass produces the J (ST) shift. Since the injured myocardium never completely depolarizes, it appears to repolarize early (hence the close resemblance to the ECG of "early repolarization"; page 55; Table 5.3).

Diastolic Injury Current (Figure 5.1B)

During diastole, the injured subepicardial zone remains partly polarized (probably due to reduced resting TMP), as in systole. Thus, there is a potential difference between it and the completely polarized remaining myocardial mass, producing a diastolic injury current oppositely oriented to the systolic injury current that shifts electrical diastole, the T-Q interval (Figure 5.1B). This interval corresponds to the ECG baseline (the TP interval) and cannot be detected by the clinical ECG, so that it appears as a J (ST) shift in the opposite direction. Unless cardiac or metabolic factors affect the QT interval, the shortened duration of activation in the injured zone tends to shorten the QTc (electrical systole corrected for heart rate).

Regression of acute inflammation eliminates or minimizes the potential difference between uninvolved or less involved myocardial mass and the injured subepicardial zone, so that the J (ST) becomes isoelectric in *Stage II*. T-wave inversion succeeding ST elevation in the same leads in *Stage III* implies a modification of the injury process such that the mean direction of repolarization (total T wave) becomes approximately opposite to normal. The T vector (axis) is reversed, but, because electrical activity is less homogeneous during repolarization, this is imperfect, i.e., less than 180°. Because activity is now prolonged in the injured zone and perhaps throughout the myocardium, the QTc tends to increase. Subsiding inflammation causes the T waves to resume their normal orientation in *Stage IV* because duration of electrical activity normalizes in the subepicardial zone, with normalization of the QTc.

Because the subepicardial myocarditis is general in typical cases, changes occur simultaneously in all leads (Table 5.1) and there are no reciprocal J (ST) deviations, in contrast to acute myocardial infarction. *Note*: Atypical cases with restricted J (ST) deviations usually do not show reciprocal changes unless there is an important element of focal/regional myocarditis (Chapter XX); in this respect they resemble some cases of atypical (Prinzmetal's) angina.

Typical Electrocardiographic Variants in Acute Pericarditis (Table 5.2)

Typical variants include (1) ST isoelectric or slightly depressed in lead III with a horizontal or semihorizontal QRS axis (Figure 5.11); with a vertical axis, ST can be isoelectric or slightly depressed in lead aVL, isoelectric in lead I (Figure 5.12). (2) Rapid evolution of Stage I to normality, i.e., return of the elevated J-"ST" to the baseline with little or no T-wave flattening and without T-wave inversion. This is a result of either a mild attack or effective suppression of inflammation. (3) Absence of any stage for unknown reasons or because of insufficiently frequent ECG monitoring (a single daily ECG usually reveals all stages). (4) Persistence indefinitely or for long periods of Stage III with T-wave flattening or inversions, indicating a more aggressive process and in some cases presaging constrictive evolution.

Atypical ECG Variants (Table 5.2)

Four *atypical variants* render the ECG diagnostically nonspecific: (1) *No ECG change* either because acute abnormalities have been missed (unusually rapid evolution or delayed ECG recording) or because superficial myocarditis is not sufficiently intense or absent. Uncomplicated uremic pericarditis, for example, even when severe, does not affect the superficial myocardium and no typical ECG is to be anticipated (page 293). In acute myocardial infarction (infarct or

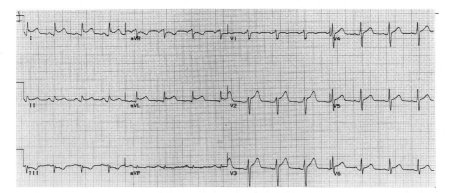

Figure 5.11   Typical variant Stage I ECG. Horizontal QRS axis (0°); J (ST) depressed in lead III; isoelectric in lead aVF with near algebraically 0 QRS. Note PR segment depressions.

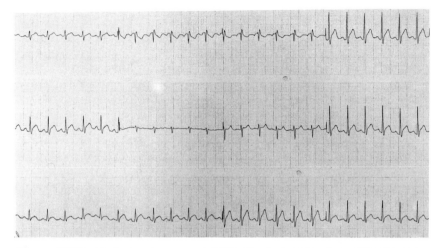

Figure 5.12   Typical variant stage I ECG. Vertical QRS axis (+75°) ST slightly depressed and T slightly inverted in aVL. Note PR segment depressions.

epistenocardiac pericarditis, Chapter 20) pericardial involvement is localized, with no generalized Stage I. (2) *PR-segment deviations alone*—by no means rare (Figure 5.5). PR segment deviations have very high sensitivity (with or without ST deviations) but undetermined specificity. For example, they may occur with atrial trauma and tumor implants without evidence of pericarditis, during tachycardias and with increased sympathetic "tone." Note: Electrocardiograms showing PR depressions are often mislabeled "ST elevation" because of an optical illusion through failing to consider that the T-P interval is the appropriate baseline. (3) *Restriction of J-ST changes to only a few leads* in any stage (Figure 5.13), which is misleading because *localized* cardiac injury is typical of *myocardial ischemia*; indeed, when the changes are most marked in the precordial leads, computer interpretations especially during Stage I often label this "anterolateral infarction" or "inferolateral infarction," depending on the relative involvement of the limb leads. With an appropriate clinical picture, however, one may suspect this variant, because pericarditic changes occur without "reciprocal" ST deviations although with unknown specificity; PR segment deviations may be absent. Such changes also suggest an element of myopericarditis. (4)*T-wave inversions before all ST junctions have returned to the baseline* (Figure 5.14). This is characteristic of myocardial infarction, which should always be considered in the differential diagnosis, especially if a typical Stage I has not been appreciated. This also can occur in myopericarditis (Chapter 9). (*Special case*: patients with antecedent T-wave inversions, espe-

Table 5.2 **Acute Pericarditis: Electrocardiographic Variants** (Patterns Deviating from Classic Stages I–IV)

Typical variants—**ECG quasispecific**
  Effect of QRS axis
    Horizontal or semihorizontal axis: J-ST isoelctric or slightly depressed in lead III
    Vertical axis: J-ST isoelectric or slightly depressed in lead aVL; may be isoelectric in I
  Rapid evolution of Stage I
    J-ST to baseline without T inversion (no Stages III and IV)
  Absence of any stage because of:
    Effective therapy
    Infrequent ECG recording
    Unknown
  Indefinite persistence of Stage III (no Stage IV)

Atypical Variants—**ECG nonspecific**
  No ECG change
  PR segment deviations without J-ST abnormalities
    (highly sensitive; specificity may be high, but unknown)
  Restricted lead involvement:
    J-ST elevations (restricted Stage I)
    T inversions (restricted Stage III)
    T inversion before J-ST returns to baseline (persistent current of injury)
      Circumcardiac tumors
      Digitalis effect
      Myopericarditis

---

cially digitalis effect, may show ST junction (J) deviations while the original T-wave abnormalities persist, with or without PR segment deviations; Figure 5.15). (5) Stage III with T-wave inversions only in some of the leads which had shown Stage I J-ST elevations (usually V3 or V4 to V6).

Atypical ECG responses are especially misleading in the absence of rubs and in the presence—or suspicion—of a primarily cardiac lesion, especially myocardial infarction. The author reported the frequency of atypical ECG changes in patients with pericardial rubs and corresponding clinical syndrome: nearly half the ECGs were atypical, meaning that they did not present with or ultimately evolve Stage I changes. Among the bare majority with typical ECG changes, these were always recorded on presentation or the first or second day thereafter. Differentiation from myocardial ischemia is crucial because *thrombolytic treatment with unrecognized pericarditis can cause hemopericardium* (page 341). And computer programs are prone to designate even some typical Stage I traces as "anterolateral infarction."

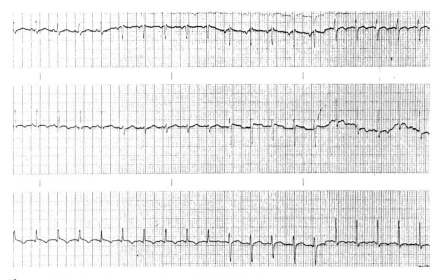

Figure 5.13 Atypical variant Stage III ECG: J points have returned to baseline in all leads except V2, but T inversions occurred only in leads II, III, aVF, V5 and V6.

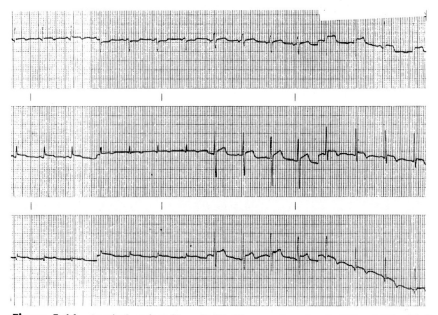

Figure 5.14 Atypical variant Stage II-III. T waves inverting in V5 and V6 with J points still above the baseline in these and the other leads.

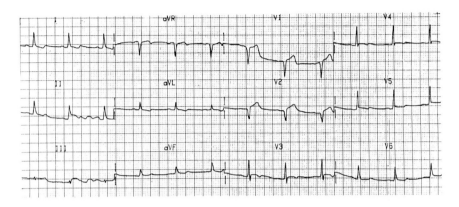

Figure 5.15 Atypical variant: modified Stage I with digitalis effect. Pericarditis identified by rub and new J-point deviations in digitalized patient. Asymmetric T-wave inversions with short QTc in many leads despite J-point elevation.

Electrocardiographic differentiation between abnormalities typical of acute pericarditis and those of acute myocardial ischemia and infarction is summarized in Table 5.3. Electrocardiographic differentiation between Stage I and the apparently normal variant ECG, "early repolarization" (Figure 5.16) is summarized in Table 5.4. Finally, minimal J(ST) deviations may be difficult to detect (Figure 5.17).

Table 5.3   ECG: Stage I Pericarditis vs. "Early Repolarization"

	Stage I pericarditis	"Early repolarization"
Sex	Either	Virtually all males
Age	Any	Usually under 40 years
Prevalence in mental institutions	Sporadic	Relatively common
J-ST evolution	Yes	No
PR segment deviations	Frequent	Occasional
	Ubiquitous	Restricted distribution
	Often conspicuous	Never conspicuous
R-S slurring	Uncommon	Nearly always
T-waves		
Amplitude	Normal	Usually tall
Summit	May be blunt	Peaked
J height/ T apex V6 (PR segment as baseline)	Usually > 25%	Usually < 25%

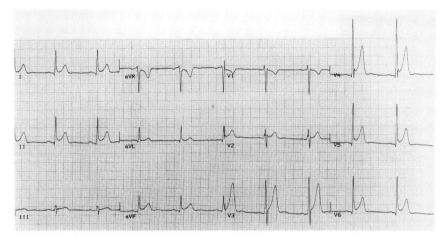

Figure 5.16 "Early repolarization," an electrocardiographic mimic of Stage I pericarditis (see Table 5.3). Voltages are large. J-point elevations occur with slurring and oscillation at J (ST) junctions. Absence of PR segment deviations is usual; when present, their distribution may be restricted.

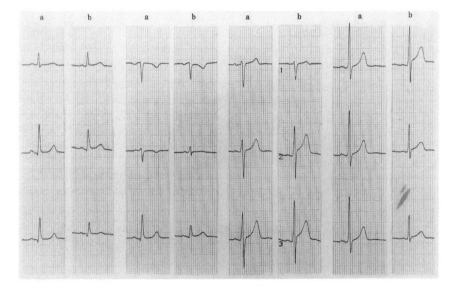

Figure 5.17 Minimal J (ST) change in a typical Stage I electrocardiogram compared lead by lead. Column a = Day 1, when pericardial rub was detected. Column b = maximum change recorded on Day 2. From left to right, columns a and b are paired from leads I, II, III, next RLF, next V1, V2, V3, finally V4, V5, V6.

Rate and Rhythm Abnormalities

Heart rate is usually rapid, between 80 and 130 beats per minute, while the acute inflammation is most intense. Slower rates may be seen in patients with autonomic problems—quite typical of uremic pericarditis, especially in the absence of tamponade.

Sinus rhythm is the rule in the absence of heart disease. Indeed, *uncomplicated acute pericarditis does not produce significant rhythm disturbances* unless there is underlying cardiac disease, either unrelated (preexisting) or related to the pericardial inflammation (myocarditis). Indeed, despite the anatomically superficial location of the sinus node, it seems virtually immune to infiltration by inflammatory cells. The rare cases in which uncomplicated acute pericarditis is accompanied by a significant arrhythmia (i.e., anything more than a few ectopic beats) are ascribable to undetected heart disease, including the occasionally significant element of myocarditis (Chapter 9).

PERICARDIAL EFFUSION; PLEURAL EFFUSION

The ECG effects of *pericardial effusion* are more difficult to asses with finality because of conflicting evidence. Low-amplitude ECGs are seen in most but certainly not all cases with effusions large enough to be detected. They may revert to normal spontaneously or with resorption of the fluid. [Long-standing effusions (Chapter 25) with compression atrophy or scarring of the myocardium may cause more or less permanent low voltage.] However, the accumulation of large amounts of pericardial fluid without voltage or other ECG abnormalities is not uncommon. Injection of fluid into animal pericardia can cause decreased voltage, which, as in many clinical pericardial effusions, disappears spontaneously or following removal of fluid. On the other hand, constriction of the right ventricular inflow tract has resulted in decreased voltage in the absence of pericardial effusion, pleural effusion or chest wall edema.

ST-T abnormalities may or may not occur during pericardial effusion. When present, they can either persist or disappear after paracentesis. Their occurrence may be related to superficial myocarditis, but in some cases their existence seems to depend upon the presence of fluid. This could result from compression or ischemia of the underlying myocardium. Clinically, ST displacements can occur with rapid fluid accumulation (as in hemopericardium), but they may be lacking with slow effusions. Experimental support for the concept of a compressive factor is derived from the effect of infusing into the pericardial cavity "nonirritants" such as saline, serum, or air. Characteristic ST segment deviations produced in this manner presumably result from "pure" compression following relatively rapid accumulation of fluid.

While it is clear that abnormal pericardial fluids are capable of altering the ECG under certain conditions, there is wide variability among cases seen in clinical practice. Experimental studies ordinarily do not deal with an inflamed sac, nor do they duplicate the clinical and physiologic settings of the human patient. Overall, the occurrence or persistence of ECG changes cannot be generally related to the presence, duration or amount of effusion.

Effusions accompanying acute pericarditis and especially noninflammatory pericardial effusion (*hydropericardium*) have little effect on the ECG unless a very large amount of fluid insulates the heart, reducing the voltages of the QRS and T waves (P-wave voltage reduction usually requires truly massive amounts of fluid) (Chapter 10). Significant hemodynamic impairment (i.e., tamponade) may reduce voltage even with smaller amounts of fluid. Pseudoinfarct patterns can be produced by reduction of small r waves in rS complexes, making them appear as deep Q ("QS") waves. In hemorrhagic fluids with sufficient hemolysis, excessive potassium concentrations can affect the ST-T waves, including T-wave peaking and reversal of previous T-wave polarity. Large effusions may abolish the ECG effects of ingesting ice water (see page 60).

Pleural effusions, particularly on the left, may contribute to voltage reduction independent of the role of the pericardial effusion. Finally, *generalized fluid retention* (as in cirrhosis and heart failure) can reduce ECG voltage with or without significant pericardial disease.

CARDIAC TAMPONADE

While all degrees of pericardial effusion can be shown to have *physiological* effects, clinical acute cardiac tamponade is defined as the overtly decompensated phase of cardiac compression resulting from an unchecked rise of intrapericardial fluid pressure. Unless massively effusive, *chronic* pericardial effusion and chronic cardiac tamponade have little effect on the ECG. Even the effects of florid acute cardiac tamponade are nonspecific. Any of the four ECG stages of acute pericarditis may be found, but most often the ST (J-junction) deviations are absent; the most frequent findings are low to flat and occasionally inverted T waves. Many patients have nearly normal ECGs, particularly some with malignancies. Critical acute hemorrhagic tamponade, especially intrapericardial rupture of a dissecting aortic hematoma or cardiac wounds, may provoke bradycardia, often of A-V junctional origin or *electromechanical dissociation* preterminally (page 159). *QRS-T voltage* tends to decrease in tamponade, at least in comparison with tracings taken before hemodynamic compromise. However, the degree of change is unrelated to severity of tamponade. Moreover, preexisting heart disease may account for high or low voltages. Very few patients will have true microvoltage and the P waves usu-

ally escape completely. While purely insulating effects of pericardial fluid require large effusions, voltage reduction in tamponade (Chapter 11) probably is
mainly due to angulation and especially compression of the heart, which reduce
its size. Indeed, occasional tamponade patients develop left axis deviation,
possibly due to ventricular displacement or greater compression of the thinner
right ventricle.

Some *T-wave abnormalities* may be due to reduced coronary flow in previously diseased coronary arteries, owing to the low aortic pressure plus massive epicardial compression of the coronary veins as well as obliteration of the
normal transmural myocardial pressure gradient (page 21). In contrast, with
normal coronary arteries, blood flow in tamponade is adequate for aerobic
metabolism (page 186). Finally, pretamponade T-wave inversions may be
pseudonormalized.

Electric alternation (Figures 5.18 and 11.6), in the appropriate clinical
setting, is virtually pathognomonic of critical cardiac tamponade (Chapter 11),
occurring in up to one-third of cases due to periodic (nearly always 2:1) os-

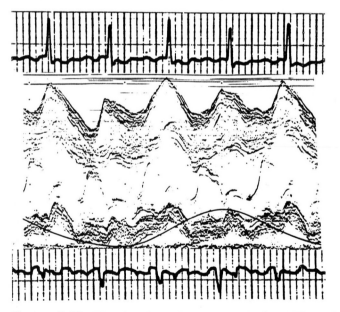

Figure 5.18 Electric alternation. Electrocardiographic strips and M-mode
echocardiogram recorded through the right ventricle, ventricular septum, the mitral valve
and the left ventricle. The whole heart alternately swings toward and away from the
anterior chest wall (RV and LV walls moving concordantly). The apparent ECG vector alternates, producing the conspicuous QRS alternation. Respiration curve near bottom of echogram shows absence of relation to breathing phase.

cillation of the heart swinging within the effusions, well seen by echo-cardiography (page 160). Although typical of large effusions, alternation may occur with as little as 200 mL of pericardial fluid in the presence of a very thick parietal pericardium. Alternation is often apparent in some or all leads as an alternate change in vectorial direction of the QRS (best seen in midprecordial leads) because *the spatial axis of the QRS alternates, due to swinging of the heart while the ECG electrodes remain in place*. (This *vector alternation* with constant cycle lengths contrasts with nondirectional *voltage alternation* seen in tachycardias like A-V nodal or accessory pathway reentry, often with slight cycle length alternation). T-wave alternation is less easily seen and may not be detectable. Rarely, the P waves alternate (best seen in leads II, aVF and/or V1); this has only been reported in critical cardiac tamponade and, taken with QRS alternation, is known as *simultaneous or "total" electric alternation*. Removal of a small aliquot of effusion fluid usually abolishes alternation, just as the same initial fluid decrement usually produces the greatest relative hemodynamic improvement. (This abrupt change in frequency, associated with small, but critical, alternation in cardiac dynamics, is *characteristic of a nonlinear system*.) Electric alternation has a critical relation to the heart rate: administration of beta-adrenergic blocking agents can slow the rate without critically changing the hemodynamics but may make electric alternation disappear. For unknown reasons, in long ECG traces electric alternation may be intermittent.

"EARLY REPOLARIZATION": MIMIC OF ACUTE PERICARDITIS (FIGURE 5.16; TABLE 5.3)

An ECG that is almost indistinguishable from the J-point deviations of ECG Stage I of acute pericarditis—found mainly in males under age 40, and strangely prevalent in mental institutions—has been called *early repolarization*. Because loose definitions of early repolarization include any number of leads, this discussion is concerned only with the full-blown, ubiquitous lead involvement. [Actually, any time the ST (J) takes off before the QRS normally reaches the baseline repolarization can be said to be "early".] Unlike stage I of acute pericarditis, this ECG does not acutely evolve. When such individuals have acute chest pain, in the absence of PR segment deviations, acute pericarditis can be clearly differentiated by ECG only with difficulty; clinical correlation is mandatory. While there is no absolute distinction, in early repolarization J-point elevations are usually accompanied by a slur, oscillation, or notch at the end of the QRS just before and including the J point. This is best seen in precordial leads with tall R and T waves. *PR segment deviations are uncommon and never marked or generalized*, as they can be in acute pericarditis. One relative differential feature, using the PR segment as a contrived baseline, is the height of the J point, especially in lead V6; if J is over 25% of the height of the apex of the T wave, pericarditis is quite likely; a lower J-point level favors early repolarization. Exercise cannot distinguish Stage I acute pericarditis from early repolarization, since in both cases the J points descend to the baseline and any PR deviations may be exaggerated.

Strangely, "early repolarization" has been ascribed to "vagotonia," "sympathicotonia" including asymmetric stellate ganglion stimulation, or latent hypertrophic obstructive cardiomyopathy. Its prevalence in mental patients and exceptional incidence in males under 40 years of age are remarkable. No conclusive mechanism or pathogenesis has been established.

NONCONSTRICTIVE PERICARDIAL SCARRING

The presence of nonconstrictive pericardial fibrosis and adhesions appears to have a negligible effect on the ECG. There are anecdotal observations of tight, thick, or immobilizing external pericardial scarring associated with QRS axis fixation during extreme postural changes and some insulation of the heart, causing local or generalized decrease in wave amplitudes. These are of such low sensitivity and specificity as to be useless. Sufficiently dense and extensive scarring over cardiac surfaces contiguous with the diaphragm and esophagus may diminish or prevent T-wave changes following ingestion of a standard dose of ice water: orientation of the T vector away from the cooled area, best noted in leads II, III, aVF, V1 and V2. Abolition of this response is also seen with large pericardial effusions.

CONSTRICTIVE PERICARDITIS

Electrocardiographic abnormalities in constrictive pericarditis are *often characteristic but none are specific*. A "typical" ECG would include mildly low-voltage QRS complexes and flattened to inverted T waves in all leads of "epicardial" derivation (page 43), as in Figure 5.19. In some patients with chronic constriction and many with acute and subacute constrictive pericarditis, the near-ubiquitous T inversions of the Stage III ECG (Figure 5.10) never improve or regress incompletely irrespective of clinical remission. Especially with chronicity, P waves can be wide and bifid (interatrial block), sometimes resembling P mitrale with a P-wave axis between +90 and –10°. P in V1 may indicate left atrial enlargement (P-terminal force ≥ 4 μV sec) or right atrial enlargement (large positive initial component) or both (Figure 5.19). On the other hand, many patients have normal ECGs or only nonspecific T-wave abnormalities. *Latent constrictive pericarditis* should be considered in such cases, especially (1) if the T waves become more abnormal or if T wave abnormalities reappear after a normal acute Stage IV evolution; (2) if T-wave abnormalities newly ap-

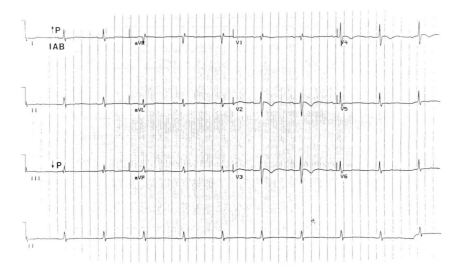

Figure 5.19   Chronic constrictive pericarditis. Low voltage in ten leads and relatively low voltage in V2 and V3, with flat (−+), inverted and frankly inverted T waves. P waves are wide (interatrial block; IAB) with P axis = 0° : flat in aVF; inverted in lead III and upright in lead I as emphasized by the arrows. Wide negative phase of biphasic P wave in V1 indicates left atrial enlargement (of which IAB is also a strong correlate).

pear or (3) if QRS voltage decreases in the absence of other causes. Pleural effusions, ascites and general fluid retention also modify the ECG in chronic constriction.

Arrhythmias

Unlike acute pericarditis, arrhythmias in constriction appear increasingly with chronicity—mainly atrial fibrillation but occasionally atrial flutter; *preoperative conversion to sinus rhythm is characteristically very difficult*. Rhythm disturbances are two to three time more common with pericardial calcification or an enlarged cardiopericardial silhouette.

QRS Abnormalities

In chronic constriction, both low voltage and myocardial atrophy are common and probably mutually related. In acute and subacute constriction (the more common contemporary forms), *QRS axes* tend to be normally oriented. In classic chronic constrictive pericarditis, the frontal QRS axis tends to be vertical, in many cases more positive than +60° and sometimes with definite right axis

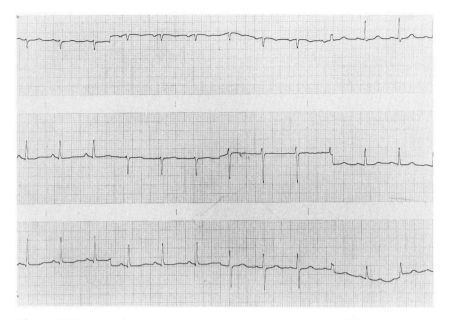

Figure 5.20   Constrictive pericarditis: nonspecific T-wave abnormalities and right axis deviation. QRS axis = +110°. P wave inverted in lead V1, typical of left atrial enlargement, as is interatrial block, shown by abnormal P duration in V1 and V4 to V6. Unlike Figure 5.19, these wide P waves are not notched.

deviation (over +90°; Figure 5.20). Verticalization increases with chronicity and accounts for the variability of axis among different reports. The tendency in chronic constriction to abnormally vertical and right deviated axis may represent disproportionate right ventricular injury and "strain," or perhaps "disuse atrophy" of the underloaded left ventricle. Rarely, *electric alternation* may occur in effusive-constrictive pericarditis with dominant parietal pericardial constriction and relatively little effusion. *QRS abnormalities typical of right ventricular hypertrophy* may evolve in patients with unequal constriction or strategically placed residual postpericardiectomy scarring that can affect the pulmonary artery, the right ventricle, the atrioventricular groove or the mitral valve. Other QRS abnormalities, including abnormal Q waves, reflect myocardial penetration by inflammation and scarring or focal atrophy. *T-wave abnormalities are quite variable* and ascribable to combinations of subepicardial inflammation and scarring, altered membrane cationic gradients, cardiac compression and any myocardial abnormalities.

After pericardiectomy QRS voltage nearly always increases with slower evolution in patients who have myocardial atrophy. Vertical or right axis orientation may persist but there is frequently at least a limited correction. T-wave abnormalities, in whole or in part, may not change, especially with chronic constriction; they often temporarily worsen due to operative trauma. P-wave abnormalities following conversion of long-standing atrial fibrillation usually are permanent either because the left atrium is not decorticated or because of irreversible abnormalities in the thin atrial myocardium, Bachmann's bundle, or the sinus node (unlike acute pericarditis; page 56). In brief, relatively few T and P abnormalities revert to normal unless constriction is recent.

KEY POINTS

1. In acute pericarditis, J-ST- and T-wave changes arise from ventricular, and PR segment changes from atrial, *superficial myocarditis*.
2. The typical stage I ECG—ubiquitous J-ST elevations except aVR and usually V1— is quasidiagnostic, especially with concomitant PR segment depressions.
3. Stages II and III and the many atypical variants resemble effects of ischemia or other cardiac abnormalities.
4. Early repolarization can closely mimic Stage I, especially in patients with Stage I without PR segment deviations.
5. In *acute* pericarditis, arrhythmias are virtually always due to associated or unassociated cardiac disease, including myocarditis.
6. Pericardial effusion, tamponade, and constriction reduce ECG voltages mainly via cardiac compression (diminished heart size and blood content) and hemodynamic changes. Insulation by fluid or scar per se usually has minimal effects.
7. Electric alternation, due to cardiac "swinging," is a common effect of large effusions and especially tamponade.
8. ECG changes associated with constriction—mainly low or inverted T waves and, in chronic cases, interatrial block—are nonspecific. After pericardiectomy, QRS voltage increases and T waves are variably affected, but interatrial block tends to be permanent.

BIBLIOGRAPHY

1. Bruce, M.A., Spodick, D.H. Atypical electrocardiogram in acute pericarditis: Characteristics and prevalence. J. Electrocardiol 1980; 13:61–66.
2. Chesler, E., Mitha, A.S., Matisonn, R.E. The ECG of constrictive pericarditis—Pattern resembling right ventricular hypertrophy.
3. Friedman, H.S., Gomes, J.A., Tardio, A.R., Heft, J.I. The electrocardiographic features of acute cardiac tamponade. Circulation 1974; 50:260–268.
4. Spodick, D.H. Electric alternation of the heart: Its relation to the kinetics and physiology of the heart during cardiac tamponade. Am. J. Cardiol. 1962; 10:155–165.
5. Spodick, D.H. Diagnostic electrocardiographic sequences in acute pericarditis: Significance of PR segment and PR vector changes. Circulation 1973; 48:575–580.
6. Spodick, D.H. The electrocardiogram in acute pericarditis: Distributions of

morphologic and axial changes by stages. Am. J. Cardiol. 1974; 33:470–474.

7. Spodick, D.H. Pathogenesis and clinical correlations of the electrocardiographic abnormalities of pericardial disease. In: Rios, G. (ed.). Clinico-Electrocardiographic Correlations. Philadelphia: Davis, 1977, pp. 201–214.

8. Spodick, D.H. Frequency of arrhythmias in acute pericarditis determined by Holter monitoring. Am. J. Cardiol. 1984; 53:842–845.

9. Spodick, D.H. Pericarditis, pericardial effusion, cardiac tamponade and constriction. Crit Care Clin 1989; 5:455–476.

6

Congenital Abnormalities of the Pericardium

Abnormal embryonic development produces a range of uncommon to rare pericardial abnormalities (Table 6.1). Rarest are *pericardial bands* obstructing the superior vena cava. *Pericardial celomic cysts* are most frequent and clinically usually least important. *Bronchogenic cysts* and *congenital pericardial defects* are most important owing tho their potential effects on the heart and vessels. Most are discovered accidentally, either at cardiac surgery or routine chest roentgenogram and often in attempting to diagnose unusual symptoms, which may or may not be related to the congenital abnormality.

CONGENITAL CYSTS AND DIVERTICULA

Pericardial (celomic) cysts are usually unilocular and smooth, without a peduncle, and contain crystal clear "spring-water" transudative fluid. They are frequently only 2 or 3 cm in diameter, most often located at the right cardiodiaphragmatic angle and clinically silent (Figure 6.1). However, cysts can be associated with chest pain, dyspnea, cough and significant arrhythmias, probably due to compression of adjacent tissues; these disappear after resection or drainage. They can be come secondarily infected and can complicate apparently unrelated pericardial effusion and tamponade. "Spontaneous" resolution is rare and probably related to traumatic rupture.

Table 6.1   Congenital Abnormalities of the Pericardium

Primary (embryonic maldevelopment)
   Pericardial absence
      Complete absence
      Left-sided (most common); total or partial
      Right-sided; total of partial
      Inferior; with diaphragmatic defects or aplasia
   Cysts
      Pericardial (celomic)
      Bronchogenic
      Hematic
   Teratoma
   Lymphangioma
   Diverticulom (related to celomic cysts)
   Pericardial bands

Secondary
   Congenitally acquired pericarditis due to maternal lupus
   Intrapericardial hernia of abdominal organs through combined
      diaphragm-pericardial defects

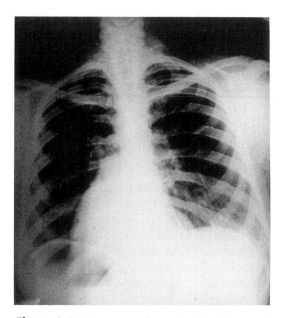

Figure 6.1   Common variety of pericardial cyst discovered on chest roentgenogram obtained for other reasons.

Cysts can occur anywhere on the pericardium. Rarely, they may become very large, with a great deal of fluid, and may even mimic pericardial effusion (Figure 6.2). Simulation of mediastinal tumors and loculated pericardial effusions and hematomas is the principal significance of unilocular and multilocular pericardial cysts (Figure 6.3) and pericardial diverticula. They may also simulate ventricular pseudoaneurysms (page 346). Diagnosis is usually made by appropriate imaging (Figure 6.4); rarely, thoracoscopy and aspiration may be unavoidable. The fluid which may contain hyaluronic acid, is yellowish or clear and watery (hence the term "springwater cysts") with Hounsfield numbers on computed tomography similar to water (typically –4).

Occasionally a *bronchogenic cyst* will be "trapped" in or on the pericardium; *benign teratomas* and *lymphangiomas,* identifiable by computed tomography have the same differential diagnosis. Usually, computed tomography, or—often with some difficulty—echocardiography will make the differential diagnosis, especially when cardiac or vascular aneurysms or other tumors must be differentiated. Thoracoscopic drainage with or without biopsy may be needed. Large bronchogenic cysts can obstruct the superior vena cava with the corresponding venous engorgement syndrome and may induce symptoms suggesting acute pericarditis. Surgical excision is necessary. A *hematic cyst* is a pouch-like dilation of an atretic left vena cava which may contain blood. *Lymphangiomatous cysts* may be a part of a more general lymphangiomatosis and may be related to lymphopericardium (page 86). *Treatment* by open or video-assisted thoracoscopic excision is required only for symptomatic and compressive, hemodynamically compromising cysts.

Pericardial diverticula are similar to cysts except that a comparable developmental anomaly has left a communication with the pericardial cavity. They are even rarer and can vary with body position, presumably due to differential filling and emptying via the communication with the pericardial cavity proper.

CONGENITAL PARTIAL ABSENCE OF THE PERICARDIUM

Any part of the pericardium may be missing, with or without a defect in the adjacent pleura, and often with some kind of associated congenital cardiac, pulmonary or skeletal abnormality. As with most pericardial diseases, there is an unexplained male preponderance. Familial occurrence is rare. The condition is often discovered accidentally at cardiac operation or during evaluation of unrelated symptoms. Most common is absence of the entire left side of the pericardium. Partial left absence and absent right pericardium are very uncommon. Absence of the inferior pericardium, with or without diaphragmatic defects or aplasia, is quite rare in adults; any associated diaphragmatic defect may permit intrathoracic, including intrapericardial, herniation of abdominal organs.

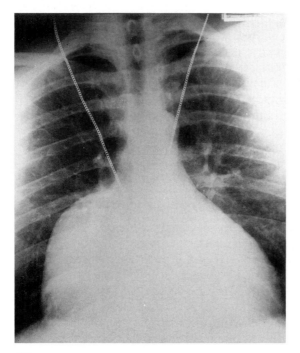

(A)

Figure 6.2   A. Posteroanterior roentgenogram of large pericardial cyst simulating pericardial effusion. B. Lateral film of Figure 6.2A emphasizing size of cyst. C. Oblique view of Figure 6.2A. Relative lucency of cyst and smoothness of contour.

Absence of the entire right or (especially) left pericardium permits homolateral cardiac displacement, visible on cardiac imaging and increased on lying on the side of the defect, *particularly on the left*, which strikingly accentuates cardiac mobility due to absent or decreased pericardial restraint. Small increases in preload, like volume loads, will cause undue ventricular dilatation, especially of the right ventricle, because of loss of pericardial restraint (page 18), and particularly with the patient in the left lateral decubitus. (This is also seen after pericardiocentesis for large effusions.) Absence of smaller parts of the left pericardium is potentially serious because of herniation and *entrapment of parts of the heart*, like the left atrium, left atrial appendage, the right atrium, the right ventricle and, with defects near the apex, dangerous protrusion through the defect of large parts of both ventricles. Moreover, *the edges of any defects may compress cardiac chambers, the great vessels, and coronary arteries and veins.* The *phrenic nerves may be displaced* to the edge of a defect, possibly contributing to symptoms.

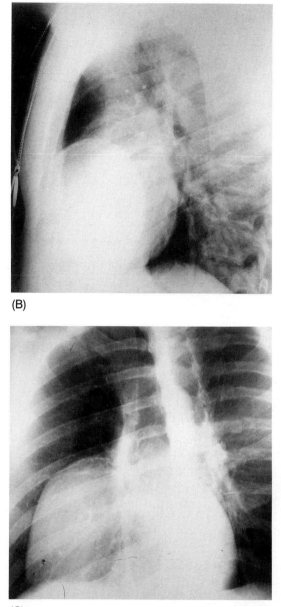

(B)

(C)

Figure 6.2 Continued

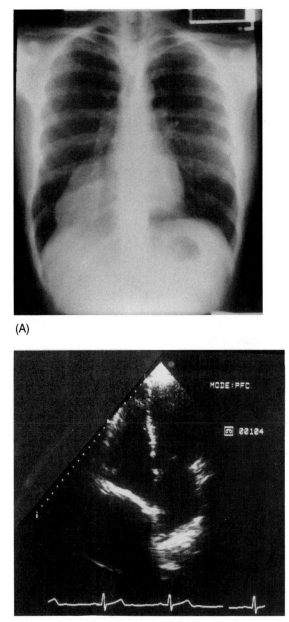

(A)

(B)

Figure 6.3   A. Multilobed asymptomatic pericardial cyst. This patient ran the Boston Marathon. B. Echocardiogram of patient in Figure 6.3A. Cyst compresses the right atrium

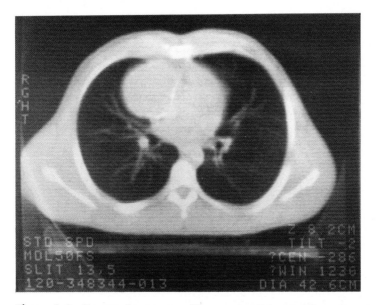

Figure 6.4 Computed tomogram of large pericardial cyst with condensed capsular rim.

Symptoms

Acute or chronic symptoms like vague, nonspecific chest pain or dyspnea, including trepopnea, may or may not be related to the pericardial defect, but exacerbation in the left lateral decubitus can lead to the detection of a left-sided defect. *Unusual torsion of the great vessels* by the unrestrained mobility of the heart may affect filling, ejection into the pulmonary artery, and aortic and coronary blood flow, all possible sources of symptoms. Torsion due to cardiac hypermobility has been associated with tricuspid chordal rupture. Typical angina and even acute myocardial infarction occur when the edge of a defect critically interrupts a coronary artery.

Physical Findings

These usually can only support the diagnosis because of nonspecificity. Most findings occur in left-sided absence and include basal ejection murmurs, wide split second heart sound, at least partly related to frequent right bundle branch block, and often bradycardia. Some patients have apical midsystolic clicks and systolic murmurs of undetermined origin that are accentuated by inspiration. Most striking in extensive left-sided defects are conspicuous precordial impulses with the apex frequently in the anterior or midaxillary line.

GRAPHIC FEATURES (TABLE 6.2)

Electrocardiogram

Sinus bradycardia is common. Usually with *complete left defects*, electrocardiographic (ECG) changes reflect the anatomic, posturally changing abnormalities and the relative volume overload of the right heart. Right axis deviation and incomplete or complete right bundle branch block are the rule; the occasional large R waves in leads V1 or V2 are mainly related to the bundle branch block. Leftward displacement of the precordial transition zone is common, with

Table 6.2   Congenital Absence of the Left Pericardium[a]: Graphic Features (Some or all Present)

Chest x-ray
    Cardiac displacement to left; increased mobility in left lateral decubitus
    Apparent right heart enlargement
    Prominent pulmonary conus
    Interposition of lung:
        Between aorta and pulmonary artery
        Between inferior heart border and diaphragm

Electrocardiogram
    Sinus bradycardia
    Right axis deviation
    Right bundle branch block: incomplete or complete
    Left displacement of precordial QRS transition
    Peaked P waves, *esp.* V1–V3
    With coronary compression by edge of defect: ischemic changes

Echocardiogram
    Cardiac hypermobility with postural changes
    Swinging movements
    Paradoxic or flat ventricular septal motion
    Marked reduction of diastolic change in dimension of right atrium
    Entrapped (herniated) structures, *esp.* left atrium; left atrial appendage

Doppler
    Increased diastolic wave velocity in superior vena cava and pulmonary artery
    Decreased systolic wave velocity in superior vena cava

Computed tomography and magnetic resonance imaging
    Absence of pericardial tissue on left
    Absent preaortic pericardial recess
    Entrapped (herniated) structures, *esp.* left atrium (decisive test)[a]

[a]Herniation of the left atrial appendage is virtually diagnostic; it is well seen on Doppler and radioisotopic blood pool examination. (Must be differentiated from congenital aneurysm of left atrium.)

poor R-wave progression sometimes mimicking anterior infarction. Conspicuous single peaked P waves in the medial precordial leads (for instance V1 to V3) reflect right atrial overload and increased right atrial proximity to the chest wall.

Imaging

In complete or extensive left pericardial absence, chest x-rays show levodisplacement of the heart and the aortic knob, with the trachea remaining midline. (Diagnostic induction of a pneumopericardium is no longer necessary.) The pulmonary artery "segment" bulges or fills in to straighten ("mitralize") the left heart borders; the right border may be so levodisplaced that the spine is clearly seen. Projections of lung between the aorta and pulmonary artery or between the left diaphragmatic leaf and the inferior cardiac border are highly diagnostic. Herniation of the left atrial appendage is virtually diagnostic of partial left defect but must be distinguished from congenital left atrial aneurysm.

Computed tomography (CT) and *magnetic resonance imaging* (MRI) show all the features and are the most reliable for actual absence of pericardial tissue, with MRI the most sensitive of all methods and capable of showing the typically absent preaortic pericardial recess, a structure that is almost always seen in normal hearts, in both partial and complete absence of the left pericardium.

Transthoracic echocardiography often requires a higher and much more lateral window than usual for the procedure; the *transesophageal* technique is superior. Echocardiography is only rarely specific enough to confirm loss of the pericardial echo but is consistent with right ventricular enlargement and volume overload, including dilation of the right heart and paradoxic or flat systolic motion of the ventricular septum, which, however, thickens normally in systole. Maximal right atrial dimensional change is radically reduced; left atrial dimensional change remains normal. Tricuspid ring excursion is correspondingly reduced; mitral excursion remains normal. *Doppler* examination of any local cardiac herniation shows low-velocity cyclic flow in and out of the herniated structure, the presence of which can be confirmed by *isotopic blood pool imaging*. In complete absence of the left pericardium Doppler interrogation of the superior vena cava and pulmonary veins shows increased diastolic wave velocity at both sites and decreased caval systolic wave velocity. These suggest accentuation of changes in systemic over those in pulmonary venous return, perhaps related to abnormal differences in right and left myocardial transmural pressures (page 21) in unilateral pericardial absence. *Radionuclide perfusion imaging* can demonstrate lung tissue between the pulmonary artery and the aorta or between the heart and the diaphragm, producing strong evidence for pericardial absence.

Catheterization and *cardioangiography* are mainly useful for differential diagnosis, identifying coronary compression and left atrial appendage herniation and also to rule in or out associated congenital cardiac abnormalities. Except for any zones of cardiac or vascular entrapment, pressures are unaffected.

The variants of congenital pericardial absence must be distinguished from lesions causing a similar appearance on imaging, like left ventricular aneurysm, left atrial aneurysm, tumors of the lung or heart, hilar adenopathy, mitral valve disease, tricuspid valve disease, atrial septal defect, pulmonic stenosis and idiopathic dilation of the pulmonary artery.

Treatment

Treatment is reserved for symptomatic patients unless an asymptomatic or threatened herniation is detected. This includes partial or complete pericardiectomy, pericardioplasty or actual incision and longitudinal extension of the defect to relieve tension on critical structures, with careful attention to preserving the phrenic nerves. Left atrial appendectomy may be necessary. As with most cardiac and pericardial operations, postoperative adhesions help to stabilize cardiac position.

COMPLETE CONGENITAL ABSENCE OF THE PERICARDIUM

Extremely rare, this is virtually always discovered by accident at operation or imaging for other conditions.

PERICARDIAL BANDS

Extremely rare, these fibrocollagenous structures tend to obstruct the superior vena cava, producing the customary "SVC syndrome." At operation there is no evidence of antecedent or concurrent inflammation.

SECONDARY CONGENITAL ABNORMALITIES

These extremely rare conditions are self-explanatory, as listed in Table 6.1.

KEY POINTS

1. Partial congenital pericardial defects have characteristic but mainly nonspecific clinical and hemodynamic consequences.
2. Principal dangers of pericardial defects, especially left-sided: herniation and entrapment of parts of the heart and adjacent vessels; coronary compression by edge of defect.

3. Congenital pericardial cysts are usually inconsequential; occasionally they simulate other masses. Large intrapericardial congenital bronchogenic cysts are more likely to encroach on adjacent structures.

BIBLIOGRAPHY

1. Bandeira FC, de Sa, VPO, Moriguti JC, Rodrigues AJ, Jurca MC, Almeida-Filho OC, Marin-Neto JA, Maciel BC. Cardiac tamponade: an unusualcomplication of pericardial cyst. J Am Soc Echocardiog 1996; 9: 108–112.
2. Churchill, E.D., Mallory, T.B. Pericardial coelomic cysts. N. Engl. J. Med. 1937; 217:958–968.
3. Fukuda, N., Oki, T., Iuchi, A., et al. Pulmonary and systemic venous flow patterns assessed by transesophageal Doppler echocardiography in congenital absence of the pericardium. Am. J. Cardiol. 1995; 75:1286–1288.
4. Maier, H.C. Diverticulum of the pericardium—With observations on mode of development. Circulation 1957; 16:1040–1045.
5. Nasser, W.K. Congenital disease of the pericardium. In: Spodick D.H. (ed.). Pericardial Disease. Philadelphia: Davis, 1976, pp. 271–286.
6. Satur CMR, Hsin MKY, Dussek JE. Giant pericardial cysts. Ann Thorac Surg 1996; 61: 208–210.
7. Vargas-Barron, J., Sanchez-Ugarte, T., Keirns, C., et al. The differential diagnosis of partial absence of left pericardium and congenital left atrial aneurysm. Am. Heart J. 1989; 118:1348–1350.

7

Acquired Pericardial Disease: Pathogenesis and Overview

SPECIAL CONSIDERATION: Polyserositis,
Hemopericardium, Chylopericardium, Cholesterol
Pericarditis, Pneumopericardium, Pericardial Disorders
During Pregnancy

DISEASES OF THE PERICARDIUM

Table 7.1 lists the nine major categories of pericardial disease. Virtually every known pathologic process, medical and surgical, is represented either as primarily involving the pericardium or with an indirect pericardial impact. Thus, a freshly diagnosed case of pericardial disease may or may not be related to other conditions recognized in any patient. Indeed, one should never be surprised to find the pericardium involved in any patient, either on its own or in the course of more generalized or neighboring disorders Moreover, the classifications in Tables 7.1 and 8.1 cannot be free of *overlapping categories, which are assigned as a matter of clarity as well as comprehensiveness.* For example, postpericardial injury syndromes like the postmyocardial infarction syndrome, belong not only to the various categories of myocardial or pericardial injury but also to the immunopathies because of their recurrent or chronic perpetuation. This is also true of "hypersensitivity states" in which the patient reacts abnormally to immunogenic stimuli like allergens and insect bites and to some medications. A category of *iatrogenic pericardiopathies* (Table 7.2) obviously overlaps traumatic, drug-induced and infectious forms; this subcategory mainly represents disorders of medical progress.

Table 7.1 Etiology/Pathogeneses of Acquired Diseases of the Pericardium[a]

Major categories[b]
- I. Idiopathic pericarditis (syndromes)
- II. Due to living agents—infectious, parasitic
- III. Vasculitis—connective tissue disease
- IV. Immunopathies/hypersensitivity states
- V. Disease of contiguous structures
- VI. Disorders of metabolism
- VII. Trauma—direct, indirect
- VIII. Neoplasms—primary, metastatic, multicentric
- IX. Of uncertain pathogenesis or in association with various syndromes

[a]Considerable overlap, e.g., categories III and IV; V and VII.
[b]See corresponding chapters for detailed outlines; see also Table 8.1

Pericardial Responses to Inflammation and Irritation

Any noxious agent impinging on the pericardium can set up responses producing clinical pericardial disease. For example, any microorganisms or their antigenic material or immunocytes activated elsewhere can reach the pericardium via the bloodstream, lymphatic vessels or adjacent organs or by traumatic (including surgical) implantation and set up infection producing an acute, chronic or subacute pericarditis. This includes perpetuation or recurrences due to persistent or intermittent immunopathic episodes or, occasionally, to reinfection. *Infectious pericardial diseases* are discussed in detail in Chapter 16. When pericarditis is sufficiently intense, a rim of inflammation of the subjadcent myocardium, usually superficial, often permits electrocardiographic diagnosis (the pericardium produces no electromotive forces of its own; Chapter 5). Whether from infection, vasculitis, irritation by tumor cells, or other pathogenetic agents, pericardial inflammatory responses are mediated by cytokines, like tumor necrosis factors and interleukins. These formidable substances nearly always also inflame the subpericardial myocardium but, curiously, spare the coronary arteries and veins.

Pericarditis and Myopericarditis

Intense inflammation involving both the myocardium and pericardium, produces *myopericarditis* in which the myocardial component is usually dominant. Clinically, it is rare for both conditions to be equally apparent (Chapter 9).

Table 7.2   Iatrogenic Pericardiopathies

Surgical
  Direct injury
  Postpericardiotomy syndrome
  Transplant
    Rejection
    Cyclosporine-associated
  Cardiac hypothermia
Instrumental trauma
  Pacemaker
    Epicardial implant
    Transvenous: perforation of heart/vessel
  Electrode catheter ablation for arrhythmias
  Endoscopic sclerotherapy of esophageal varices
  Transseptal catheterization of left ventricle
  Percutaneous left ventricular puncture
  Sternal bone marrow tap (historical)
  Kirchner wire (for sternoclavicular joint)
  Cerebral ventricular-atrium tubing (Torkildsen shunt)
Cardiac resuscitation
Iatrogenic pneumopericardium
Drug reactions and complications

Procainamide (lupus)	Penicillin
Hydralazine (lupus)	Dantrolene
Phenylbutazone	Cromolyn sodium
Methysergide	Doxorubicin
Diphenylhydantoin	Cyclosporine
Isoniazid	? Minoxidil
Anticoagulants (hemopericardium)	Antithrombotics (hemopericardium)

Radiation

Diseases of Neighboring and Contiguous Structures

Abnormalities of the myocardium, the pleura, the lungs, the diaphragm, the esophagus and the mediastinal lymph nodes may directly involve the pericardium by contiguity or by hematogenous or lymphogenous transmission and may remain silent or become clinically obvious. Sometimes pericarditis is the first clue to the disease in the offending organ. Transmural myocardial infarction involves the pericardium frequently, but pericardial involvement is diagnosed in fewer than half the cases. Tuberculous pericarditis when not due to hematogenous or lymphogenous implantation can be introduced by adjacent infected mediastinal lymph nodes. Pneumonias may eventually affect the pericardium directly if there is empyema. However, there may be simultaneous infection in both organs by the same microorganism or parasite via vascular transmission.

Neoplasia, Primary and Metastatic

Each of the tissues of the pericardium with the exception of the elastic tissue can give rise to primary malignancies and benign tumors, producing irritative (inflammatory) and physical effects that are usually misinterpreted. This is less true for metastatic malignancies. *If a primary neoplasm is already recognized, symptoms of any pericardial disease should always be considered suspect for metastases or a complication of treatment.* Occasionally, pericardial involvement is the first sign of the primary tumor.

PERICARDIAL FAT NECROSIS

Pericardial fat necrosis is included here only for completeness. This rare condition causes nondescript though sometimes sharp chest pain, usually in the left lower chest, which, because of its pleuritic fluctuation in some cases, suggests pleuritis or pericarditis. It may be suspected if the chest radiograph shows a particularly smudgy-looking pericardial fat pad near the cardiac apex. (At this writing, computed tomography and magnetic resonance studies are not available.) The lesion appears to have been successfully treated by anti-inflammatory agents or surgical resection.

PERICARDIAL EFFUSION

Strictly speaking, the term "pericardial effusion" refers to excess pericardial fluid produced by the pericardium itself, that is, its serosa, due to inflammation or other irritation. Clinically, "pericardial effusion" is identified as any excessive pericardial contents due to inflammatory exudation, systemic fluid retention, bleeding, gas (including air), pus or combinations of these. *Note: Pericardial effusions arise mainly if not entirely from the visceral pericardium.*

Hydropericardium (Transudates)

When there is systemic fluid retention, as in cardiac failure and other conditions that stimulate renal solute (particularly sodium) and water retention, pericardial fluid sometimes increases. Usually this is detected only by imaging, mainly by echocardiography, or at autopsy; the fluid is a transudate comparable to excessive pleural fluid accumulated under similar circumstances. Occasionally, hydropericardium can be first recognized as enlargement of the cardiac silhouette which may already be increased if there is cardiac disease. Acquired immunodeficiency syndrome (AIDS), though sometimes associated with acute fibrinous pericarditis (Chapter 8), more often leads to hydropericardium. There are no recognized clinical consequences except with exceptional massive hydropericardium, which may compress lung and other adjacent structures or cause misdiagnosis of a primarily pericardial lesion.

Inflammatory/Irritative Effusion (Exudates)

Most significant pericardial effusions are exudates appearing when the rate of inflammatory exudation exceeds the resorptive capacity of the serosa, particularly its lymphatics and veins, which may be obstructed by the inflammatory disease itself and compressed by the effusion itself. Pericardial diseases can damage or destroy some of all of the serosa; however, even if it is relatively intact, it may be overwhelmed by the sheer quantity of liquid. In most cases with significant effusion, serosal cell damage and desquamation combine with injury and compression of the microvasculature to impede reabsorption. Since large molecules are poorly transported by the pericardium, the tendency to fluid accumulation may be exaggerated by the oncotic effect of the protein-rich serous exudate. Yet it is not clear why inflammatory processes of apparently similar character may remain dry in one patient and pour out up to liters of fluid in another.

Pericardial effusions give rise to four functional states:

1. Slow production of small amounts of fluid, which remain undetected during life.
2. Clinically demonstrable effusion without apparent symptoms or signs of cardiac compression.
3. Smaller or larger effusion at a rate appropriate to compress the heart significantly but eventually checked by compensatory mechanisms.
4. Cardiac tamponade (although, as we shall see, *tamponade is a dynamic continuum*).

In items 1 and 2 above, either the normal residual capacity of the pericardium is not significantly exceeded or the fibrosa has an adequate opportunity to stretch. In either circumstance the clinical course is essentially that of clinically "dry" pericarditis (Chapter 8). On the other hand, *any degree of cardiac compression* may radically alter the situation by provoking far-reaching physiologic reactions, which may or may not succeed in compensating the effects of continuously increasing intrapericardial pressure that is proceeding in parallel with increased pericardial contents. Physiologically, *there is an indistinct border between compensated, even gently compressing pericardial effusion and overtly progressive tamponade of the heart*. Clinically, many significant effusions become stabilized at some level by cardiovascular, neuroendocrine and renal compensatory mechanisms (Chapter 12), while frank tamponade is a first-class emergency. Any effusion can become chronic or constantly threaten overt tamponade by further progression or precipitation due to intercurrent events like bleeding. However, in some cases with noncritical cardiac compression, including some with liters of effusion, effective cardiac performance, at least at rest, may not be compromised. Thus, clinical details and management of cases without critical cardiac compression may differ considerably from those of outright tamponade (Chapter 11). Yet, even in patients who never develop corresponding clinical syndromes, *physiologic effects of effusions from minimal to very large are detectable with the appropriate instrumentation* (page XX)

In the absence of adhesions or loculations, intrapericardial fluid accumulation proceeds in a characteristic sequence, beginning inferiorly and proceeding anteriorly and laterally. Accumulation may occur principally to one side, usually the left, where the parietal pericardium is thinnest. Except for the pericardial oblique sinus, which is a part of the *pericardial reserve volume* (Chapter 3), and except in massive effusions, virtually no fluid collects directly behind the heart due to the thickness of the posterior pericardium and its shell-like clasp of the left atrium. Further limiting retrocardiac fluid penetration is posterior pericardial tautness from the pericardium's attachment to the great vessels above, the pulmonary veins, and the diaphragm below. Yet anterior intrapericardial scarring—e.g., after cardiac surgery, may anchor the heart, preventing retrodisplacement and permitting fluid to enter the posterior pericardial recesses much earlier.

When abnormal pericardial contents include bleeding, thrombosis, neoplastic tissue, pus, gas or combinations of these, the clinical picture may be modified significantly, as may the texture of the effusion on imaging.

POLYSEROSITIS

Polyserositis means multiple serous membrane inflammation—and "polyserositis" is a descriptive term rather than a disease. Many of the conditions causing pericarditis can simultaneously or sequentially inflame other serous sacs. Like pericarditis, polyserositis may make its debut at any inflammatory stage from acute, which can be dramatic or insidious, to chronic. Symptoms and signs referable to one or another serosa may dominate the clinical picture, yet pericardial involvement can be most distressing because of the quality of certain pericardial pain syndromes, the emergent situation of cardiac tamponade or the steady deterioration of cardiac constriction (e.g., *tuberculous serositis*). In other instances, physiologically unimportant pericardial adhesions are the result. The *vasculitis–connective tissue disease group* is most likely to produce true polyserositis (exudates), while *AIDS* produces a capillary leak syndrome with noninflammatory transudative polyserosal effusions much more often than true polyserositis. During cardiac tamponade or constrictive pericarditis, noninflammatory transudates across membranes other than the pericardium can falsely suggest multiple membrane involvement by a primary process, such as Pick's disease ("Pick's pericarditic pseudocirrhosis"). Classically, Pick's occurs in patients diagnosed as having hepatic cirrhosis owing to ascites and hepatomegaly but belatedly proving to have constrictive pericarditis.

HEMOPERICARDIUM (TABLE 7.3)

Hemopericardium is always important because it signifies either frank bleeding into the pericardium, as in cardiac rupture, intrapericardial rupture of dissecting hematoma or intramural hemorrhage of the aorta, erosion of vessels by a tumor or by an aggressive inflammatory process, or bleeding diatheses including administration of thrombolytic agents to patients with pericarditis. While many inflammatory effusions are accompanied by at least microscopic bleeding, *detectable bleeding can occur in effusions of almost every etiology and sometimes cannot be distinguished by inspection from frank blood.* Unless overwhelmed by the rate of bleeding, the distinct fibrinolytic and anticoagulant properties of the pericardial serosa (page 24) as well as the beating action of the heart (which tends to defibrinate blood) nearly always keeps most or all of the blood liquid and well mixed with the other pericardial contents. It must be emphasized that frank blood (by hematocrit), and particularly clots, nearly always indicates major bleeding, which must be dealt with at its source. Indeed, clots are recognizable by echocardiography as hyperechoic objects in a pericardial effusion and usually mandate *surgical* rather than needle drainage. Moreover, *any significant amount of blood in the pericardial fluid, especially in the presence of damaged serosa, has the potential for forming adhesions and loculations.* These are common after blunt cardiopericardial trauma, penetration of the myocardium by catheters and of the heart and pericardium by penetrating wounds; the latter include cardiac surgery, especially valve replacement and coronary bypass. Postsurgical intrapericardial hematoma can occur anywhere but most often over the right atrium. Yet, in the absence of an obvious physical or inflammatory cause, malignancy is probably the major etiology of hemopericardium.

Subacute and chronic hemopericardium may be the result of trauma, bleeding disorders or vascular anomalies; frequently the etiology is untraceable. Even following wounds of the heart, tamponade may be sufficiently delayed to qualify as chronic, possibly because of late displacement of a sealing thrombus or tearing of adhesions. Persistent enlargement of pericardial contents may occur due

Table 7.3 Hemopericardium

A. Frank blood
  I. Wounds
      Penetrating
          Catheters
          Pacemaker wires
          Ablation of arrhythmogenic tissue
          Chest (cardiac) wounds
          Esophageal wounds/erosion
          Intracardiac injections during resuscitation
          Cardiac laceration
          Pericardiocentesis
          Removal of epicardial wires
          Amniocentesis (fetal tamponade)
      Blunt chest trauma
          Impacts/deceleration
          Resuscitation
  II. Cardiac abnormalities
          Chamber rupture
          Hemorrhagic infarct
  III. Neoplasms—malignant/benign
          Erosion of pericardial vessels
          Pericardial irritant coagulation disorders
          Vascular tumors
  IV. Aortic disease
          Dissecting hematoma ("aneurysm")
          Intramural hemorrhage (IMH)
  V. Hemorrhagic diatheses
          Reperfusion/thrombolysis
              +Pericarditis
              +Hemorrhagic infarct
          Primary coagulation disorders
          Scurvy
B. Bloody pericardial effusion
  I. All from section A above
  II. Idiopathic pericarditis
  III. Infection (all forms)
  IV. Parasitoses
  V. Noninfective inflammation
  VI. Uremic pericarditis
  VII. Vasculitis—connective tissue disease group

to indrawing of fluid "attracted" by the osmotic effects of split proteins (e.g., fibrinolysis) and other molecules that increase the total number of intrapericardial particles.

In either chronic or subacute bleeding, the danger of adhesions, potentially leading to constriction, is such that pericardiectomy must be considered. Indeed both loculated and clotted hemopericardium (massive or localized) have caused typical constrictive pericarditis syndromes and hemodynamics. Usually the pericardium contains large quantities of old, chocolaty blood, which may be loculated and mixed with evidence of more recent hemorrhage. Organization of bloody sludge and clots, rich in fibrin, is a substrate for constriction, the pericardial tissue itself often showing inflammatory changes, including granulomas and evidence of old and recent hemorrhage.

CHYLOPERICARDIUM

Chylopericardium is the result of copious extravasation of chyle owing either to a neoplasm, particularly lymphangiomatous hamartoma (congenital lymphangioma) involving the pericardium, or abnormal communication between the pericardium and thoracic duct. Many cases, however, are of unexplained origin, although they may follow cardiac and other thoracic surgery, suggesting damage to lymphatic channels. (Significant anatomic variability in the mediastinal lymphatics and thoracic duct makes this likely.) Chylopericardium tends to be large and chronic with an element of chronic tamponade and has rarely been implicated as the cause of constrictive pericarditis. The fluid is milky and alkaline, with electrolyte, protein, glucose and cholesterol levels similar to those of blood serum. Fat studies are typical of chyle, including the presence of chylomicrons on ultracentrifugation. In the neoplastic group, the pericardium can refill so rapidly that reaccumulation may be visible during operation.

Although the posterior pericardial lymph drains around the esophagus to the thoracic duct, no visible communication may be demonstrated between the pericardium and the alimentary tract, especially in nonneoplastic patients. Yet some communication is indicated in chylopericardium by (1) intrapericardial appearance of ingested lipophilic dyes (e.g., Sudan III mixed in corn or olive oil); (2) frequently successful treatment by ligating the thoracic duct; (3) lymphangiography, including technetium-99m lymphangiography, demonstrating a relationship between the thoracic duct and the pericardial cavity; and (4) computed tomography or magnetic resonance imaging densities consistent with fat. (It is important to recognize that if the patient has not eaten for some time, chylous fluid may become clear).

Cases that have no relation to surgical or other procedures or to an erosive malignancy are often referred to as *primary chylopericardium*. (Note: Chyle

more often extravasates directly into the pleural spaces. Even a primary pericardial mesothelioma may cause chylothorax without chylopericardium.) While
chylous pleural and peritoneal effusions usually cause no adhesions, chlyo-
pericardium can be associated with pericardial inflammation and scarring. These
may follow repeated drainage, which may end the chylopericardium but obli-
gates indefinite assessment for constrictive pericarditis. Because chyle is bactericidal, the inflammation is unlikely to be infectious.

Conservative management includes pericardial drainage and a low-fat diet
with an increased ratio of medium-chain triglycerides. More often, low thoracic
duct ligation plus a pericardial window or resection, preferably through a left
thoracotomy, is required. Pericardial-peritoneal shunt drainage has been successful in children with the advantage of local anesthetic and subxiphoid incision.

CHOLESTEROL PERICARDITIS

Also known as "gold-paint pericarditis," *cholesterol pericarditis* is characterized by a high concentration of cholesterol and other lipids in pericardial fluid
and often cholesterol crystals in pericardial tissue. Cholesterol effusions tend
to be large and subacute or chronic and of multiple etiology. Total pericardial
fluid cholesterol approaches or exceeds blood cholesterol (usually normal), with
values often over 500 mg/dL, accompanied by increased total lipids (usually
well over 300 mg/dL). Cholesterol is found in all *myxedematous effusions,* but
without crystal formation and usually in concentrations well below the elevated
serum level characteristic of this disease. Exceptional cases, however, are indistinguishable from other forms of cholesterol pericarditis, with precipitation
of cholesterol crystals due to unusually high pericardial fluid concentrations
(page 299).

Cholesterol effusions are cloudy or turbid, brown, yellow, orange, amber,
or opalescent and occasionally port wine or coffee colored. When there are
many flakes of crystallized cholesterol, they develop a satiny sheen, imparting
a "gold paint" appearance. There may be evidence of recent or remote hemorrhage with leukocytes, mainly lymphocytes, in varying numbers. Specific
gravity is nearly always over 1.020, while the electrolyte, total protein concentrations and albumin:globulin ratios approximate those of blood. The pericardium is often thickened by scarring, frequently with variable amounts of fibrin
and yellowish nodules, plaques and papillomatous masses of cholesterol lining
the interior. The epicardium may be visibly inflamed and constrictive epicarditis
is not uncommon. Microscopically, there is often intense fibrosis, inflammation with many cholesterol clefts and crystals and other lipid crystals in plates,
needles and rhomboids. Phagocytes take up considerable lipid material, and

some iron pigment and histocytes with foamy cytoplasm can be seen. Crystals and clefts are often surrounded by foreign-body giant cells and elements of a chronic granulomatous inflammation.

Cholesterol-laden effusions and precipitation of crystals have been found in association with pericarditis in *tuberculosis, rheumatoid arthritis and after traumatic hemopericardium* as well as in *myxedema.* In the inflammatory lesions, *granulomas* (granulomas normally contain cholesterol) are probably the source of the cholesterol, as is *blood*; since bleeding can occur in most forms of pericarditis, blood may be a common denominator. In "formes frustes," high concentrations of cholesterol are not accompanied by crystal formation. However, *aging of serous effusions causes a significant fall in an initially high tendency to keep cholesterol in solution.* Thus, any chronic effusion might result in cholesterol precipitation, particularly in the presence of a rich source of cholesterol, such as hemorrhage.

These usually very large effusions have been documented for as long as twenty years. Unfortunately, paracentesis frequently results in rapid refilling and may be followed by epicardial constriction (which can occur rapidly) or unremitting chronic cardiac tamponade (Chapter 25). Curiously, repeated drainage often yields fluid of widely varying, including extremely low, cholesterol concentrations. Conservative treatment is drainage, but definitive treatment is pericardial resection and management of any underlying disease.

LYMPHOPERICARDIUM

This rare lesion is related to either local or, more commonly, generalized lymphangiectasis. The fluid has characteristics of lymph and, like many cases of chylopericardium, may contain a predominance of lymphocytes.

PNEUMOPERICARDIUM AND PNEUMOHYDROPERICARDIUM (SEE ALSO CHAPTER 21)

In adults, *pneumopericardium* usually occurs in conjunction with either hemopericardium or some type of effusion (Table 7.4). It may follow wounds or fistulous communications due to primary disease or instrumentation of the esophagus, the bronchi, the stomach or other viscera, which can also produce *pyopneumopericardium.* Pericardial infection by gas-producing organisms duplicates the picture. Some cases may be due to malignant destruction of tissue but also to penetrating and nonpenetrating trauma of the chest and upper abdomen or following single lung transplantation. After pneumonectomy, pneumopericardium may be produced by gas instilled to prevent mediastinal shift. Laparoscopy can admit air via peritoneopericardial communications prob-

Table 7.4 **Pathogenesis of Pneumopericardium and Pneumohydropericardium**

A. **Traumatic**
  1. Penetrating
     1. Missiles, blades
     2. Fractured ribs
  2. Blunt
     1. Lung/pericardial injury
     2. Fractured ribs
  3. Penetration—esophagus, stomach, intestine, peritoneum
     1. Swallowed objects
     2. Penetrating ulcer
     3. Penetrating malignancy
B. **Infectious**
     1. Lung/pleural/tracheobronchial infection penetrating pericardium
        a. Empyema, gangrene, abscess
        b. Tuberculosis
        c. Fungal infection
        d. Purulent infection
        e. Other
     2. Suppurative pericarditis
        a. Perforation of lung
        b. Sinus through chest wall
        c. Gas-producing microorganisms
C. **Iatrogenic**
     1. Pericardicentesis
     2. Diagnostic pneumopericardium (rare today)
     3. Pericardiotomy
     4. Pneumonectomy
     5. Therapeutic pneumothorax
     6. Positive pressure ventilation (mainly infants)
     7. Laparoscopy

ably of embryonic origin. Infants and occasional adults on respirators develop pneumopericardium due to alveolar rupture by high-pressure air and oxygen dissecting its way into the pericardium via weak points in the pericardial reflections over the great vessels (page 11). When due to indirect (blunt) trauma, pneumopericardium occurs by three main mechanisms: (1) direct tracheobronchial-pericardial communication, (2) pneumothorax with a pleuropericardial tear and (3) penetration along pulmonary venous perivascular sheaths from ruptured alveoli to the pericardium (Chapter 21)

On *chest roentgenography* an air fluid level indicates that this is a *pneumo-hydropericardium*. An upright chest x-ray may show air in the transverse sinus (page 10) in the posteroanterior projection, a lucent triangle anterior to the aortic root in the lateral projection and often subcutaneous emphysema. *Iatrogenic pneumohydropericardium* (Figure 7.1) results when air, carbon dioxide or other gas is deliberately introduced after drainage of pericardial fluid to obtain more detailed pictures of the pericardium and the cardiac surfaces. Since the introduction of sophisticated cardiopericardial imaging techniques like magnetic resonance imaging, this procedure (which was once thought to also prevent adhesions) is no longer useful. Rarely, unusual conditions resemble a pathologic pneumohydropericardium (Figure 7.2A and B). *Tension pneumo-pericardium* due to increasing air or gas produces *pneumotamponade*, often with marked cyanosis and hypotension. It is diagnosed and imaged like fluid tamponade (Chapter 11).

Pneumopericardium and hydropneumopericardium can produce audible clicks and splashes and an "air gap" sign on M-mode echocardiograms: a cyclic band of interfering echoes with a dropout of posterior structures (also seen

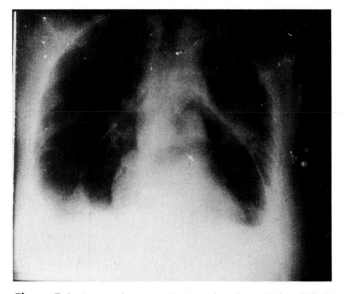

Figure 7.1 Iatrogenic pneumohydropericardium. Fluid—450mL—was drained to relieve tamponade and 450mL of air was introduced, demonstrating some residual fluid below and essentially normal pericardium (perhaps some thickening on the left). Pericardial passage over the aortic arch is well demonstrated.

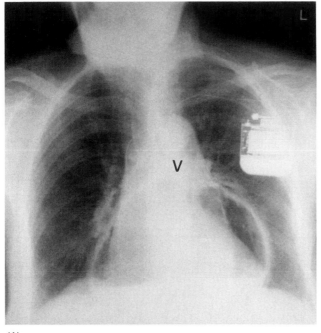

(A)

Figure 7.2 A. False pneumohydropericardium. Large diaphragmatic hernia. Heart outlined by fundus of stomach, containing gas and fluid. Striking resemblance to Figure 7.1 except that the false "pericardium" passes well below the aortic arch (arrowhead). B. Same patient as in Figure 7.2A. Opacification of esophagus and stomach obliterates heart shadow.

in pneumomediastinum). However, diagnosis of pneumopericardium is by direct imaging.

Pericardial Disorders During Pregnancy

The etiopathogenetic mix of pericardial disorders is what would be expected in nonpregnant women, although increasing numbers of pregnancies in patients in their midthirties to midforties require differential diagnosis from other diseases more prevalent at those ages. As in nonpregnant patients, idiopathic pericarditis is usually benign, but can cause tamponade and eventuate in chronically recurrent pericarditis, particularly after corticosteriod therapy (Chapter 24), or chronic pericardial effusion (Chapter 25)

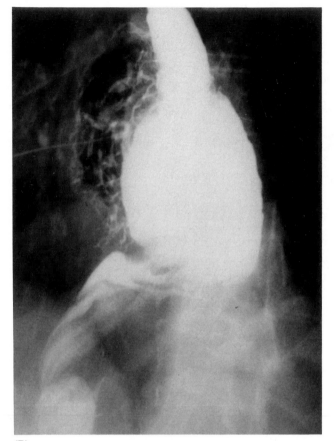

(B)

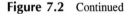

Figure 7.2 Continued

Pericardial diseases occur only sporadically in pregnant women. While a variety of etiologic forms and every functional type and complication occur, there is no evidence that pregnancy increases susceptibility to the causative processes. Indeed, although serious tamponade has been observed, the physiologic 40 to 50% increase in blood volume during pregnancy may moderate its physiologic and clinical expression (effect of hypervolemia; page 181). For the same reason, acute myopericarditis with an intense myocardial component (Chapter 9) could more easily cause congestive failure—a form of peripartum cardiomyopathy. On the other hand, many pregnant women develop a minimal to moderate-sized, clinically silent hydropericardium by the third trimester

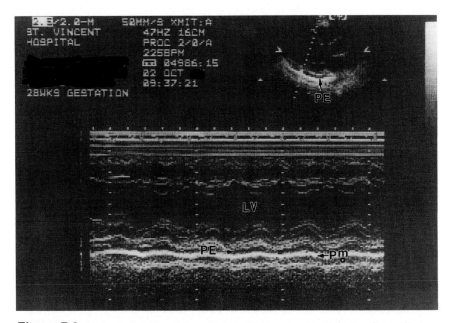

Figure 7.3 Hydropericardium of pregnancy. Typical small, clinically silent effusion discovered at 28 weeks. PE = pericardial effusion. pm = pericardium. LV = left ventricle.

(Figure 7.3), presumably physiologic and unrelated to any abnormalities of blood proteins or cells; this could combine with less than usual exudation by any acute pericarditis to cause cardiac compression.

Significant symptoms, electrocardiographic changes or physiologic impairment warrant hospitalization for diagnosis and at least initial management. Most pericardial disorders run their accustomed courses during pregnancy and are managed as in nonpregnant patients: nonsteroidal anti-inflammatory drugs (NSAIDs) for most acute pericarditis, antibiotics and drainage for suppurative pericarditis; NSAIDs or corticosteroids for lupus and other vasculitides; drainage of tamponading fluid; and pericardectomy for constrictive pericarditis, recurrent pericardial effusion and resistant bacterial pericarditis. Even after pericardectomy, there are, as a rule, normal deliveries of normal infants; premature labor has been only occasional, and patients have gone on to one or more additional successful pregnancies.

Fetal Pericardial Fluid can be detected by echocardiography after 20 weeks' gestation and is normally of 2mm or less depth. Over 2mm should raise questions of hydrops fetalis, Rh disease, hypoalbuminemia or an immunopathy. However, "idiopathic" pericardial effusions may occur in an otherwise normal fetus.

KEY POINTS

1. Virtually every category of disease affects the pericardium.
2. *Diseases of neighboring tissues* involve the pericardium directly, often silently, sometimes with serious consequences and frequently complicating diagnosis.
3. *"Pericardial effusion"* includes *exudates* due to a variety of irritative/inflammatory processes and *transudates* that are usually complications of systemic disorders. Systemic inflammations also cause *polyserositis*.
4. Small effusions can be accommodated by the pericardial reserve volume without detectable clinical consequences.
5. *Hemopericardium* can occur in almost every kind of pericardial lesion and has adhesion-producing, including constriction-producing potential.
6. *Chylopericardium*, usually due to surgical trauma of the thoracic duct, is occasionally of unknown ("idiopathic") or neoplastic origin.
7. *Cholesterol pericarditis*, whether of unknown origin or due to myxedema or granulomatous disorders like tuberculosis and rheumatoid arthritis, provokes large, rapidly recurring effusions and occasionally—except in myxedema—constrictive pericarditis.
8. *Pneumopericardium* and *pneumohydropericardium* are usually due to pathologic communication between the pericardial cavity and gas-filled organs and rarely due to gas-producing microorganisms, or they are deliberately or accidentally iatrogenic. In infants, the principal cause is complications from the use of mechanical respirators.

BIBLIOGRAPHY

1. Brawley, R.K., Vasko, J.S., Morrow, A.G. Cholesterol pericarditis: Considerations of its pathogenesis and treatment. *Am. J. Med.* 1966; 41:235-248.
2. Chan BBK, Murphy MC, Rogers BM. Management of chylopericardium. J. Pediat Surg 1990; 25:1185-1189.
3. Enein, M., Abou-Sina, A.A., Kassem, M., El-Tabbakh, G. Echocardiography of the pericardium in pregnancy. Obstet. Gynecol. 1987; 69:852-853.
4. Kim S, Sahn SA. Postcardiac injury syndrome. An immunologic pleural fluid analysis. Chest 1996; 109: 570 - 572.
5. Miller, W.L., Osborn, M.J., Sinak, L.J., Westbrook, B.M. Pyopneumopericardium attributed to an esophagopericardial fistula: Report of a survivor and review of the literature. *Mayo. Clin. Proc.* 1991; 66:1041-1045.
6. Santora, L., Elkayam, U. Pericardial disorders and pregnancy. In: Elkayam, U., Gleicher, N. (eds.). Cardiac Problems in Pregnancy. New York: Liss, 1982, pp. 115-129.

7. Spodick, D.H. Infective pericarditis: Etiologic and clinical spectra. In: Reddy, P.S. (ed.). *Pericardial Disease*. New York: Raven Press, 1982, pp. 307–312.
8. Spodick, D.H. Diseases of the Pericardium. In: Parmley, W.W., Chatterjee, K. (eds.). Cardiology. Vol. 2. Philadelphia: Lippincott, 1995, chap. 43.
9. Spodick, D.H. Pericarditis in systemic diseases. Cardiol. Clin. 1990; 8:709–716.

8

Acute, Clinically Noneffusive ("Dry") Pericarditis

GENERAL CONSIDERATIONS

The term "dry pericarditis" (*pericarditis sicca*), strictly speaking, indicates pericardial inflammation without pericardial effusion—that is, with a strictly fibrinous inflammatory exudate, containing variable numbers of inflammatory cells (Figures 8.1 to 8.3). Since most pericardial irritation evokes at least some fluid—often discoverable by sensitive imaging, notably echocardiography—*clinically dry pericarditis* encompasses those cases in which excess pericardial fluid is virtually absent or clinically unimportant: *no signs or symptoms are ascribable to increased pericardial fluid*. Clinically dry pericarditis is the form of acute pericarditis most commonly recognized by most physicians because it epitomizes acute pericarditis of the most common etiologies, mainly the acute infectious pericarditides and especially viral pericarditis, which includes most cases of "idiopathic" pericarditis (Chapter 23). Virtually all etiologic forms of acute pericarditis can present in this manner (Table 8.1). In some (e.g., rheumatoid pericarditis; pages 317–318) the acute phase is usually missed or discovered by accident. Consequently, the patient's history is that of the etiologic illness, like various viral syndromes; exceptions include cases where acute pericarditis is the first sign of systemic disorders, e.g., systemic lupus erythematosus, various malignancies, tuberculous pericarditis. Thus, with in-

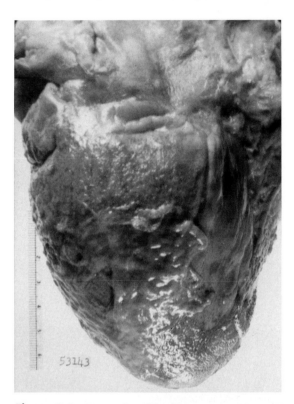

Figure 8.1 Dry pericarditis. Heart covered by exuberant fibrin masses apparently patterned by cardiac movements (From Spodick, Acute Pericarditis, 1959; author's copyright.)

fectious pericarditis, the onset may be preceded by local and systemic signs of infection. In many of these, as in the vasculitis–connective tissue disease group (Chapter 19), there is also an immunopathic component, although initially the pericarditis may be infective. The classic example is of acute viral pericarditis, responsible for the majority of cases of "idiopathic" acute pericarditis and nearly always preceded by a recent respiratory, gastrointestinal or "flulike" illness. Accordingly, the symptoms and signs of acute pericarditis will often be modified by or coexist with those of the inciting illness. Finally, a specific etiologic diagniosis (i.e. nonidiopathic) is most often determinable in "sicker" patients and those with nonserous fluids who develop tamponade.

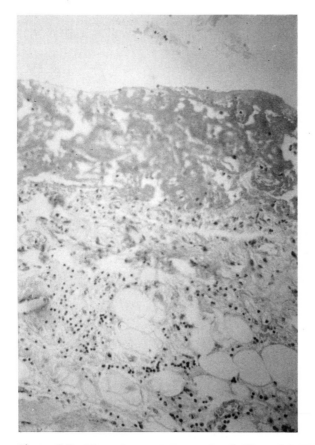

Figure 8.2   Photomicrograph from patient in Figure 8.1. Thick fibrin layer with scattered inflammatory cells overlies epicardial fat, which is densely infiltrated by leukocytes—mainly polymorphonuclears with some lymphocytes. (From Spodick, Acute Pericarditis, 1959; author's copyright.)

SYMPTOMS

Onset

Clinically dry pericarditis of any etiology may begin abruptly or insidiously, although certain varieties tend to be characterized by one or the other mode of onset. Bacterial and viral pericarditis, for example, often strike with dramatic symptoms, while the advent of uremic or tuberculous pericarditis often goes unnoticed by the patient. Diagnosis may be suggested by symptoms alone when the onset is abrupt; it may depend partly or entirely on objective manifestations

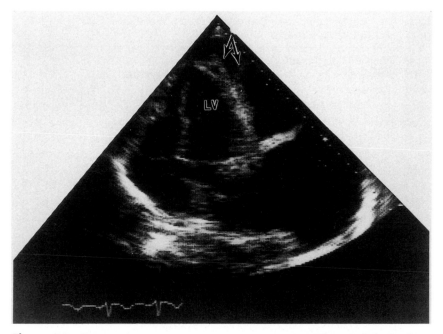

Figure 8.3 Echocardiogram in a patient with acute pericarditis and clinically silent pericardial effusion ("clinically dry" pericarditis). Arrows show fibrin masses along the left ventricular epicardium.

when the onset is insidious. Viral pericarditis, for example, can declare itself painfully by awakening the patient in the early hours of the morning or by crescendoing pain over several hours, while tuberculous pericarditis often presents as a fever of unknown origin.

Pain (Table 8.2)

Over the large range of etiologies (Table 8.1), pain is the commonest single symptom although absent in many cases; thus, rheumatoid pericarditis is nearly always silent, while most acute infectious pericarditis only rarely lacks pain. Pain can be due to potentiation of the algesic properties of bradykinin by pericardial prostacyclin (Chapter 3), inflammation of the pericardium itself, the phrenic nerves, the adjacent pleura and, probably, sympathetic nerves accompanying the coronary vessels in the epicardium. There is no good evidence for concomitant coronary spasm despite the superficiality of the main coronary arteries and the often striking electrocardiographic (ECG) changes (Chapter 5). All varieties of pain—sharp, "sticking," dull, aching and pressurelike—char-

Table 8.1 Etiologies of Acute Pericarditis (Note: Most Cause Both "Clinically Dry" and Effusive Pericarditis)

I. **Idiopathic pericarditis**
II. **Pericarditis due to living agents: infections, parasites**
    A. Bacterial
        1. Suppurative (any organism)
        2. Tuberculous
    B. Viral
        1. Coxsackie virus
        2. Influenza
        3. AIDS (HIV)
        4. Hepatitis B, A, ?C
        5. Other
    C. Mycotic (fungal)
    D. Rickettsial
    E. Spirochetal
    F. *Spirillum* infection
    G. *Mycoplasma pneumoniae*
    H. Infectious mononucleosis
    I. *Leptospira*
    J. *Listeria*
    K. Lymphogranuloma venereum
    L. Psittacosis (Chlamydiaceae)
    M. Parasitic
III. **Pericarditis in the vasculitis–connective tissue disease group**
    A. Rheumatoid arthritis
    B. Rheumatic fever
    C. Systemic lupus erythematosus (SLE)
    D. Drug-induced SLE
    E. Scleroderma
    F. Sjögren's syndrome
    G. ?Whipple's disease (*Tropheryma whippleii* organisms)
    H. Mixed connective tissue disease (MCTD)
    I. Reiter's syndrome
    J. Ankylosing spondylitis
    K. Inflammatory bowel disease
    L. Serum sickness
    M. Wegener's granulomatosis
    N. Vasculitis, e.g. temporal/giant cell arteritis
    O. Polymyositis (dermatomyositis)
    P. Behcet's syndrome
    Q. Familial Mediterranean fever
    R. Dermatomyositis
    S. Panmesenchymal reaction of steroid hormone withdrawal
    T. Polyarteritis

Table 8.1 Continued

    U. Churg-Strauss syndrome
    V. Thrombohemolytic thrombocytopenic purpura
    W. Other
  IV. **Pericarditis in immunopathies and "hypersensitivity" states**
    A. Drug reactions
    B. Serum sickness
    C. Allergic granulomatosis
    D. Giant urticaria
    E. Other sensitivity reactions
  V. **Pericarditis in disease of contiguous structures**
    A. Myocardial infarction
        1. Acute myocardial infarction
        2. Postmyocardial infarction syndrome
        3. Postpericardiotomy syndrome
        4. Ventricular aneurysm
    B. Dissecting aortic aneurysm
    C. Pleural and pulmonary diseases
        1. Pneumonia
        2. Pulmonary embolism
        3. Pleuritis
  VI. **Pericarditis in disorders of metabolism**
    A. Renal failure
        1. Uremic (chronic/acute renal failure)
        2. "Dialysis" pericarditis
    B. Myxedema
        1. Cholesterol pericarditis
    C. Gout
    D. Scurvy
  VII. **Neoplastic pericarditis**
    A. *Secondary* (metastatic, hematogenous, or by direct extension): carcinoma, sarcoma, lymphoma, leukemia, carcinoid, other
    B. *Primary* mesothelioma, sarcoma, fibroma, lipoma
 VIII. **Traumatic Pericarditis**
    A. Direct
        1. Pericardial perforation (*esp.* pneumopericardium)
           a. Penetrating chest injury
           b. Esophageal perforation
           c. Gastric perforation
        2. Cardiac injury: direct trauma
           a. Cardiac surgery (see also V.C above)
           b. During catheterization
               i. Pacemaker insertion
              ii. Electrode catheter ablation for arrhythmias

(*continued*)

Table 8.1 Continued

iii. Diagnostic

iv. Percutaneous transluminal coronary angioplasty with coronary dissection

v. Fistulas between pericardium and neighboring organs

3. Indirect trauma

a. Radiation pericarditis

b. Nonpenetrating chest injury

4. "Foreign-body" pericarditis

IX. **Pericarditis of uncertain pathogenesis and in association with various syndromes**

A. Postmyocardial and pericardial injury syndromes (?immune disorders)

B. Pericardial fat necrosis

C. Inflammatory bowel disease

1. Colitis (ulcerative; granulomatous)

2. Segmental enteritis (Crohn's disease)

D. Löffler's syndrome

E. Thalassemia (and other congenital anemias)

F. "Specific" drug reaction (Psicofuranine, ?Minoxidil, ? others)

G. Pancreatitis

H. Sarcoidosis

I. Cholesterol pericarditis not associated with myxedema or granulomata

J. Fat embolism

K. Bile fistula (to pericardium)

L. Wissler's syndrome

M. "PIE" syndrome

N. Stevens-Johnson syndrome

O. Gaucher's disease

P. Diaphragmatic hernia

Q. Atrial septal defect

R. Giant cell aortitis

S. Takayasu's syndrome

T. Castleman's disease (giant lymph node hyperplasia)

U. Fabry's disease

V Kawasaki's disease

W. Degos' disease

X. Other

acterize individual cases with intensities varying from 1 to 10 on a scale of 10, although usually less than 5. Initially, pain of acute pericarditis tends to be sharp, precordial and *pleuritic, exacerbated by inspiration and recumbency* and only rarely exacerbated by sitting up—a posture often assumed by the patient for relief). At any intensity, the pleuritic characteristics of the pain are the most

Table 8.2   Pain in Acute Pericarditis Vs. Acute Ischemia

	Acute pericarditis	Acute ischemia (AP, MI)
Onset	More often sudden	Usually gradual, crescendo
Main location	Substernal or left precordial	Same or confined to zones of radiation
Radiation	May be same as ischemic, also trapezius ridge(s)	Shoulders, arms, new, jaw, back; not trapezius ridge(s)
Quality	Usually sharp, stabbing; "background" ache or dull and oppressive	Usually "heavy" (pressure sensation) or burning
Inspiration	Worse	No effect unless with infarction pericarditis
Duration	Persistent; may wax and wane	Usually intermittent; <30 min each recurrence, longer for unstable angina
Body movements	Increased	Usually no effect
Posture	Worse on recumbency Improved on sitting, leaning forward	No effect or improvement on sitting
Nitroglycerin	No effect	Usually relief

distressing to the patient. *Pain onset*, frequently perceived as sudden, particularly when it interrupts patients' sleep, is only occasionally related to exertion, and this may be coincidental, whereas, once established, pain becomes worse with exertion. Characteristic *pain relief from sitting up and leaning forward* may be related to the biomechanical characteristics of the parietal pericardium (Chapters 2 and 3) : these maneuvers may reverse the increased pericardial tissue tension caused by inspiration and truncal extension.

Pain radiation may occur in all the distributions common to angina as well as to the epigastrium, creating a problem in differential diagnosis when the pain is not pleuritic or has a pressing quality and particularly when it radiates to the jaw or one or both shoulders. *Shoulder pain must be distinguished from pain in one or both trapezius ridges*, usually the left. *Trapezius ridge pain* is transmitted through the phrenic nerves; it is *virtually pathognomonic for pericardial irritation*. Indeed, in some patients, pain is perceived only in a trapezius ridge. The patients, therefore, must be asked to *point to the areas of pain perception*, since patients *and most physicians* characteristically confuse the trapezius ridge with the shoulder. Pain may also be appreciated in the midposterior thorax or below the left scapula. Rarely, pain appears to throb with each heartbeat, especially at relatively slow ventricular rates, as in uremic pericarditis (page 294). Pain may be exacerbated on palpation of the abdomen or even when the blood

pressure cuff is inflated. In contrast, palpation of the chest wall can elicit local tenderness, revealing costochondritis, Tietze's syndrome or other *chest wall
syndromes*, including rib fractures in patients with traumatic pericarditis (direct
trauma; pages 369–381). Finally, some patients do not describe "pain" but
rather vague *precordial distress*, with or without inspiratory or postural exacerbation. Some patients with *myopericarditis*, particularly of Coxsackie viral
origin, may have considerable skeletal muscle myalgia.

Abnormal Breathing

Patients tend to adopt a rapid, shallow breathing pattern because of the pleuritic pain and its exacerbation by body movement, cough and inspiration. True
dyspnea is not due to the pericardial lesion itself but occurs where dry pericarditis is part of another cardiac insult, like rheumatic carditis (page 320) or
superimposed on preexisting heart disease. Thus, *the shallow tachypnea of
patients attempting to splint their chest movements against exacerbation of pain
should be distinguished from true dyspnea.*

Other Symptoms

A *nonproductive cough* is common and exacerbates pleuritic pain. When "idiopathic" or infectious pericarditis follows a respiratory infection, the cough
may antedate chest symptoms. *Productive coughing* occurs due to associated
illnesses, as when pericarditis results from spread of empyema, pneumonia or
lung cancer. *Hiccough* is relatively rare and probably due to inflammation of
the diaphragmatic pleura or phrenic nerves. *Odynophagia,* rarely the only sign
of pericarditis, occurs because of the apposition of the esophagus and the posterior parietal pericardium; odynophagia and *dysphagia* result from pericardial
inflammation or effusion and when pericardial disease is due to the spread of
esophageal inflammation (page 361), trauma (page 362) or malignancy (page
363). Some patients have *symptomatic extrasystoles* and *palpitations*, probably
due to anxiety, since uncomplicated acute pericarditis appears not to cause
arrhythmias (page 56). *Faintness* and *dizziness* are uncommon in the absence
of cardiac tamponade but can occur when there is considerable pain, tachycardia
or constitutional reaction. Occasional patients have *gastrointestinal symptoms*,
including nausea, anorexia and even vomiting in the first few days, which tend
to be self-limited or disappear with sedation and suppression of pain if they are
not due to concomitant extrapericardial disease.

SYSTEMIC REACTION

Fever, usually below 39°C, is very common and may herald the clinical onset as a result of pericarditis itself or of associated or accompanying diseases.

Pericarditis of myocardial infarction, for example, may appear mainly as a secondary temperature rise. Tuberculous pericarditis, frequently painless, may present as a "pyrexia of unknown origin." Elderly patients lacking mechanisms for cytokine liberation may not be febrile and some with systemic diseases like renal failure may be hypothermic. *Chills* (rigors) are likely to accompany spiking fevers, as in suppurative pericarditis and some cases of idiopathic (presumably viral) pericarditis. *Weight loss* may occur because of anorexia or odynophagia. *Weakness* and even depression accompany some cases with marked systemic manifestations. *Anxiety* is common in patients with very painful pericarditis or disagreeable precordial sensations, and especially in those with pre-existing heart disease. *Pallor* may be a clue to systemic illness, like tuberculosis, uremia or neoplasia; it is apt to be especially "whitish" in rheumatic pericarditis. In some persons severely ill from antecedent or accompanying disease, symptoms and constitutional reaction provoked by acute pericarditis may be submerged in the total picture or suppressed by treatment already in progress.

OBJECTIVE MANIFESTATIONS

The *pericardial rub*—three (Figure 8.4) or fewer (Figure 8.5) friction sounds per cardiac cycle—described in detail in Chapter 4, is the cardinal sign of pericarditis. Rubs may be transient or intermittent and often last from hours to 2 or more days. Their discovery often results from fortuitous times of auscultation or diligent reexamination when pericarditis is suspected. Rubs are common in the presence of even large pericardial effusions. Unusually persistent rubs indicate a tendency to chronicity or continuing pericardial irritation, as from malignant infiltration. *Echocardiograms* in clinically dry pericarditis may show fibrin either as epicardial masses with or without a small effusion or with a ragged, "sunburst" appearance along the cardiac perimeters. All very sick patients and those with high fever, as well as any with a suspicion of effusion, should have an echocardiogram. *Electrocardiographic abnormalities*, discussed in detail in Chapter 5, range from normal to nonspecific to typical Stage I ST segment deviations, usually with PR segment deviations (Figure 8.6A and B). Like the pericardial rub, the *Stage I ECG change* is virtually diagnostic of acute pericarditis, always requiring differentiation from certain mimics, and particularly when there are *typical ECG variants* (page 50). *Atypical ECG variants* (pages 51–55) may be supportive in the presence of other evidence but are not diagnostic, especially if there is sufficient accompanying myocarditis; (myopericarditis, Chapter 9) or other heart disease. Occasionally ECG abnormalities are the only evidence of pericarditis, especially in patients without pericarditic symptoms, e.g., many postoperative patients. Finally, *any arrhythmias are not due to the acute pericarditis itself* (page 56). This is equally true of any

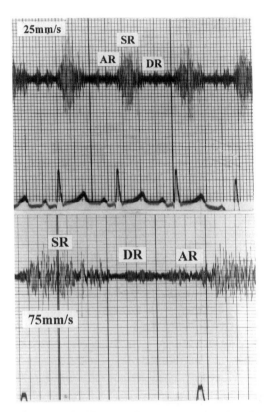

Figure 8.4 Phonocardiogram at 25 mm/sec (top: electrocardiographic speed) and further analyzed at three times as fast, showing typical triphasic pericardial friction. AR = atrial rub; SR = ventricular systolic rub; Dr = ventricular diastolic rub.

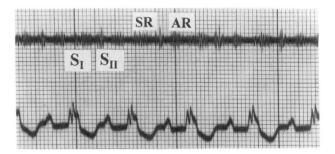

Figure 8.5 Biphasic pericardial friction: ventricular systolic and atrial rubs only. Atrial systole begins very shortly after ventricular systole ends (T wave) with a long PR interval leaving no "space" for a ventricular diastolic rub if there were one.

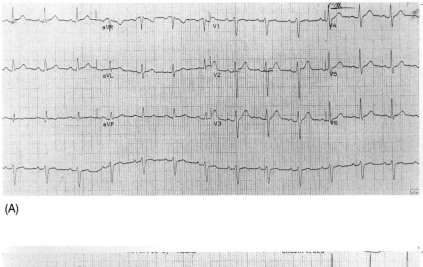

(A)

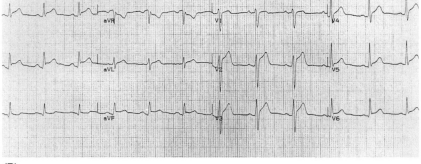

(B)

Figure 8.6 A. Acute pericarditis—day of onset. No J (ST) deviations except for lead V2. PR segment deviations only. In V2, due to PR segment depression, minimal J (ST) elevation gives an illusion of greater elevation but is seen as slight when compared to the T-P baseline. B. Same patient as in Figure 8.6A: second day. Classic stage I: ubiquitous J (ST) elevation except a VR and V1. PR deviations much less marked. (*PR segment deviations usually precede J (ST) deviations in acute pericarditis.*)

cardiac enlargement demonstrated by imaging. *Pleural effusions*, mainly on the left, are frequent in acute pericarditis, both "dry" and "wet" (Figure 8.7). Right and bilateral effusions occur much less often.

   Leukocytosis is the rule, the dominant cell type being the result of the etiologic agent or any primary illness accounting for pericarditis. For example, bacterial pericarditis (pages 265–268) tends to provoke higher neutrophil counts and tuberculous pericarditis a predominance of lymphocytes. Uncommon dis-

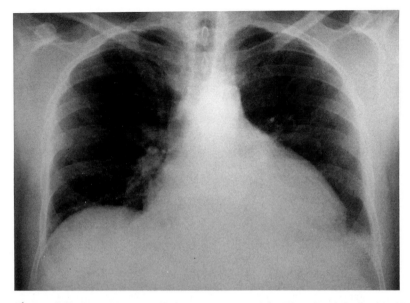

Figure 8.7 Roentgenogram during acute pericarditis. There is a left pleural effusion. the right costophrenic angle is clear. For unknown reasons, left pleural effusions are common in acute pericarditis.

eases with *eosinophilia* will have increased circulating eosinophils; some of these are parasitoses (pages 282–285); others are immunopathic vasculitides, including allergies. *Leukopenia* is uncommon and may be due to bone marrow depression by associated disease (e.g., systemic lupus erythematosus), drugs, or radiation and chemotherapy for malignancy. A few patients, usually with a mild clinical course, have normal white blood cell counts.

Other acute phase reactants, like the erythrocyte sedimentation rate (*ESR*) and C-reactive protein (*CRP*), show mild to marked elevations, the level usually reflecting the intensity of the pericarditic process, its inciting disease or subepicardial myocardial involvement. *Serum enzyme elevations* derived from myocardium—like CPK-MB, SGOT, serum aldolase, LDH, and probably troponin—reflect the degree of myocardial involvement by subepicardial myocarditis since they are not derived from the pericardium itself. Patients with the greatest degree of ST segment deviation tend to develop the largest CPK rises, although the correlation is imprecise; some patients do not have significant enzyme rises despite ECG changes. Like white blood cell counts and all acute-phase reactants, enzymatic changes are thus important components of the clinical picture but are not specific for diagnosing pericarditis.

TREATMENT: GENERAL CONSIDERATIONS

In general, treatment of all forms of acute pericarditis is aimed at relieving symptoms and eliminating etiologic agents. Most patients are hospitalized for complete diagnosis and observation for complications, particularly effusion and tamponade. *Anti-inflammatory and symptomatic treatments* resemble those of other conditions producing comparable symptoms and thus are aimed at pain, fever and malaise. The agents used and intensity of such therapy must be individualized and commensurate with the degree of the patient's distress. *Nonsteroidal anti-inflammatory drugs (NSAIDs)* are the mainstay, possibly because many inhibit pericardial synthesis of prostaglandin I_2 (page 24); 325 to 650 mg of aspirin every 4 to 6 hr is often sufficient. Any NSAID that is effective may be used. However, indomethacin should be avoided in adults unless all other options fail, since it reduces coronary flow and has deleterious effects on myocardial infarcts. At this writing, *ibuprofen* has the best side-effects profile; it increases coronary flow and has the largest dose range. Depending on clinical severity and response of symptoms, treatment may initially require ibuprofen 300 to 800 mg every 6 to 8 hr and can be increased if necessary. In many mild cases, particularly of "idiopathic" (usually presumably viral) pericarditis, 1 to 4 days of treatment appears to adequately attack the inflammation and the symptoms. Finally, all patients should be monitored for side effects (Table 8.5); since all NSAIDs induce gastrointestinal mucosal changes it is wise to combine these with misoprostol or another mucosal protectant. Anecdotal evidence is increasing that *colchicine added to a NSAID or even as monotherapy is effective both for the initial attack and to prevent recurrences.* It is well tolerated at 0.6 mg every 12 hr with or without a loading dose (2 to 3 mg), but it must be moni-

Table 8.3 Clinical Factors[a]: Acute Pericarditis Vs. Acute Ischemia

	Acute pericarditis	Acute ischemia (AP, MI)
Myocardial enzymes	Normal or elevated	Elevated (infarct)
Pericardial friction	Rub (most cases)	Rub only if with pericarditis
Abnormal S3	Absent unless preexisting	May be present
Abnormal S4	Absent unless preexisting	Nearly always present
S1	Intact	Often dull, mushy after first day
Pulmonary congestion	Absent	May be present
Murmurs	Absent unless preexisting	May be present

[a]Electrocardiographic differences in Table 8.4

Table 8.4   ECG: Acute Pericarditis Vs. Acute Ischemia

	Acute pericarditis	Acute ischemia (AP, MI)
J-ST	Diffuse elevation usually concave, without reciprocal depressions	Localized deviation usually convex (with reciprocals in infarct)
P-R segment depression	Frequent	Almost never
Abnormal Q waves	None unless with infarction	Common with infarction ("Q wave" infarcts)
T waves	Inverted after J points return to baseline	Inverted while S-T still elevated (infarct)
Arrhythmia	None (in absence of heart disease)	Frequent
Conduction abnormalities	None (in absence of heart disease)	Frequent

tored for side effects. A well controlled trial is needed. (See also Chapters 23 and 24).

Corticosteroid therapy should be avoided unless it is aimed at a specific inciting illness like one of the connective tissue diseases or when all else fails. If their use is unavoidable, corticosteroid agents should be used in minimally effective doses and carefully tapered on an individual basis. There are always at least three dangers, particularly with viral, "allergic" or "idiopathic" pericarditis: (1) that too early use of a corticosteroid will increase viral multiplication and virulence—this is also possible but less likely with some NSAIDS; (2) steroid suppression of early eosinophilic responses may obscure diagnoses (e.g., parasitoses); (3) that the patient will become "hooked" with recurrences every time a corticosteroid (usually prednisone) is discontinued (Chapter 24). For patients with a protracted need for prednisone, ibuprofen or another NSAID should be introduced during the tapering period; after the steroid is satisfactorily discontinued, the nonsteroidal agent should be tapered. Colchicine appears to improve therapeutic results and to facilitate the tapering ("weaning") process. It can also be useful in the initial attack and may prevent subsequent recurrences. Patients should thereafter be observed indefinitely for one or more recurrences. Opiates should be used only if there is severe pain at the onset of the illness. If patients require anticoagulants—for example, those with prosthetic cardiac valves—heparin, with effects rapidly reversible by protamine sulfate, should be used under strict observation while the pericarditis is in progress.

**Table 8.5 Principal Side Effects
of Nonsteroidal Anti-Inflammatory
Drugs (NSAIDs)**

Hypersensitivity
Gastrointestinal
    Gastric or duodenal ulceration
    Dyspepsia and gastritis
    Diarrhea
    Hepatitis
Central nervous
    Dizziness
    Headache
    Tinnitus (salicylates)
    Aseptic meningitis
Cardiovascular
    Edema
    Hypertension
    Heart failure
Respiratory
    Pneumonitis
    Asthma
Hematologic
    Neutropenia
    Thrombocytopenia
    Hemolytic anemia
    Aplastic anemia
Renal
    Precipitation of acute renal failure
    Interstitial nephritis
    Hematuria
    Nephrotic syndrome
    Papillary necrosis

DIAGNOSTIC AND DIFFERENTIAL DIAGNOSTIC
CONSIDERATIONS (TABLES 8.3, 8.4, 8.6 AND 8.7)

Acute pericarditis must be recognized and differentiated from syndromes producing similar symptoms and signs, bearing in mind that pericarditis may be
(1) part of a more generalized disease, (2) an apparently "isolated" illness or
(3) part of a disorder affecting a neighboring organ like the heart or lung, and
(4) occasionally the presenting syndrome of numerous disorders. *Presence of*

Table 8.6   Clinically "Dry" Acute Pericarditis: Principal Differential Diagnoses

Manifestation	To be differentiated
Electrocardiogram	
Stage 1	Acute myocardial infarction
	Early repolarization
Stage 2	Ischemia/infarction
Stage 3	Ischemia/ infarction/myocarditis
Pain	Myocardial ischemia
	Angina
	Infarction
	Pleuritis
	Pneumonia
	Chest wall pain
	Pulmonary embolus (usually small)
Tachypnea	Pleuropulmonary disease
	Cardiac failure
Pericardial rub	Murmurs
	Pleural rub
	Chest wall sounds
	"Conus rubs"
	Pulmonary embolism
	Acute hyperthyroidism (Means-Lerman "scratch")
	Pacemaker rub (endocardial)

any disorder associated with pericarditis should always raise the possibility of pericarditis. Pain isolated to or referred to one or both trapezius ridges strongly compels consideration of pericarditis as long it is not confused with shoulder pain, which also occurs in pericarditis and other conditions resembling it. Central pleuritic chest pain should always raise the question of acute pericarditis if pleurisy can be ruled out. (Note: Both may occur simultaneously.)

Table 8.7   Major Conditions That Can Simulate Pericarditis Without Effusion*

Acute myocardial infarction
  Extension and/or reinfarction
Angina pectoris
Chest wall syndromes
Pulmonary embolism
Pneumonia and/or pleuritis
Chest pain in patients with early repolarization

*Each may also occur with pericarditis.

When the pain of acute pericarditis resembles that of *cardiac ischemia* (Table 8.2), it yet may be longer lasting, sharper, not precipitated by effort and unresponsive to vasodilator therapy. Purely ischemic pain does not have the frequently pleuritic quality of infarction or postinfarction forms of pericarditis (pages 100–101; Table 8.2). Angina pectoris produces ECG changes nearly always marked by depressed rather than elevated ST segments except in some patients with variant (Prinzmetal's) angina. Tables 8.2 to 8.4 summarize the crucial differentiation of pericarditis from ischemia and infarction.

On strictly ECG grounds, up to one-third of cases of acute pericarditis may resemble ischemic heart disease because of atypical ECG evolution (pages 51–53). Particularly because of the frequency of contemporary computer misinterpretation of "myocardial infarction" in patients with acute pericarditis, it is essential to read over all ECGs to avoid antithrombotic and anticoagulant therapies that are so successful for coronary thrombosis but potentially catastrophic, via hemopericardium, in pericarditis. Yet, it is interesting that numerous patients with pericarditis, despite full anticlotting therapy, do not bleed and may even develop nonhemorrhagic serous effusions, suggesting that any pericardial bleeding is more related to the vascularity of the pericardial inflammation. Finally, various clinical instances of *pulmonary embolism* can mimic acute pericarditis, particularly those with pleuritic pain. The ECG is most often nonspecifically altered and the pleural rub, if any, as well as the pain, may be remote from the precordium. In those cases with pleuritic anterior chest pain, rubs may be deceptive; the rest of the clinical picture should support one or the other diagnosis. Rarely, pulmonary embolism provokes a purely pericardial (page 28) or pleuropericardial rub, pericardial effusion (usually small) or an unusual pericardial response resembling the postmyocardial infarction syndrome (page 360).

A *pericardial rub* (pages 27–33), recognized as such, is virtually pathognomonic for acute pericarditis. Chronic rubs are well recognized but comparatively uncommon (page 29). Clearly triphasic rubs are distinguishable from murmurs because no murmurs are truly triphasic. Pericardial rubs are otherwise distinguished by their superficiality and often by their grating or scratching quality, which, taken together, are usually quite different from murmurs. Even biphasic pericardial rubs can usually be distinguished on these grounds from continuous murmurs. Monophasic rubs, particularly the most common one, the ventricular systolic rub, can mimic murmurs of mitral and especially tricuspid regurgitation and ventricular septal defect, principally because *rubs*—not only monophasic rubs—*tend to be most intense at or to occur only at the left mid- to lower sternal border*, where the most intense rubs can be palpable. Features assisting differential diagnosis include the frequent association of a pericarditic syndrome, the short-term changeable nature of rubs and their occasionally unpredictable precordial distribution, as well as the frequent absence of findings of associated heart disease. Although rubs are typically louder in inspiration, particularly when there is some increase in pericardial fluid, the atypical respiratory behavior of many rubs (no change or increase in expiration) generally will not resemble that of a similar murmur.

Electrocardiographic abnormalities are quasidiagnostic when they undergo typical evolution in three of their four phases (pages 41–45). *A typical stage I alone is virtually diagnostic*, although it is easily confused with the normal ECG variant "early repolarization" (pages 59–60). The characteristic widespread ST segment changes are distinguishable from most acute myocardial ischemia and infarctions, which nearly always involve "regional" lead groupings with associated reciprocal ST segment deviations in other leads; reciprocal ST depressions virtually never occur in uncomplicated acute pericarditis. Absence of reciprocals also characterizes "regional" atypical variant ECG changes in pericarditis (page 51). Q waves do not occur in pericardial disease without associated or preexisting myocardial disease. If an ECG is first recorded in stage III, in which almost all T waves are inverted (pages 41; 44), the distinction between a primarily pericardial or myocardial disorder must be made from other data.

KEY POINTS

1. Most acute pericarditis is *clinically* "dry": without (nonimaging) evidence of significant pericardial effusion.
2. Acute pericarditis of any pathogenesis may be painful (usually *pleuritic*) or painless. Pain in, pain referred to or pain radiating to one or both *trapezius ridges* is quasi-specific for pericardial origin.
3. Pericardial rubs and ECG stage I and its typical variants are each virtually diagnostic.
4. Nonsteroidal anti-inflammatory drugs are the mainstay of treatment. A corticosteroid should be used only for specific etiologies or if all else fails and the patient is not recovering. Colchicine appears to have great promise as monotherapy or added to a a NSAID both for the initial attack and to prevent recurrences.
5. Principal differential diagnoses of symptomatic acute pericarditis: most variants of myocardial ischemia, including infarction; pleurisy; pulmonary embolism; chest wall syndromes.

BIBLIOGRAPHY

1. Anguita M, Zayas R, Ruiz M, Torres F, Gimenez D, Valles F. Diagnosing specific causes of primary acute pericarditis. Cardiol Rev 1996; 13:28–31.
2. Bruce, M.A., Spodick, D.H. Atypical electrocardiogram in acute pericarditis: Characteristics and Prevalence. J. Electrocardiol. 1980; 13:61–66.
3. Spodick, D.H. Pain mechanisms in pericardial disease. Bull. Tufts-N. Engl. Med.

Center, 1957; 3:191–194.

4. Spodick, D.H. The normal and diseased pericardium: Current concepts of pericardial physiology diagnosis and treatment. J. Am. .Cardiol. 1983; 1:240–251.

5. Spodick, D.H. Electrocardiographic changes in acute pericarditis. In: Fowler, N.O. (ed). The Pericardium in Health and Disease. Mt. Kisco, NY: Futura, 1984, pp. 79–98.

6. Spodick, D.H. Pitfalls in the recognition of pericarditis. In: Hurst, J.W. (ed.). Clinical Essays on the Heart. New York: McGraw-Hill, 1985, pp. 95–111.

7. Spodick, D.H. Critical care of pericardial disease. In: Rippe, J.M., Irwin, R.S., Alpert, J.S., Fink, M.P. (eds). Intensive Care Medicine, 2d ed. Boston: Little, Brown, 1991, pp. 282–295.

8. Spodick, D.H. Diagnosis and management of acute non-effusive pericarditis. Cardiol. Board Rev. 1994; 11:13–16.

9. Spodick, D.H. Pericarditis. In: Rakel, R.E. (ed.). Conn's Current Therapy 1995. Philadelphia: Saunders, 1995, pp. 289–292.

9

Myopericarditis/Perimyocarditis

Pericarditis is often accompanied by some degree of myocarditis and vice versa, the preponderant influence of either one dominating the clinical picture. They are only rarely approximately of equal intensity in their clinical or pathologic expression. thus, most syndromes are primarily myocarditic or pericarditic. The terms "myopericarditis" and "perimyocarditis" are used interchangeably or to indicate the dominant form: for example, "myopericarditis" indicates a primarily pericarditic situation; it represents the majority of clinically appreciated cases. In children, perimyocarditis, like myocarditis, is more common than in adults. Indeed, the myocardial element is in general more prominent in younger people, probably because viruses are a major cause of acute pericarditis and myocarditis. While precision would be served by using each term selectively, "myopericarditis" not only represents the majority of recognized cases but is somewhat more euphonious and is used here in both senses (Table 9.1 lists recognized forms of myopericarditis by etiology).

Finally, there is a high incidence, often unappreciated, of myocarditis with or without pericarditis that is increasingly seen in a form usually masquerading as acute myocardial infarction. Indeed, it can have its own "infarction"-associated forms of pericarditis (pages 20).

PATHOGENESIS

Disorders with frequent myocarditis, pericarditis and myopericarditis include immunopathies, the vasculitis–connective tissue disease group (Chapter 19) and

Table 9.1 Myopericarditis (Perimyocarditis): Principal Etiologies

A. **Infectious**
   I. **Viral**
      Enteroviruses (*esp.* Coxsackie B and A)
      Echoviruses
      Epstein-Barr virus (EBV; *esp.* infectious mononucleosis)
      Influenza A and B
      Cytomegalovirus (CMV)
      Rhinoviruses/picornaviruses
      Adenoviruses
      Hepatitis B
      Vaccinia
      Herpes
      Varicella; varicella zoster
      Mumps
      Rubeola
      Rubella
      Poliomyelitis virus
      HIV
      Rhinoviruses
  II. **Bacterial**
      Streptococcus: acute rheumatic fever (ARF); nonrheumatic streptococcal myopericarditis
      Staphylococcus
      Mycobacterium (*esp. M. tuberculosis*; atypical forms, *esp.* in AIDS)
      Salmonella
      Brucella
      Haemophilus influenzae
      Mycoplasma
      Neisseria (esp. meningitidis)
      Gram-negative rods
      Chlamydia (esp. C. psittaci; C. trachomatis; LGV)
      Yersinia
      Legionella
      Campylobacter
      Other
 III. **Fungi**
      Aspergillus
      Candida species
      Cryptococcus
      Actinomyces
      Histoplasma
      Bastomyces

(*continued*)

Table 9.1 Continued

    IV. Rickettsiae
        R. rickettsi (Rocky Mountain spotted fever)
        Coxiella burnetii (Q fever)
        Other
    V. Parasites: protozoal and metazoal
        Toxoplasma gondii
        Echinococcus
        Trichinella spiralis
        Schistosoma species
        Amebae
        Babesia microti
        Other
    IV. Spirochetes
        Leptospira
        Borrelia (esp. B. burgdorferi; Lyme disease)
B. **Infections in Immunosuppressed states** (esp. AIDS, therapeutic
      immunosuppression)
C. **Immunopathic**
    Any acute damage followed by recurrences (*esp.* enteroviral;
      cytomegalovirus)
    Vasculitis–connective tissue disease group (see below)
    Inflammatory bowel diseases
    Postmyocardial/pericardial injury syndromes
    Insect stings
    Reiter's disease
D. **Vasculitis–connective tissue disease group**
    Acute rheumatic fever (ARF)
    Sarcoid
    Systemic lupus erythematosus (SLE)
    Churg-Strauss syndrome (with eosinophilia)
    Rheumatoid arthritis
       Adult
       Juvenile
       Still's disease (juvenile and adult)
       Other
E. **Therapeutic irradiation** (? including immunopathic effects)
F. **Sarcoidosis**
G. **Kawasaki's disease**
H. **Giant-cell myocarditis**
 I. **Drugs** (including hypersensitivity reactions)
    Methyldopa
    Methylsergide
    Sulfonamides

Table 9.1 Continued

Cytosine arabinoside
Anthracycline derivatives (*esp.* doxorubicin; daunorubicin)
Phenylbutazone
Cocaine
Other
J. **Other**
Ulcerative colitis
Wegener's granulomatosis
Behçet's disease
β-Thalassemia

drug-related pericarditis (Chapter 22). Yet viral and other infections appear to be the dominant types encountered clinically; indeed, an almost identical list of agents provokes acute infectious pericarditis and myocarditis. It is important to remember that myocarditis, classically considered generalized, can be localized due to one or multiple myocardial zones.

Several pathogenetic mechanisms for myopericarditis are implied in Table 9.1. *Cardiotropic viruses* can inflame the myocardium and pericardium hematogenously, whereas *bacterial and other organisms* do so either hematogenously, via lymphatics, or by direct involvement from pericardial infection, just as in severe endocarditis and mediastinitis. Acquired immunodeficiency syndrome (AIDS) of any pathogenesis (pages 279–282) frequently involves the myocardium, pericardium or both.

Some inciting agents may produce circulating "toxins" or, perhaps more commonly, *immunopathic mechanisms* that appear necessary for ongoing myopericarditis even in the absence of a viral genome. Viruses especially provoke antibodies to myolemmal and sarcolemmal membranes (AMLABs and ASABs respectively); such viruses may be both etiologic and pathogenic because of their cytolytic or cytotoxic properties. The AMLABs and ASABs are part of B-cell-driven immune responses. They fix complement, are cytotoxic and cross-react with corresponding viruses due to molecular mimicry. *Drug-induced myopericarditis* probably is pathogenetically related, via "allergic" or hypersensitivity mechanisms. Some immunologic component cannot be excluded in *radiation-induced myopericarditis,* but direct injury of both structures is also apparent. Immune mechanisms are epitomized by *inflammatory bowel disease* (pages 325–326), since there is no myopericardial contiguity to bowel. Indeed, almost any kind of acute pericardial or myocardial damage can induce an immunopathy with recurrences; these are most common in enteroviral and cytomegalovirus infections.

Persistence in the myocardium and pericardium of *enteroviruses (the commonest viral cause of acute myopericarditis)*, especially Coxsackie B-specific IgM responses, as in recurrent chronic relapsing pericarditis, may be related to suppression of immunity during the acute process when an anti-inflammatory agent is used too early.

Many members of the *vasculitis–connective tissue disease group* (Chapter 19) (classically including acute rheumatic fever) regularly produce myopericarditis. However, in most of them, the pericarditic component is the important form, although myocardial involvement may be demonstrable by functional abnormalities or frank myocardial failure.

Enteroviruses are the commonest viral cause of acute myopericarditis (and of related chronic cardiomyopathies). They are increasingly recognized by sensitive and specific hybridization and related studies. These detect viral RNA sequences and enterovirus-specific IgM and IgA in patients with acute and recurrent pericarditis and myopericarditis consistent with persistent enteroviral, particularly Coxsackie B, infection. (Coxsackie viruses rarely if ever attack the pericardium without also attacking the subjacent myocardium.) The influence of host genetic factors is indicated by associations between enterovirus IgM and the HLA A2 and DRz allotypes.

Occasionally inflammation spreads by contiguity from a primarily pericarditic process to the myocardium, comparable to myocardial extension of infective endocarditis. Each may also occur simultaneously. Spread from mediastinitis to the pericardium and myocardium is also recognized. Modern control of *bacterial infections* now make these rare and mainly represented by tuberculosis and aggressive organisms causing endocarditis. *Pericardial tuberculosis* often involves the myocardium, which becomes inflamed and ultimately fibrotic; both active and burned out tuberculous inflammation are evident in constrictive pericarditis. In contrast, pure uremic pericarditis may have a brisk inflammatory process in the pericardium and epicardial fat without invading the myocardium (page 294). On the other hand, *inflammatory bowel disease* —including Crohn's disease, ulcerative colitis, Whipple's diseases and *Yersinia* infection—can involve the pericardium or myocardium or both simultaneously through immunopathic mechanisms.

EVIDENCE OF MYOCARDIAL INVOLVEMENT IN PERICARDITIS (TABLE 9.2)

In the absence of other heart disease, there are certain signs that are more or less attributable to myocardial involvement by the pericarditic process. The *electrocardiographic (ECG) changes* of acute pericarditis, typical and especially atypical (Figures 9.1 and 9.2), as well as significant prolongation of the QT (JT) interval indicate myocarditis even when myocardial involvement is clini-

Table 9.2 **Clues to Significant Myocarditis in Patients with Acute Pericarditis**

1. *Any* acute electrocardiographic contour change, especially if localized or with atypical evolution.
2. Any significant arrhythmia, especially ventricular (in absence of other heart disease).
3. Evidence of myocardial dysfunction (in absence of other heart disease):
   a. Postpericardiocentesis abnormal S3 (in absence of constrictive pericarditis).
   b. Postpericardiocentesis cardiac failure, especially pulmonary edema.
   c. Abnormal imaging and catheterization studies:
      (1) Cardiomegaly
      (2) Abnormal hemodynamics (in absence of constrictive pericarditis).
      (3) Wall motion abnormalities.
4. Sinus tachycardia:
   a. Out of proportion to fever, anemia, and/or chest pain.
   b. Persistence after resolution of 6 through 10, below.
5. Skeletal muscle myalgias, especially during viral pericarditis (suggests a myotropic organism).
6. Pericarditis with transudative effusion fluid.
7. Nonpleuritic substernal chest pain with or without radiation (other than to trapezius ridges).
8. Elevated serum levels of cardiac enzymes, especially in presence of elevated serum myoglobin or ortroponin.
9. Antimyosin-indium 111 scintigraphy.
10. Myocardial production of tumor necrosis factor in absence of septic shock and congestive heart failure.

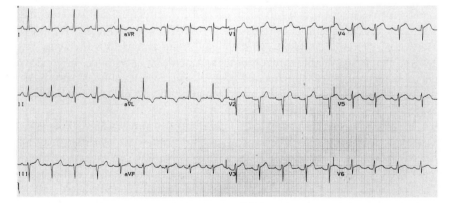

Figure 9.1 A 36-year-old women with myopericarditis. Electrocardiogram is atypical for uncomplicated pericarditis mainly because of T-wave inversions in leads I and aVL. Elsewhere there are characteristic J (ST) and PR segment deviations.

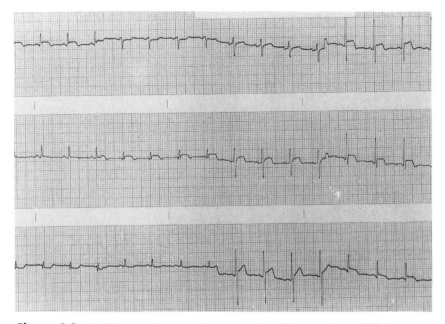

Figure 9.2 A 25-year-old man with myopericarditis. Atypical ECG for acute pericarditis Stage II: T waves inverting while J (ST) remains elevated. Leads III and aVF suggest "reciprocal" ST-T changes.

cally insignificant, since the pericardium does not create electromotive forces. (Conversely, the absence of acute ECG changes in uncomplicated uremic pericarditis are consistent with the usual absence of myocardial inflammation in that disorder.) Reciprocal J (ST) changes and abnormal Q waves (Figure 9.3) in the absence of infarction probably represent significant myocarditis involving regions of the myocardium disproportionately. Significant arrhythmias or conduction disturbances appear to be absent even in severe pericarditis without independent or related diseases of the myocardium or valves; myocarditis qualifies as such a related myocardial disease.

In some patients, following even mild idiopathic (presumably viral) pericarditis, transient myocardial *functional and wall motion abnormalities* may be detected for months; in severer cases global LV or RV dysfunction or eventual dilated cardiomyopathy are strong evidence of a myocarditic component. The occasional patient who, after drainage of a pericardial effusion, develops myocardial dilation and acute cardiac failure ("pericardial shock," page 175) in the absence of antecedent heart disease almost certainly has had a significant myocarditic component, just as do those with any cardiac dysfunction during

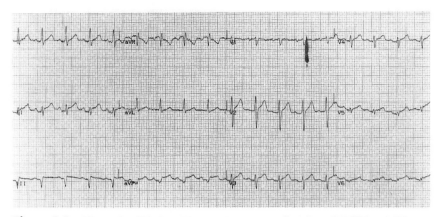

Figure 9.3 Myopericarditis in a 32-year-old man. Typical Stage I J (ST) and PR segment deviations. Pathologic Q wave in aVF (and III). Patient had reduced left ventricular function but completely normal coronary arteries.

apparently isolated pericarditis. Similar weight must be given to transient cardiac enlargement, usually first recognized by chest x-ray, in the absence of increased pericardial fluid, and to any true dyspnea with or without the characteristic pleuritic respiratory splinting of acute pericarditis. Patients with acute pericarditis and faster heart rates (generally over 100 beats per minute) and especially the persistence of tachycardia after the fever and chest pain of acute pericarditis have subsided show strong indications of a myocarditic component. During acute pericarditis, particularly of viral origin but also with *Mycoplasma* and *Borrelia* (Lyme) infections, the occurrence of skeletal muscle pain (myalgia) and tenderness suggests a myotropic organism that may also involve the myocardium. Such simultaneous involvement is more common in viral myocarditis of young adults and children. Conditions like trichinosis are overwhelmingly if not solely myocarditic, although the pericardium can be involved simultaneously.

Increased serum levels of *cardiac enzymes* in the presence of normal levels of myoglobin suggest that the pericarditic process has affected only cell membranes in the myocardium, causing them to leak these substances without necrosis—probably the mildest detectable form of myopericarditis; elevated serum *myoglobin* indicates severe (cytoplasmic) damage. Although the characteristic *ECG changes* of acute pericarditis (pages 41–50) can occur without abnormal enzyme release; in more severe cases with significant myopericarditis, CK-MB increases (> 10 u/1) particularly during pericarditic ST (J) elevations (Figure 9.4) and is often more marked with higher ST elevations and with deeper subsequent T-wave inversion. (Comparably, with greater ST (J) devia-

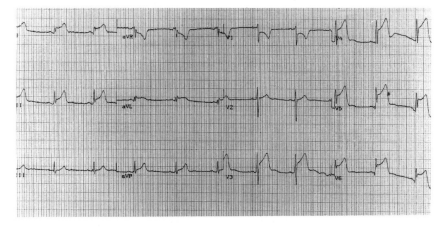

Figure 9.4 Myopericarditis in a 34-year-old man with typical Stage I ECG but exceptionally marked J (ST) deviations. Serum CPK-MB was elevated and left ventricular function significantly abnormal.

tions, technetium 99m stannous pyrophosphate is more often positive, even in early pericarditis.) Monoclonal antimyosin antibodies labeled with indium 111 are markers of myocarditis, as is detection of the proinflammatory cytokine tumor necrosis factor (TNF) in the absence of congestive failure and septic shock.

Pericarditis with pericardial effusions that are closer to *transudates*, particularly in the presence of undue dyspnea, suggest significant myocardial involvement, whereas *exudates* indicate at least a strong pericardial component. *Imaging methods* and cardiac *catheterization* can demonstrate transiently or permanently reduced myocardial function; i.e., diffuse or localized abnormal ventricular wall motion, just as in myocardial infarctions. With significant myocarditis, *nuclear magnetic resonance* (*NMR*) shows focal myocardial edema in such zones of segmental or generalized wall motion abnormality. (This is obviously related to the increasing awareness that myocarditis frequently mimics acute myocardial infarction.) One sensitive test to detect myocardial involvement is identification of increased left ventricular end-systolic wall stress. Finally, auscultation of a *third heart sound* ("ventricular gallop") not previously present is evidence either for such myocardial inflammation or some degree of constrictive pericarditis, including the mild, transient constriction that follows many cases of acute pericarditis (page 254).

CLINICAL CONSIDERATIONS

In general, with myopericarditis, a pericardial rub or significant effusion is less common than with pure or dominant acute pericarditis. Another rough correlation is the degree of chest pain, which also can parallel the release of CK-MB.

Although ECG J-ST changes always indicate some myocardial involvement during acute pericarditis, their absence may be due to either reduced sensitivity of the ECG or, as in pure uremic pericarditis, a unique sparing of the myocardium even by intense pericardial inflammation (page 294). However, although cardiac enzymes "leak" in well over one-half of those with ECG abnormalities, even with marked changes, cardiac enzymes may be normal or only slightly increased. Thus, enzyme rises frequently parallel the degree of ECG change, but the correspondence is rough and, indeed, in occasional patients enzyme levels fall while the ST (J) is still elevated. On the other hand, a clue to the presence of a myocarditic component during apparent pericarditis is the occasionally *convex* elevated J-ST segment, in contrast to the typical concave ST elevation characteristic of acute pericarditis (page 41). Probably some of the quite frequent *atypical variant ECG* evolutions during pericarditis, (pages 50–53), particularly T-wave inversion while the J point is still elevated and the rare reciprocal ST changes, represent a strong myocarditic component. Indeed, these are much more characteristic of myocardial infarctions, so that it is worth reiterating that myocarditis masquerading as acute infarction is increasingly recognized and likely to involve both local ECG and wall motion abnormalities. Hence, the pericarditic component, absent a rub and pleuritic pain, would not be recognized (as is the case in most true transmural myocardial infarcts with pericarditis; page 336). Patients will occasionally have mixed forms of pain of both ischemic and pleuritic types—with the dominance of one kind suggesting the dominant lesions—e.g., an increase of squeezing chest pain during apparent pericarditis indicating myopericarditis with an important degree of myocarditis. Skeletal muscle pains and tenderness, particularly during Coxsackie and other picornavirus infections, suggest a myotropic—hence cardio-myotropic—organism.

If *cardiac asynergy* is palpable or otherwise demonstrable (e.g., by imaging), this can only be due to a myocardial abnormality. Naturally, a *biopsy* obtained either by catheter (*endomyocardial biopsy*) or by thoracoscope (*epimyocardial biopsy)* will identify myocardial inflammation if an adequate specimen is obtained, preferably from the left ventricle, from which biopsies are more often positive. Epimyocardial biopsies are much more productive than endomyocardial biopsies for diagnostic cellular filtrates by light microscopy and immunohistochemistry. An active immune process will yield MHC Class I expression and tissue binding of IgG, IgA, IgM and C_3. Occasionally, biopsy is revealing in patients with malignancies, who can develop myocardial and pericardial inflammation without neoplastic tissue necessarily invading either structure.

MANAGEMENT

In the absence of myocardial failure, no measures for management of myopericarditis differ from those for acute pericarditis (pages 107–109). In both cases, there are no adequate controlled clinical trials. Patients may respond to anti-inflammatory agents. However, corticosteroids should be avoided unless all else fails and the patient is severely ill. They should be particularly avoided near the onset of viral illness because they can stimulate virus replication and paralyze immune responses, favoring exacerbation and chronicity. (This has not been ruled out for nonsteroidal agents.) Even with clinical improvement, corticosteroid therapy seems to be the forerunner of unpredictable pericarditic recurrences with stubborn steroid dependency in some patients. Immunosuppressive agents have not yet been of conclusive value and could be injurious. Hyperimmune globulin has been used for CMV-associated myopericarditis.

PROGNOSIS

Prognosis for recovery is generally good if the myocarditis is not intense, particularly in the infective types. Otherwise, varying degrees of myocardial damage can produce congestive heart failure and, ultimately, dilated or restrictive cardiomyopathy.

KEY POINTS

1. Some degree of myocarditis nearly always accompanies most forms of clinically significant pericarditis, with one dominating the clinical picture.
2. Recognizable myopericarditis is most often viral and more frequent in younger patients; enteroviral infections are commonest.
3. In patients with pericarditis, cardiac dysfunction, significant arrhythmia or disproportionate sinus tachycardia may indicate myocarditis (in absence of preexisting heart disease).
4. Immunopathic mechanisms for myopericarditis are increasingly recognized in primary conditions anatomically remote from the heart (e.g., certain gastrointestinal inflammations) as well as in infectious forms of myopericarditis.
5. Electrocardiographic abnormalities atypical for pericarditis, like localized and reciprocal ST-T deviations, convex elevated ST segments and T-wave inversions while J points remain elevated, strongly suggest degrees of myocardial involvement in the inflammatory process.

BIBLIOGRAPHY

Dec, G.W., Waldman, H., Southern, J., et al. Viral myocarditis mimicking acute myocardial infarction. J. Am. Acad. Cardiol. 1992; 20:85–89.

Frisk, G., Torfason, E.G., Diderholm, H. Reverse radioimmunoassay of IgM and IgG antibodies to Coxsackie B viruses in patients with acute myopericarditis. J. Med. Virol. 1984; 14:191–200.

Heikkila, J., Karjalainen, J. Evaluation of mild acute infectious myocarditis. Br. Heart J. 1982; 47:381–391.

Maisch, B. Cardiocytolysis by sera of patients suffering from acute perimyocarditis. In: Bolte, H.-D. (ed.). Viral Heart Disease. Berlin: Springer-Verlag, 1984, pp. 121–129.

Peters, N.S., Poole-Wilson, P.A. Myocarditis—Continuing clinical and pathologic confusion. Am. Heart J. 1991; 121:942–947.

Sodeman, W.A. Acute pericarditis: Its role in diagnostic interpretation. Chest 1970; 57:477–479.

Spodick, D.H. Infection and infarction: Acute viral (and other) infection in the onset, pathogenesis and mimicry of acute myocardial infarction. Am. J. Med. 1986; 81:661–668.

10

Pericardial Effusion and Hydropericardium Without Tamponade

PATHOGENESIS AND CLINICAL CHARACTERISTICS

Most pericardial effusions "weep" from the visceral pericardium. Irritative and inflammatory effusions are associated with local production of substances like cytokines, tumor necrosis factors and interleukins. Like most body fluids, pericardial fluid is in dynamic equilibrium with the blood serum, including free exchange of water and electrolytes, with surprising pericardial permeability to some large as well as smaller molecules. However, the inflamed pericardium may obstruct these exchanges. Exudation of proteinaceous material and larger molecules due to irritation and inflammation and dissolution of intrapericardial thrombi osmotically impedes reabsorption of the exudate and attracts additional fluid. Very large effusions usually follow *venous and lymphatic obstruction* in the pericardium and often in the subjacent myocardium. Indeed, myocardial lymph drainage normally occurs via the pericardium and probably contributes to effusions.

Some fluid probably exudes in every case of acute pericarditis. *Symptomatic effusions* are more likely to be discovered because of early definitive echocardiography. *Asymptomatic effusions* are only occasionally suggested by physical examination; typically, the first clue is by chest x-ray (Figure 10.1). A

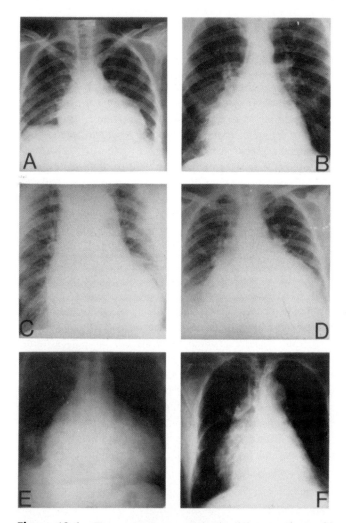

Figure 10.1   Chest roentengograms in six different patients with pericardial effusion. Cardiopericardial silhouettes vary. All show loss of normal arcuate contours. No shape pathognomonic. A and B. Indistinguishable by x-ray from cardiomegaly. C. Wide mediastinum in patient with large hydropericardium due to congestive heart failure. D and E suggest pericardial effusion due to "sac of water" shape; bilateral pleural effusions in D. F. Featureless protrusion of silhouette to right and straight left border suggest pericardial fluid. B and C. Vascular engorgement of lungs due to congestive heart failure causing hydropericardium type effusion. A, D, E, and F. Typical clear lung fields of uncomplicated pericardial effusion.

minimum of 250 mL of fluid is needed to fill the pericardial reserve volume (page 19) to the point of detectably increasing the cariopericardial x-ray shadow. Even rather large accumulations of fluid may not significantly embarrass the heart as long as the rate of exudation is slow enough to permit the pericardium to stretch. Surprisingly small increments and even the normal 15 to 35 mL can be identified by echocardiography and other imaging methods. In general, increased pericardial fluid is either *hydropericardium* (transudate), "true" *pericardial effusion* (exudate; *pyopericardium* if with pus), *hemopericardium,* or mixtures of these, all lumped as "pericardial effusion" (Table 10.1). Exudates characteristically have more cholesterol, protein and LDH than transudates, with cholesterol levels over 45 mg/dL, protein concentration more than half the serum level and LDH over 200 U/L and more than 0.6 the serum LDH. The protein level is the least specific. (The serum-effusion albumin gradient may have greater validity.) However, *the exudate-vs.-transudate characterization often has no firm basis, with no decisive distinction in many cases.* For example, in patients with improving congestive heart failure, more rapid reabsorption of water than protein and LDH may convert the hydropericardium to a *pseudoexudate* by those standards.

The physical presence of excess pericardial contents has been loosely associated with vague chest symptoms, such as pressure sensations and aches. Rapid accumulation of fluid, usually exudate, may stretch the pericardium, which could be painful. However, extremely large effusions—over 1 L—(usually chronic) may make their physical presence known by *encroachments on neighboring structures,* manifest as *dyspnea* and especially *dyspnea on exertion,* produced by displacement and compression of lung tissue causing a restrictive pulmonary defect; *dysphagia* from esophageal compression; *cough* from bronchial encroachment; *hiccups* from esophageal compression and involvement of the vagi and phrenic nerves; and *hoarseness* from compression of the recurrent laryngeal nerve.

ETIOLOGY: GENERALITIES

The etiology of *exudative pericardial effusions* of all sizes essentially corresponds to that of pericardial inflammation and irritation (Table 7.1); large exudative effusions are most common with tumors, tuberculous pericarditis, cholesterol pericarditis, myxedema, vasculitis/connective tissue disease, uremic pericarditis and parasitoses. Unusual conditions must always be considered, including, for example, the eosinophilic syndromes, endomyocardial fibrosis and the increasing patient population with cardiac transplants (in whom infections can be related to chemotherapy, especially cyclosporine, or, arguably, to rejection episodes). *Hydropericardium,* usually of small to moderate size, is related to cardiac failure and fluid retention. Small to moderate clinically silent

Table 10.1 Exudative vs. Transudative Fluids in Pericardial Effusion NB. - Frequently No Clear Distinction

	Exudate	Transudate
Appearance	Clear, ground-glass or turbid; purulent or hemorrhagic, rarely chylous (milky); basic tint: straw or amber; usually contains fibrin shreds	Clear; basic tint: straw or amber
Specific gravity	>1.015 (usually >1.017)	<1.017, usually <1.015
Cholesterol	>45 mg/dL	<45 mg/dL
LDH	>200 IU/L	<200 IU/L
Total protein	>30 g/L	<30/mL[a] (usually <20 g/L)
Seromucin	Positive	Negative
Coagulation	Frequent	None
Cells	Usually many: mesothelial and inflammatory (leukocytes usually are lymphoctyes; sometimes few to many polymorphonuclears; rarely eosinophils); Neoplastic cells in malignant pericarditis. "Lyphocytic Effusion" = 50% lymphocytes	Few (mesothelial)
Glucose concentration	Less than blood sugar glucose, *esp.* in cases with many leukocytes or other cells	Usually = blood glucose concentration
Microorganisms	In infectious pericarditis if still viable	Absent
Magnetic Resonance Imaging (MRI)[b]	Signal intensity like (or stronger than) mycocardium. Hemopericardium: especially intense intensity related to *protein content*	Typically very low signal intensity

[a] Noninflammatory effusions in myxedema may contain large amounts of protein.
[b] MRI is variable because of signal loss from dephasing effects of fluid motion. *Cell content* affects T_1 and T_2 relaxation parameters.

hydropericardium develops in many pregnant women by their third trimester (page 89) (Pregnant patients sporadically develop any kind of pericardial disease.) Occasional patients with chronic cardiomyopathies accumulate large hydropericardiums. *Myopericarditis* tends to produce mixed forms; depending on severity, any hydropericardium due to heart failure variably dilutes the inflammatory effusion. *Drug-related effusions* (Chapter 22) may be difficult to recognize in the presence of a disease which is itself capable of involving the pericardium. Effusions are relatively common in the uncommon *postpulmonary embolism pericardial syndrome* (page 360) and, like the post-cardiac injury syndromes, may appear from days to many weeks later, confounding the diagnosis, especially if the embolism was unrecognized.

HYDROPERICARDIUM AND CLINICALLY NONCOMPRESSING EFFUSIONS

Hydropericardium, usually of relatively small volume, occurs mainly in conditions of fluid retention, like congestive heart failure (Figure 10.1B and C), in which it is surprising that hydropericardium is not more frequent, as is, for example, pleural effusion. Yet, if all pericardial effusions are lumped, congestive failure is probably the most common cause of small to moderate-sized effusions. Hydropericardium is usually discovered by accident when evaluating the chest or heart by x-ray, echocardiography, or other imaging method. In general, patients with heart failure and hydropericardium have larger right ventricles than those without hydropericardium. This may be related to obstruction of venous and lymphatic drainage in those with chamber enlargement.

"Noncompressing" exudative pericardial effusions due primarily to pericardial lesions may (1) be entirely asymptomatic, (2) present pericarditic pain or symptoms and signs of the condition causing an accompanying pericarditis or both, or (3) show subclinical, asymptomatic, but significantly increased respiratory fluctuation in ventricular function as demonstrated by sensitive techniques like systolic time intervals.

By definition, clinically "noncompressing" effusions produce no significant change in blood pressure or cardiac output and no pulsus paradoxus (as defined; Chapter 13). Noncompressing exudative pericardial effusions thus may have no detected manifestations or may be the only sign of pericarditis. Most show the symptoms and signs only of a clinically "dry" pericarditis, or such pericarditic signs are present initially with later appearance of slow or rapid effusion. If a primary extrapericardial disease is responsible for the pericarditis, the signs and symptoms of that condition may dominate the picture. If the pericardial effusion is truly an inflammatory exudate, a pericardial rub will be audible at some time in the majority. A few patients have slight inspiratory exaggeration of the normal fall in systolic blood pressure (possibly a "borderline" tamponade). The

Bamberger-Pins-Ewart sign is common with very large effusions, i.e., an area of dullness and bronchial breathing between the tip of the left (rarely the right) scapula and the vertebral column.

Physical examination in conditions associated with hydropericardium is of little use in identifying increased pericardial fluid, since the results are nonspecific and undependable; indeed, even with cardiac tamponade, heart sounds may not be muffled and increased precordial flatness or dullness by percussion is untrustworthy. However, inflammatory and irritative effusions frequently do not disguise pericardial rubs (Figure 10.2).

The *electrocardiogram (ECG)* (Table 10.2) is of little or no direct help, although occasionally in very large nontamponading effusions there may be electric alternation (page 58), a sign that is otherwise (usually) quasipathognomonic of critical tamponade. Reduced ECG voltage is nonspecific and undependable; only massive effusions, as in severe myxedema, produce striking reduction in ECG amplitude, which in many patients may be equally related to associated myocardial or hemodynamic abnormality. On the other hand, a relatively large effusion that reduces voltage can reduce small r waves in rS complexes to convert them to deceptive "QS" complexes—a pseudoinfarct pattern.

IMAGING

Roentgenography can be suggestive but is nonspecific (Figure 10-1). *The shape of the heart shadow on fluoroscopy or on static films cannot decisively distinguish between true cardiomegaly and pericardial effusion. Recognition of excess pericardial contents usually requires echocardiography or other special imaging modalities.* These methods also permit definition of cardiac size and function, which must be determined by echocardiography, contrast x-ray ex-

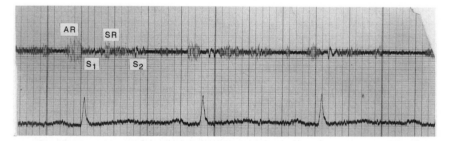

Figure 10.2 Biphasic pericardial rub during large effusion with tamponade. Heart sounds (S1, S2) are of small amplitude. Atrial systolic rub (AR) is most intense sound; ventricular systolic rub (SR) is less intense; each rub is of greater magnitude than the heart sounds.

Table 10.2 Pericardial Effusion: ECG Abnormalities

Reduced QRS-T voltage, *esp.* with tamponade; myocardial disease
    Reduction of small r waves in rs complexes: deep "Q"
    (QS) = pseudoinfarct
Electric alternation
    Very large effusion [QRS-T alternation uncommon]
    Tamponade
        QRS-T alternation (2:1) common: large effusion or any size
        with stiff pericardium.
        P-QRS-T alternation rare, apparently pathognomonic
        Preterminal bradycardia; electromechanical dissociation
Hemopericardium
    Preterminal
        Bradycardia-sinus; junctional
        Peaked T waves ("hyperkalemic" effect of hemolysis)
        Reversed polarity of previously inverted T waves

---

amination, radiation-scanning procedures, computed tomography (CT) or magnetic resonance imaging (MRI). In the absence of such more specific examinations, a "water-bottle" cardiac silhouette on x-ray (Figure 10.1D and E) or an unusually wide mediastinal shadow (Figure 10.1C) is highly suggestive, particularly when the lung fields are not congested. *Unilateral left or left larger-than-right pleural effusions* are common in both "wet" and "dry" pericarditis (Figure 8.7). On a well-penetrated ordinary lateral film, pericardial fluid is suggested by the presence of lucent *pericardial fat lines* well within the cardio-pericardial outline (Figure 10.3). *Radionuclide* "opacification" of the cardiac blood pool (Figure 10.14) can demonstrate effusions but is usually rendered unnecessary by echocardiography, CT and MRI.

ECHOCARDIOGRAPHY OF PERICARDIAL EFFUSION (TABLES 10.3 TO 10.5)

On the *echocardiogram* both normal pericardial fluid and small amounts of excess fluid are seen posteriorly, between the left ventricular wall and the parietal pericardium in systole only (Figure 10.4). With progressive accumulation, posterior fluid appears in both systole and diastole (Figure 10.5), and with larger effusions fluid appears anteriorly (anterior to the right ventricle). Not infrequently, fluid can be found behind the left atrium (i.e., in the oblique sinus of the pericardium), but usually only with very large, often tamponading effusions (Figure 10.6). A number of cardiac and extracardiac conditions may simulate this finding (Table 10.5). The best echo scan planes are the parasternal short axis and the apical four chamber to demonstrate the posterior and circum-

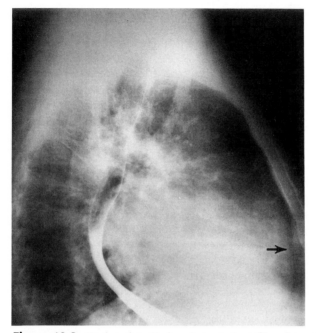

Figure 10.3   Pericardial effusion. Lateral chest film. Arrow indicates vertical lucent "stripe": a pericardial fat line.

ferential extent of the fluid. The subcostal plane is best for fluid loculated over the right atrium. Postoperative changes may degrade image quality and structural recognition. In such circumstances the location of the descending aorta should aid identification. *Pleural effusions*, especially on the left, frequently accompany pericardial effusions (Figure 10.7A and B). The best scan plane for these is the parasternal long axis, where pericardial fluid will be anterior and any pleural fluid posterior to the descending aorta (Figure 10.8). Some pleural effusions act as a "window" improving echocardiographic definition of pericardial and cardiac targets.

Size of effusions by echocardiography may be generalized as follows. *Small*: echo-free space in systole and diastole < 10 mm. *Moderate*: echo-free space in systole and diastole and ≥ 10 mm, at least posteriorly. *Large*: echo-free space ≥ 20 mm. As fluid increases, movement of the parietal pericardium decreases (compare Figures 10.4 and 10.5). Very large effusions compress the heart to where the whole structure becomes visible (uncommon in normal adults; Figure 10.9). NB. - *Effusion size is a powerful predictor of prognosis in hospitalized patients.*

Anterior pericardial fluid tends to unmask brisk pulsations of the right ventricular and atrial walls (Figure 10.10A and B). Small anterior effusions are

Table 10.3 **Echocardiographic and Doppler Effects of Pericardial Effusion and Cardiac Tamponade** (Varying Sensitivities and Specificities)

A. Pericardial Effusion
1. Echo-free space:
    Posterior to LV (small-to-moderate effusion)
    Posterior and anterior (moderate-to-large effusion)
    Behind left atrium (large-to-very large effusion and/or anterior adhesion)
2. Decreased movement of posterior pericardium-lung interface
3. Brisk RV wall movements unmasked with anterior fluid
4. "Swinging heart" (large effusions, usually tamponade)
    RV and LV walls move synchronously
    Periodicity 1:1 or 2:1 (one or two swings per cardiac cycle) 2:1
    characteristic of definite tamponade
    Pseudoparadoxic motion of LV posterior wall
    Mitral/tricuspid pseudoprolapse; occasional true prolapse
    Mitral systolic anterior motion (SAM)
    Alternating mitral E-F slope and aortic opening excursion
    Aortic valve: midsystolic closure involvement
    Pulmonic valve: midsystolic notch
5. Hemopericardium: clotted blood identifiable
6. Inspiratory decrease in left ventricular ejection time (with effusion less than
    with tamponade)
B. Cardiac tamponade—*changes of effusion* plus:
1. RV compression
    RV diameters decreased, especially outflow tract ($\leq$ 7 mm)
    Early diastolic collapse of RV
2. RA free wall indentation (collapse) during late diastole and/or isovolumic
    contraction lasting at least one-third of the cardiac cycle.
3. LA free wall indentation (cases with fluid behind LA)
4. LV free wall paradoxic motion
5. SVC and IVC congestion (unless volume depletion); IVC >2.2 cm with
    <50% inspiratory collapse
6. Exaggerated *inspiratory effects* (especially with pulsus paradoxus with
    reciprocal right-heart–left-heart effects during inspiration and expiration)
    RV expands
    IV septum shifts to left
    LV compressed
    Mitral
        D-E amplitude decreased
        E-F slope decreased or rounded
    Open time[a] decreased; delayed mitral opening
    Aortic valve: opening decreased[a]; premature closure
    Echographic stroke volume decreased
7. Notch in RV epicardium during isovolumic contraction

Table 10.3 Continued

8. Course oscillations of LV posterior wall
9. Pseudohypertrophy: apparent wall thickening due to compression
C. **Doppler Studies: any degree of tamponade**
1. Major changes on first beats during inspiration and expiration
2. Generally reduced flows/stroke volumes
3. Exaggerated inspiratory augmentation of right-sided and decrease of left-sided flows
4. Respiratory *variation* in superior and inferior vena caval flow velocities marked in tamponade, less increased with effusion; double-peaked superior vena cava systolic wave. Decreased expiratiory diastolic SVC flow.
5. Hepatic vein expiratiory effects
   a. marked atrial reversal (AR wave)
   b. marked decrease or reversal of diastolic forward flow
   c. (occasional) systolic flow reversal
6. (Transesophageal echocardiograms)—expiratory increase in pulmonary vein diastolic forward flow
7. Marked inspiratory decrease in left ventricular ejection time (LVET); increased RVET
8. Marked inspiratory increase in LV isovolumic relaxation time (LVIVRT); decrease RVIVRT
9. Hepatic vein velocity difference between systole and atrial reversal < 0 cm/sec.

[a]Often difficult to define during pericardial effusion with tamponade; mitral valve opens late and may open only with atrial systole during inspiration.
Abbreviations: IV, interventricular; IVC, inferior vena cava; LA, left atrium; LV, left ventricle; RA, right atrium; RV right ventricle.

best identified in the subcostal scan plane between the right atrium and liver. With large amounts of posterior fluid, there is decreased amplitude of movement of the posterior parietal pericardium-lung interface (Figure 10.5). With large posterior effusions, only rarely is there no anterior pericardial fluid, a situation usually due to anterior adhesions and frequent after cardiac surgery (Chapter 21). *With only an anterior echo-free space, posterior adhesions might be present although epicardial fat is a more likely explanation;* occasionally, an infiltrative lesion, often malignant, is responsible. Other conditions producing real or apparent anterior echo-free spaces include pericardial cyst or tumor, thymus, and extracardiac masses. In contrast, right heart enlargement may encroach on any anterior space. Finally, large amounts of epicardial fat occasionally simulating posterior and circumcardiac effusions must be specifically recognized by CT scan or MRI.

Table 10.4   Pericardial Effusion: False-Positive M-Mode Echocardiogram

1. Faulty technique
   a. Faulty transducer location (interfering echoes from spine, aorta, mitral annulus, coronary sinus, pulmonary veins)
   b. Decreased gain, increased reject (false-positive separation between epicardium and pericardium posteriorly or between anterior chest wall and anterior right ventricular wall or both)
2. Enlarged left atrium
3. Summation artifact
4. Intrapericardial
   a. Tumor
   b. Adhesive/fibrotic pericardial disease
   c. Subepicardial fat
   d. Pseudoaneurysm
   e. Other (e.g., cyst, abscess)
5. Extrapericardial
   a. Anterior mediastinal mass or cyst
   b. Posterior lung consolidations
   c. Extrapericardial fluid (left pleural effusion)
   d. Foramen of Morgagni hernia
6. Combinations of 1–5

Table 10.5   Conditions Mistaken for Pericardial Effusion by Echocardiography

A. Extracardiac
   1. Mediastinal tumors, *esp.* anterior
   2. Descending aorta (M-mode echo)
   3. Foramen of Morgagni hernia
   4. Hiatal hernia (resembles pneumohydropericardium)
   5. Pleural effusion
   6. Ascites (subcostal scan plane)
B. Pericardial
   1. Infiltrative lesions, usually malignant
   2. Pericardial tumors/masses
   3. Pericardial cysts and diverticula
C. Cardiac
   1. Subepicardial fat, *esp.* if inflamed or hemorrhagic
   2. Giant left atrium (M-mode)
   3. Mitral annular calcification (M-mode)
   4. Prominent coronary sinus
   5. Cardiac tumors
   6. Ventricular pseudoaneurysms

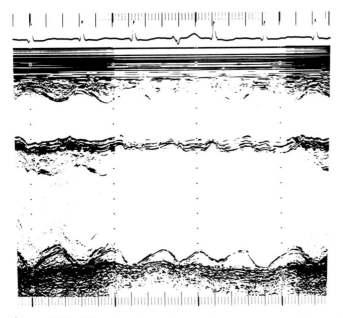

Figure 10.4 M-mode echocardiogram showing minimally increased pericardial fluid visible in systole only. Damping maneuver (most of center of tracing) reveals strong echo of the posterior epicardium.

With very large effusions two-dimensional echocardiography may show the heart to oscillate ("swing") within the pericardium (Figure 10.11; Table 10.3A); here, M-mode echocardiograms are valuable to show the right ventricular anterior wall and the left ventricular posterior wall to move synchronously. With some degree of cardiac tamponade, often critical, this swinging reverses direction on alternate beats instead of on every beat (Figure 5.18). Large effusions, especially with some degree of swinging, may cause *prolapse* or *pseudoprolapse* (Figure 10.12) of the mitral and other valve leaflets in systole as well as mid-systolic notching of the aortic or pulmonary valves and systolic anterior motion of the mitral valve. Prolapse tends to be early or late and at heart rates over 120 beats per minute, pansystolic. Finally, on echocardiograph, especially M-mode tracings, the descending aorta and other structures can be mistaken for a pericardial effusion (Figure 10.13; Tables 10.4 and 10.5).

Transesophageal is superior to transthoracic echocardiography for identifying metastases, pericardial thickening and clots, although it tends to underestimate the volume and distribution of effusion fluid.

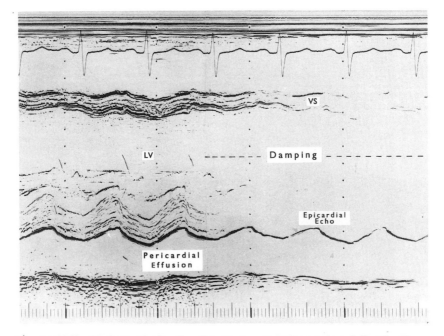

Figure 10.5 Moderate-sized pericardial effusion; fluid in systole and diastole. Damping isolates epicardial echo.

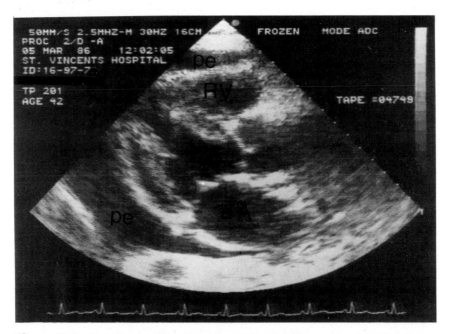

Figure 10.6 Two-dimensional echocardiogram showing large pericardial effusion (pe) anterior to right ventricle (RV) and posterior to left atrium (LA) as well as left ventricle.

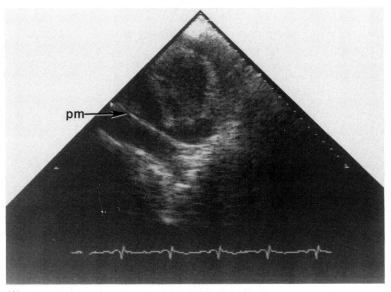

(A)

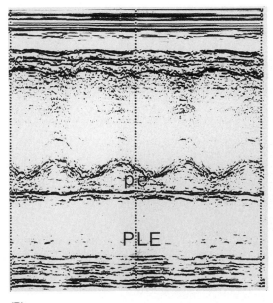

(B)

Figure 10.7   A. Two-dimensional echocardiogram of left ventricle in transverse plane. Pericardium (pm) is "sandwiched" between the pericardial effusion (above) and the pleural effusion (below). B. M-mode echocardiogram showing pericardium "sandwiched" between a large pleural effusion (PLE) and a small pericardial effusion (pe).

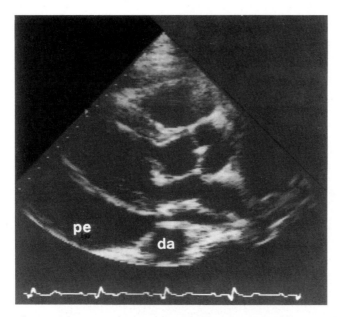

Figure 10.8 Two-dimensional echocardiogram showing large pericardial effusion (PE) penetrating behind and compressing the left atrium but anterior to the descending aorta (da).

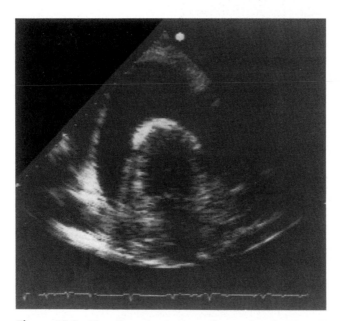

Figure 10.9 Two-dimensional echocardiogram in apical four-chamber scan plane. The heart is compressed (especially the right ventricle) and entirely visible.

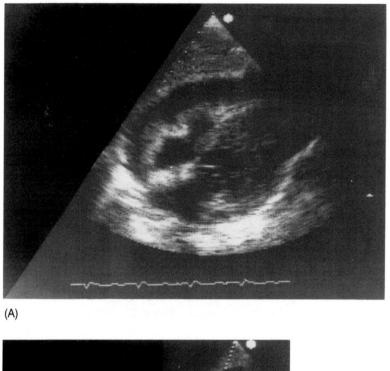

(A)

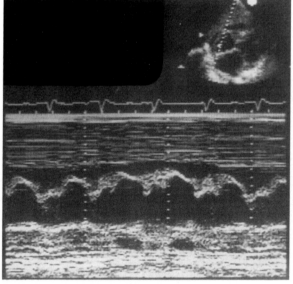

(B)

Figure 10.10 A. Subcostal two-dimensional echocardiogram. Characteristic pulsations of right epicardial borders unmasked by adjacent fluid. B. M-mode tracing of border motion in Figure 10.9A. There is a cycle-to-cycle "ripple" appearance.

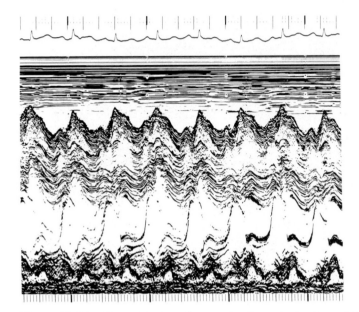

Figure 10.11 M-mode echocardiogram showing swinging heart. The anterior right ventricle and posterior left ventricle move synchronously anteriorly and posteriorly in each cardiac cycle. This 1:1 swinging is a sign of a large effusion without significant pericardial adhesions and does not produce electric alternation.

OTHER IMAGING MODALITIES

Echocardiography is the mainstay of diagnosis. Pericardial effusions have been made radioopaque by directly infusing roentgenographic contrast media for fluoroscopy or films (Figure 10-14), but this procedure is not clinically productive. *Computed tomography* (Figure 10.15) and *MRI* (Figure 10.16) may be used when echo-Doppler results are equivocal. However, uniform pericardial thickening on CT may be due to an effusion and may only be identified by ultrasound or MRI. With all methods, technical care is indispensable to avoid confusing pericardial thickening with effusion.

MANAGEMENT, INDICATIONS FOR DRAINAGE, PERICARDIAL BIOPSY

In the absence of tamponade (Chapter 12) or pyopericardium (page 265), there are few absolute indications for drainage. Successful treatment of the inciting cause should resolve hydropericardium or any noncompressing pericardial ef-

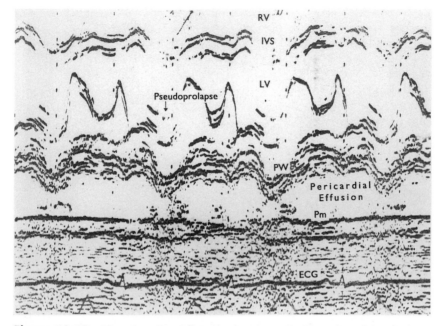

Figure 10.12 M-mode echocardiogram showing mitral pseudoprolapse in large nontamponading effusion with a variant of cardiac swinging at a relatively slow heart rate. The ventricular septum (IVS), the closed mitral valve ("pseuodprolapse" and arrow) and the left ventricular posterior wall (PW) move synchronously giving an illusion of mitral prolapse. Pm = pericardium.

fusion. Very large nontamponading effusions can be drained to relieve dyspnea, presumably due to compression of lung and other thoracic structures. Rarely, it becomes necessary to actually demonstrate fluid by pericardial paracentesis *(pericardiocentesis)*.

Pericardial drainage (Table 10.6) occasionally may be required for etiologic diagnosis by examining what fluid can be obtained, and when one suspects malignancy or a systemic disease; for example, *pericardial biopsy* can be obtained simultaneously. Pericardiocentesis by needle drainage alone frequently is unrewarding for diagnostic purposes, although modern chemical and bacteriologic methods are improving the results (Table 10.7, 10.8). Adequate fluid with an adequate *pericardial biopsy* is better and much more safely obtained surgically, either by *subxiphoid incision* or by *video-assisted thoracoscopic pericardial resection and drainage*. This is highly safe and effective and also permits removal of thrombi, adhesions and fibrinous material, minimizing the chances for recurrence and cicatrization (Chapter 14). *Percutaneous balloon*

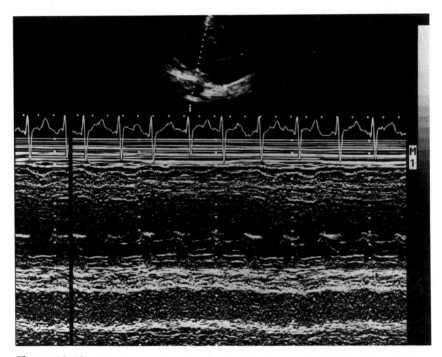

Figure 10.13 False impression of pericardial effusion on M-mode (bottom of figure). Inset shows two-dimensional tracing cursor through left ventricle and descending aorta. There is no pericardial effusion.

periocardiotomy may be used, but is best for palliation in malignant tamponade (Chapter 18). Of course, direct surgical approaches may be unavoidable to drain loculated effusions. Patients with effusions who have pain as a principal symptom may require resection, which will resolve the effusion; it may or may not end the pain (see Chapter 24). The decision for operative intervention depends on (1) clinical evaluation that urgency of diagnosis and the patient's prognosis warrant aggressive management and (2) the probable yield of the diagnostic sample. Thus, persistent illness without an etiologic diagnosis warrants obtaining tissue as well as fluid surgically: *biopsy samples* should be examined histologically, cultured for all likely organisms and stained for mycobacteria and fungi; immunologic investigation of tissue and fluid may be necessary if these are inconclusive (Chapter 16).

   All patients, especially those with underlying cardiac disease, should be monitored for postdrainage decompensation due to latent acute cardiac dilation that had been restrained by the pericardial fluid.

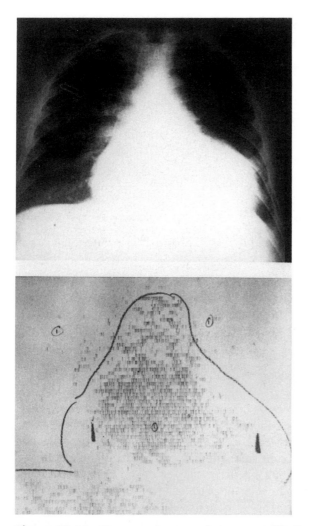

Figure 10.14 Top: roentgenogram shows nonspecifically enlarged cardiopericardial silhouette with clear lung fields. Bottom: radionuclide scintigraphy shows cardiac blood pool surrounded by a nonscintigenic border, which is the pericardial effusion also separating the heart from the liver (right bottom of scan).

TECHNIQUE OF PERICARDIOCENTESIS

In patients in whom emergent tamponade does not permit time for the preferred surgical approach, classic needle pericardiocentesis will be unavoidable. The technique has been refined over many years and if time permits, imaging meth-

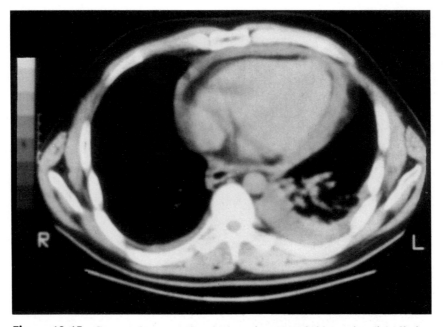

Figure 10.15   Computed tomography: the heart is surrounded by pericardial effusion highlighted by abundant epicardial fat (black layer).

ods, like two-dimensional echocardiography, (2DE), and computed tomography (CT) are now used routinely, to locate the effusion and guide needle insertion. (A Japanese instrument combines a pericardiocentesis needle with an echocardiographic 3.5 MHz probe.) Larger effusions produce higher success rates; small effusions (less than 5 mm anteriorly) may be missed by the needle and are associated more frequently with complications such as penetration or laceration of cardiac structures. Thick. viscous fluids like pus and partly clotted blood, are difficult to aspirate. Patients with severe hemorrhagic diseases may tend to bleed from the slightest inadvertent wound.

Overall the subxiphoid approach appears to be the safest route, although sites on the chest wall opposite the deepest anterior and inferior fluid (as determined by imaging) may be used. The procedure is best performed in an environment where periocardiocentesis kits and rescuscitation and monitoring equipment are available.

Needles and Catheters: Needles should be at least 5 cm long with short bevels. In desperate situations a long spinal needle may be used. A 16-gauge

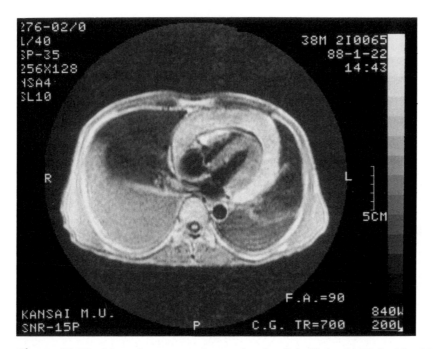

Figure 10.16   Magnetic resonance image of pericardial effusion highlighted by thin band of epicardial fat. (courtesy of Doctor Hitoshi Koito, Osaka, Japan).

Rochester-type needle or a No.16 intravenous cannula can be used with their companion catheters so that the needles can be withdrawn. (If for any reason only a needle is used for continuous drainage, place a surgical clamp on its shaft at the surface of the patient's skin to prevent further penetration).

Table 10.6   Pericardial Drainage

Surgical (including biopsy)
Subxiphoid incision
With endoscopic and digital inspection
Creation of pericardioperitoneal "window"
Insertion of pericardioperitoneal shunt
Video-assisted thoracoscopy
Thoracotomy with open pericardial inspection and resection
Percutaneous
Needle (classic pericardiocentesis)
Needle with catheter
Balloon catheter for pleuropericardial or peritoneopericardial window

Table 10.7   Examination of Pericardial Fluids

Basic tests
1. Hematocrit and cell count
2. Stains: Gram, Ziehl-Nielsen, special
3. Cultures
4. Viral cultures; identification of appropriate immunoglobulins
5. Glucose; protein
6. Cytologic examination

Additional tests for anticipated diagnoses
    a. Lactate dehydrogenase
    b. Rheumatoid factor; antinuclear antibody
    c. Quantitative complement levels
    d. Cholesterol
    e. Pathologic examination of cell blocks; cytochemical staining
    f. pH
    g. Amylase
    h. Adenosine deaminase (ADA)
    I. Carcinoembryonic antigen (CEA)

Electrocardiographic Equipment: Cardiac arrhythmia during the procedure will be detected by an ECG monitor. I do not recommend direct monitoring from the needle itself.

Pressure Monitoring Equipment: Blood pressure should be monitored with a cuff or catheter. A balloon flotation catheter can be used to monitor right atrial pressure, while the intrapericardial needle or catheter permits measuring pericardial pressure. Invasive monitoring usually is not necessary unless the accuracy of diagnosis of uncomplicated tamponade is in question. However, it may reveal unanticipated effusive-constrictive pericarditis (Chapter 15). With uncomplicated tamponade, right atrial and pericardial pressures are approximately equal and fluctuate in parallel during respiration.

Resuscitation Equipment: Standard "crash cart" items including a defibrilator, endotracheal tubes, emergency medications and oxygen are desirable.

TECHNIQUE

An intravenous drip containing isotonic saline or dextrose in water is desirable and can be begun in parallel with preparations for emergency pericardiocentesis. A local anesthetic like procaine is used to anesthetize the needle track.

Ideally the patient should be recumbent or with the chest elevated 30 degrees from the bed. Using the subxiphoid approach, insert the needle into the left xiphocostal angle perpendicular to the skin and 3-4 millimeters below the left costal margin. Advance it perpendicularly, the depth of penetration depending on the amount of soft tissue until the inner aspect of the rib cage is reached. Next, depress the needle's hub so that the needle points "northeast" toward the patient's left shoulder. Using a cautious "worm gear" turning action, advance the needle 5-10 mm (or more) until it reaches the pericardial fluid. Repeated injection of small amounts of procaine will clear the needle and provide anesthesia to deeper tissues.

If no fluid appears, depress the needle's hub further so that its point is slightly closer to the inner aspect of the rib cage (in obese patients, this may require indenting the abdominal wall). Advance the needle again. If fluid is still not encountered and the needle is not touching the heart, withdraw the needle slightly and elevate its hub so that it is in the same "northeast" axis but more posteriorly; advance the needle by "worm gear" action until fluid is reached. Failure to obtain fluid requires a "mirror image" of this approach: redirect the needle toward the patient's right shoulder. If unsuccessful, try a direct anterior-posterior, slightly cephalad, route to seek fluid beneath the heart.

Frequently, puncturing the parietal pericardium imparts a "give" to the fingers, although fluid is often reached without any change of sensation. The fluid is under pressure, often coming out in spurts with each heartbeat; these are audible as "pings" from within a syringe attached to the needle hub; however, even high pressure fluids may dribble out. Contact with the epicardial surface of the heart imparts a "ticking" sensation to the fingers; if this occurs, withdraw the needle slightly and aspirate by syringe.

The first aliquot of fluid should confirm that the needle is intraperiacardial. If the fluid is bloody it is possible that the needle has penetrated the heart. (Another reason for confirming the needle's position is that left pleural effusions and pericardial cysts are occasionally tapped). A microhematocrit apparatus will compare the hematocrit of the first aliquot of bloody fluid with that of peripheral blood. Unless a massive hemorrhage is present intrapericardial blood will not clot because of various antithrombotic pericardial constituents (Chapter 2) and because the whipping action of the heart tends to defibrinate blood. Despite this, in some patients with anemia (common in uremia and malignancy) the hematocrit of the pericardial fluid and that of peripheral blood may be similar, and further confirmation of the needle's location is needed. Saline may be injected and monitored by 2-DE using an apical four-chamber view. It is often difficult to see the needle tip, but the saline bubbles are easily detected. If the needle is in the pericardial cavity no bubbles will appear in the heart. Fluoroscopy will also confirm the position of the needle tip but may require a small amount of contrast material, air or carbon dioxide. Stethoscopic auscultation will yield a bubbling sound during the injection of these gasses.

Confirmation of the needle position permits insertion of a catheter which also permits measuring initial pericardial pressure (in most emergencies this is not necessary and wastes time). The catheter minimizes the chances of cardiac trauma and permits prolonged drainage as a safeguard against refilling. The catheter is inserted by the Seldinger technique: disconnect the syringe from the needle and advance the flexible tip of a short guidewire through the needle into the pericardial space (ideally under imaging guidance). Withdraw the needle and dilate the needle track by advancing a dilator over the guidewire. Finally, insert a soft, multihole 60 cm. pigtail catheter (#6 to #8 French) over the guidewire, monitoring its progress with a fluoroscope if possible. (Alternatively an introducer sheath may be placed over the guidewire and the catheter inserted through it). While advancing the catheter, gradually remove the guidewire. Begin draining the pericardial fluid. If an introducer sheath was used to facilitate catheter insertion, cover the site of skin penetration with antiseptic ointment and apply a sterile dressing (to be changed regularly under sterile technique during drainage). Bloody and viscous fluids may obstruct the catheter, therefore leave a few milliliters of heparinized or plain saline in the catheter unless there is a contraindication. (Table 10.8)

With critical tamponade, the first small aliquot of fluid should make an obvious difference hemodynamically and clinically; in severely ill patients it may take longer for clinical recovery. Atrial and pericardial pressures and the degree of pulsus paradoxus (Chapter 14) should decrease simultaneously. Any electrical alternation (Chapters 5 & 11) should decrease or disappear. Blood pressure and cardiac output should increase (cardiac output may lag the blood pressure increase) The atrial pressure waveform should regain its y descent, amputated by tamponade.

Followup care

Monitor patients for recurrent tamponade, which may result from blockage of the catheter or reaccumulation of fluid. This is particularly important with bloody fluids or frank hemorrhage because of clot formation. Clots can later dissolve producing osmotically active fragments, thus renewing tamponade. Evidence of reformation of fluid includes hypotension, a new increase in venous pressure and recurrence of pulsus paradoxus; confirmation is by imaging.

Complications

The major complications of pericardiocentesis occur during tapping and are caused by needle contact with the heart, particularly laceration of a coronary vessel or a chamber wall or perforation of the myocardium. Injuries to coronary veins, the right atrium or the right ventricle are the most dangerous because these are thin-walled and likely to bleed briskly producing a severe hemo-

Table 10.8   Drainage Methods (esp. purulent/hemorrhagic effusions)

	Advantages	Disadvantages
1. Subxiphoid tube drain	Relatively small procedure. Good for thin pus.	Loculi and clots not drained.
2. Subxiphoid tube and irrigation	Thrombolytics (UK;SK) can prevent tube blockage and attack clots.	May not be sufficiently extensive.
3. Pericardial window and pleural drain	Loculi and clots removed. Permits pericardioscopy.	Frequent window closure.
4. Pericardiotomy with tube	Evacuation of clots. Resection of loculi.	Thoracotomy or thoracoscopy.
5. Partial pericardiectomy with pericardial tube	Reaccumulation less likely.	Thoracotomy or thoracoscopy.
6. Anterior pericardiectomy or anterior interphrenic pericardiectomy	Thorough evacuation. Inspection.	Thoracotomy. Completed surgical procedure.
7. Total pericardiectomy	Later constriction very unlikely.	Thoracotomy. Extensive surgical procedure.
8. Balloon pericardiostomy	Palliation of malignant effusions. Avoids surgery.	May be complicated.

pericardium. "Simple" perforation of the myocardium, particularly the left ventricle without laceration is not rare, especially from the subxiphoid "northeast" and subcardiac routes, but is well tolerated unless vital structures like conduction tissue are traumatized. The left atrium is virtually immune to injury. However, hypotension, probably of reflex origin, can occur at any point so that atropine should be on hand. Rare penetrations include stomach, colon and lung (with pneumothorax). Arrhythmias may occur, particularly in patients with pre-existing heart disease. Direct contact of the needle with the ventricular surface may produce ventricular ectopic beats; with the atrial surface, atrial ectopic beats.

KEY POINTS

1. Pericardial effusions "weep" from the visceral pericardium and may increase greatly due to osmotic attraction of fluid and impedance of venous and lymphatic drainage.
2. Effusions are either (a) inflammatory exudate, (b) hydropericardium (transudate), (c) pyopericardium (pus-containing), (d) hemopericardium (pure blood) or (e) variable mixtures of two or more of these.

3. Very large effusions compress various adjacent structures, accounting for a variety of nonspecific symptoms like breathlessness and hoarseness.

4. Physical examination is untrustworthy, although pericardial rubs may be heard at some time in most inflammatory effusions. Imaging methods other than plain roentgenography identify effusions and permit simultaneous assessment of cardiac chamber size and function.

5. Echocardiography is the mainstay of clinical diagnosis. In absence of pericardial adhesions, an echo-free zone must be present at least posteriorly. Computed tomography and MRI are more definitive but needed only for equivocal echo results.

6. Nontamponading and noninfected pericardial fluids only occasionally require diagnostic testing. Drainage may be done by cautious needle pericardiocentesis, but video-assisted thorascoscopic surgery is safer, surer and permits generous biopsy or resection.

BIBLIOGRAPHY

Ciliberto, G.R., Anjos, M.C., Gronda, E., et al. Significance of pericardial effusion after heart transplantation. Am. J. Cardiol. 1995; 76:297–300.

Isner, J.M., Carter, B.L., Roberts, W.C., Bankoff, M.S. Subepicardial adipose tissue producing echocardiographic appearance of pericardial effusion. Am. J. Cardiol. 1983; 51:565–569.

Spodick, D.H. The normal and diseased pericardium: Current concepts of pericardial physiology diagnosis and treatment. J. Am. Coll. Cardiol. 1983; 1:240–251.

Spodick, D.H. The technique of pericardiocentesis. J. Crit. Illness 1995; 10:802–812.

Wayne, V.S., Bishop, R.L., Spodick, D.H. Dynamic effects of nontamponading pericardial effusion: Respiratory responses in the absence of pulsus paradoxus. Br. Heart J. 1984; 51:202–204.

Suehiro S, Hattori K, Shiba T, Sasaki Y, Minamura H, Kinoshita H. Echocardiography-guided pericardiocentesis with a needle attached to a probe. Ann Thorac Surg 1996; 61:741–742.

11

Cardiac Tamponade: Clinical Characteristics, Diagnosis and Management

GENERAL CONSIDERATIONS

Pericardial lesions of hemodynamic significance include cardiac tamponade, constrictive pericarditis, effusive-constrictive pericarditis and entrapping partial pericardial defects (congenital and traumatic). Tamponade is numerically most important.

Cardiac tamponade is defined as significant compression of the heart by accumulating pericardial contents; these include effusion fluids, pus, blood, clots and gas, singly or in combinations. *Pericardial disease of almost any etiology can produce cardiac tamponade.* This becomes especially important in the occasional patient who presents first with tamponade, since the range of pericardial diseases makes the initial assessment a selection by diagnostic probability, always anticipating etiologic and pathogenetic surprises. Since *tamponade is a pathophysiologic continuum* (Chapter 12), patients may be said to be mildly to floridly tamponaded, the latter being a life-threatening emergency and the former a stage that can progress in that direction. The clinical onset—initial symptoms and signs—mirrors the rate of physiologic impairment. The terms "medical" and "surgical" tamponade are very loosely applied to convey a sense of urgency—they imply nothing else. In general, *"surgical tamponade,"* typified by intrapericardial hemorrhage of any kind, can quickly overwhelm cardiovascular compensatory mechanisms (page 187). With cardiac wounds and rupture of an aortic dissecting hematoma or mural hemorrhage into the pericardium, as little as 150 mL of rapidly added pericardial contents (usually blood) can be lethal in minutes. This contrasts with primarily inflammatory or irritative bloody pericardial effusions in which relatively slowly escaping blood entering the pericardium can be prevented from clotting by the pericardium's fibrinolytic activity (page 24) and the "whipping" action of cardiac beating, which defibrinates blood. (Note: Almost every form of pericarditis, though especially pericardial neoplasia, can provoke variably hemorrhagic effusions.) Primarily inflammatory or irritative processes are usually part of *"medical tamponade,"* in which fluid exudes at a wide range of rates, so that critical cardiac compression may first appear at anywhere from 200 mL to well over a liter (Figure 11.5). Finally, *disorders that thicken or scar the pericardium, like intense or repeated inflammation, sharply reduce the amount of effusion or bleeding that will cause critical cardiac compression.*

SYMPTOMS

The onset of symptoms, ranging from insidious to rapid to sudden, is related to the tempo of physiologic impairment (Chapter 12). A patient first discovered to have many hundred milliliters of fluid did not produce this "overnight," since the interplay of the rate of exudation and the rate of pericardial "give" permits time for widespread compensatory responses to keep effusions subclinical longer than in "surgical tamponade." *Florid tamponade*, whether "surgical" or "medical," is a form of cardiogenic shock, and the diagnosis may be elusive if the patient is first seen in this state. Of course, anyone with obvious *chest or abdominal wounds* should be investigated for pericardial bleeding and observed as a candidate for rapid or delayed cardiac tamponade (Chapter 21).

   Patients may or may not have symptoms of an inciting pericardial disease, notably *chest discomfort*, but in patients presenting unconscious, obtunded or with convulsions there may be no useful history. Cerebral venous congestion and reduced arterial flow, particularly in elderly patients, may make them poor informants. *Tachypnea* is common, even with small effusions, while *dyspnea* on exertion progressing to *air hunger at rest*, and occasionally orthopnea, are the common complaints. Indeed, severe tamponade frequently provokes air hunger, syncope and even convulsions. *Cough* and *dysphagia* are not uncommon and can be deceptive early complaints. *Most patients are weak, faint and anorexic.* Because there are thus no symptoms specific for tamponade, any of the foregoing warrants a determined search utilizing appropriate bedside and laboratory evidence. Of course, large effusions without hemodynamic compromise can cause breathlessness (page 128). *Anemia* is another cause or exacerbating factor for dyspnea and weakness. Finally, *insidiously developing tamponade* may first present as one of its complications, like renal failure.

PHYSICAL FINDINGS; SIGNS

Physical examination, as already noted (Chapter 10), is of little use in determining the presence of the pericardial effusion itself, although occasionally there is a *Bamberger-Pins-Ewart sign* with very large effusions (page 131). *Tachycardia* (>100 beats per minute is the rule) although many patients have heart rates between 90 and 100, and the rate is even lower in many uremics. With effusions during acute pericarditis, most patients retain their *pericardial rub.* Indeed, *contrary to common belief, pericardial rubs are frequently present and may even be quite loud with inflammatory effusions of all sizes.* On the other hand, the heart sounds themselves may be distant due both to insulation by the surrounding fluid and reduced heart function. *Heart sounds* are often better heard over the base of the heart or the epigastrium, often with a diminished first sound (S1) and sometimes with relative accentuation of the pulmonic component of the second heart sound ("P2"). Sometimes the precordium is quiet and an apex beat not palpable. In patients with preexistent cardiomegaly or anterior and apical pericardial adhesions, quite active pulsations may be palpated.

Significant tamponade produces absolute or relative *hypotension.* (Indeed, tamponade must be considered in the differential diagnosis of any unexplained hypotension.) In surgical tamponade, *shock* levels are usual but, in early medical tamponade, systolic blood pressure is commonly between 90 and 100 mm Hg. Moreover, occasional patients are hypertensive, especially those with preexisting hypertension; in them, "normal" levels may actually be low. Hypertensive blood pressures characterize patients with exaggerated compensatory adrenergic responses and greatly increase peripheral resistance (*hypertensive tamponade*). *Cool extremities, nose and ears*, sometimes with *peripheral cyanosis*, are due to vasoconstriction and relative circulatory stasis. *Central cyanosis* is rare and may be due to right to left shunting, usually through a patent foramen ovale, which disappears after relief of tamponade.

If the patient is not hypovolemic, and especially if the rate of accumulation of fluid has been sufficiently slow for expansion of blood volume, *jugular venous distention* may be anywhere from just visible to striking, depending on the patient's neck tissues (leaner and younger necks are more revealing). *Peripheral venous distention* may also be seen in the forehead, scalp and ocular fundi. In rapid "surgical tamponade," especially acute hemopericardium, only *jugular pulsations without distention* may be visible, since there has been no time for compensatory blood volume expansion. Since most patients, especially those with medical tamponade, have heart rates between 85 and 120, jugular pulsations may be slow enough to accurately determine that there is an *x descent*, but *absent or greatly attenuated, y descent* (Figure 11.1). Indeed, if a venous level can be accurately discerned at some upper-body elevation from the horizontal, the single definitely negative phase (*x descent*) may be seen in

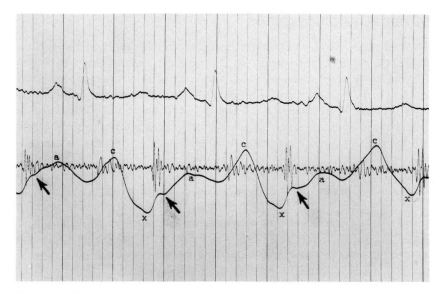

Figure 11.1 Jugular venous pulse tracing with ECG and phonocardiogram. *a* and *c* wave are clear (and the *z* depression between them). There is a clear *x* descent during ventricular systole but no *y* descent in early diastole; arrows indicate where it would have begun. (Right atrial pressure curves would be virtually identical). There is no third heart sound (made impossible by tamponade physiology; see Chapter 12).

midsystole if the heart rate is not too fast. (Quite slow atrial rates are not rare in uremia with tamponade but are uncommon in other forms). The *x* descent can also be timed as occurring between the two heart sounds if both are clearly audible. It is imperative to realize that *these are not outward pulsations; x and y in compressive pericardial disease are "collapses" from a high standing level.* The neck veins may also show the normal fall in pressure level during inspiration. (An inspiratory *increase*—Kussmaul's sign—is typical of constriction; when seen with tamponade, or after pericardial drainage, it is usually due to epicardial constriction (page 253). Rarely this may be seen without explanation, comparable to genuine pulsus paradoxus in constriction; ultimately these riddles will be explained.)

Pulsus Paradoxus

A most important physical finding is *pulsus paradoxus* (analyzed in Chapter 13), defined as a systolic fall in arterial pressure of at least 10 mm Hg. During normal breathing, the majority of patients with cardiac tamponade have some degree of pulsus paradoxus, and this is often readily palpable in peripheral arteries (Figure 11.2). At very low cardiac outputs, however, an arterial catheter or a sphygmomanometer will be needed. This phenomenon is perceived as a relatively marked fall in systolic arterial pressure during inspiration that returns in expiration. With a pronounced "pulsus," there may in fact be no Korotkoff sound in inspiration—indeed, the aortic valve may fail to open in inspiration—with complete inspiratory loss of pulsations in muscular arteries, like the radial. (The more elastic carotid pulse is not as easily evaluated.) This may first be appreciated when taking the radial pulse and watching the patient's abdomen during *normal breathing*. (Note: Breathing should not be exaggerated, since that can exaggerate the pressure drop.) As the abdomen rises, the pulse either weakens or disappears. To quantify the blood pressure change noninvasively, a blood pressure cuff is inflated to 15 mm Hg above the apparent highest systolic level. The cuff is slowly bled of air until the first beats are heard (the sequence goes something like "bump-bump-bump, silence-silence-silence, bump-bump-bump"; the "bumps"—Korotkoff sounds—are expiratory.) The cuff is then deflated to where all beats are heard. *The difference between these pressures gives the "size" of the pulsus.* The proportion of the pulse pressure—peak systolic pressure minus diastolic pressure—occupied by the measured pulsus, i.e., the "size" of the pulsus divided by the pulse pressure, can be loosely proportional to the cardiac impairment. Naturally, if a patient is first discovered with pulsus paradoxus, the pericardial variety must be differentiated from *other conditions that can produce pulsus paradoxus*, like massive pulmonary embolism, profound hemorrhagic shock and other forms of severe hypotension, and obstructive lung disease—especially during asthmatic attacks. In pulmonary disease, *both* the systolic and diastolic levels fluctuate with respiration, whereas

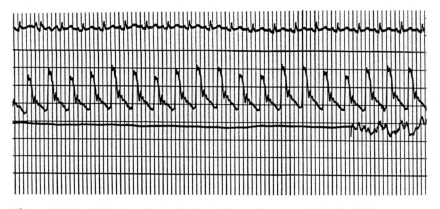

Figure 11.2 Pulsus paradoxus during early cardiac tamponade. Brachial artery systolic pressure falls excessively during normal breathing (142 to 124 mm Hg); diastolic pressure is steady at 76 mm Hg. ECG shows marked PR segment depression.

in tamponade only the systolic level fluctuates (Figure 11.2). Conditions in which *pulsus paradoxus may be absent* or undetectable despite tamponade are those that alter tamponade physiology and respiratory mechanisms (Table 11.1).

One phenomenon will be *absent*: *a third heart sound* (Figure 11.1); its presence would call into question the diagnosis of tamponade. By eliminating rapid filling, tamponade eliminates one of the hemodynamic necessities for a third heart sound. [Indeed, in severe tamponade, inspiratory ventricular filling may only occur when atrial systole opens the atrioventricular (A-V) valves.] Two *uncommon exceptions* occur in some cases of effusive-constrictive pericarditis with mixed hemodynamics: (1) an abnormal S3 (page 35) and (2) Kussmaul's sign (inspiratory distention of the neck veins; page 245).

Renal Effects

Patients with tamponade become *oliguric*, as with any other profound hypotension. Despite high central circulatory pressures, *atrial natriuretic factor cannot increase* due to the absence of myocardial stretch. Moreover, tamponade itself tends to signal reduced sodium and fluid output by the kidney with consequent fluid and electrolyte retention.

ELECTROCARDIOGRAPHY (CHAPTER 5; TABLE 10.2)

The *electrocardiogram (ECG)* can be entirely normal, but most often is non-specifically altered (mainly ST-T abnormalities). It may show acute pericarditis at ECG Stages 1, 2 or 3 (Chapter 5). *Electric alternation* of the QRS complex (Figure 11.3), less often including the T (Figure 11.4) and much less often the P wave, is quasidiagnostic. This is *vector* alternation, not voltage alternation as seen in certain tachycardias, in which the amplitude but not the direction alternates and there is often a slight R-R alternation. P-QRS or P-QRS-T al-

Table 11.1   Cardiac Tamponade Without Pulsus Paradoxus[a]

Ventricular hypertrophy	Severe hypotension
Left ventricular failure	Dehydration
Aortic regurgitation	Pre-terminal tamponade with bradycardia
Aortic stenosis	Cardiac rupture
(LV paradoxus)	Arrhythmias
Atrial septal defect	Breathing rate/rhythm abnormalities
Isolated chamber compression	Low-pressure tamponade

[a]See also Chapter 13, page 198.

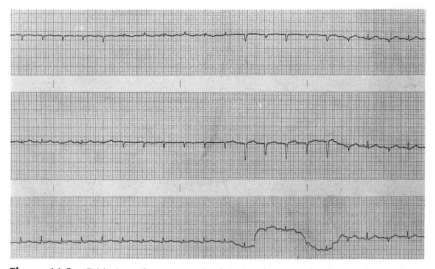

Figure 11.3 Critical cardiac tamponade: 2:1 electric alternation in a patient with true low voltage and right axis deviation. Alternans is seen in all leads but best seen in leads V4, V5 and V6—the last panel of the trace—with complete reversal of QRS direction, indicating alternate anterior and posterior vector shift in the horizontal plane (to which the limb leads are relatively insensitive).

ternation (*simultaneous alternation*) has been reported only in critical cardiac tamponade. Any *low voltage* (Figure 11.3) is due to reduced heart size or to cardiac disease and is common in transplanted hearts. Significant vagally mediated *bradycardia* (overriding normal baroreceptor reflexes) and ultimate *electromechanical dissociation* (EMD) occur in end-stage tamponade, most often in rapid hemopericardium of any etiology, in which critical cardiac compression prevents filling and therefore cardiac output, while the ECG is continuously generated.

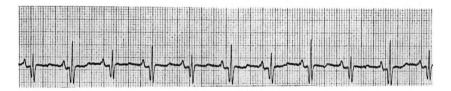

Figure 11.4 Cardiac tamponade: single ECG monitor lead with marked 2:1 QRS alternation and subtle but definite alternation of the abnormal T waves (had they been of greater voltage, alternation might be more marked).

IMAGING: PRIMARY RELIANCE ON ECHO-DOPPLER CARDIOGRAPHY

All imaging methods can demonstrate pericardial effusion (Chapter 10). *Chest x-rays* show an enlarged cardiopericardial silhouette with clear lungs (in the absence of pulmonary disease). *Echo-Doppler Cardiography*, ideally, though not necessarily, transesophageal (TEE), can eliminate the need for invasive hemodynamic measurement by giving a dynamic, real-time picture and therefore physiologic as well as anatomic data consistent with tamponade (detailed in Table 10.3). Some features are blunted in hypervolemic patients. *Echo-Doppler signs are somewhat less accurate in patients with pulmonary hypertension and of greatly reduced sensitivity after cardiac surgery.*

If the effusion is large enough, the heart may be seen to swing freely in it (Figures 11.5 and 11.6); this is the basis of electric alternation on the ECG. Swinging during tamponade is rarely associated with a mechanical pulsus alternans, usually of small degree, detected as slightly alternating strength (amplitude) of peripheral pulse waves owing to alternating systolic blood pressure levels; the intensity of the first heart sound may also rarely alternate. These may be partly related to alternate torsion of the heart's vascular pedicle—the roots of the aorta and pulmonary artery—within the pericardial fluid.

With large and many moderate-sized effusions, compression by pericardial fluid permits the entire adult heart outline to be seen, particularly in the four-chamber scan plane (Figure 11.5). Cardiac compression may also falsely suggest myocardial hypertrophy (*pseudohypertrophy*). With hemopericardium, clot-

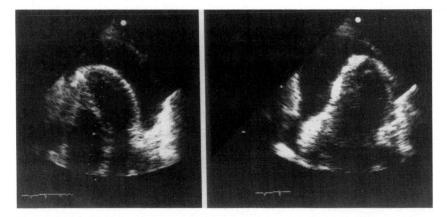

Figure 11.5 Swinging heart in pericardial effusion: cause of electric alternation. Two-dimensional echocardiogram of large pericardial effusion compressing heart. Left frame: swing to right with smaller QRS. Right frame: swing to left with larger QRS.

ted blood may be detected. If there is no underlying heart disease, all cardiac chamber sizes are restricted, but especially the right ventricular inflow and outflow tracts. On the left, decreased filling correlates with delayed mitral valve opening and prolonged left ventricular isovolumic relaxation time, worse in inspiration. Yet, in the absence of heart disease, systolic function appears grossly good, with excellent echocardiographic shortening and ejection fractions in tamponaded ventricles, although they operate at reduced volumes and hence small stroke outputs. Thus, the heart is *underloaded*—"underpreloaded" and "underafterloaded"—and is obviously working hard but prevented by reduced inflow from keeping up with circulatory demands. *Collapse of the right ventricular free wall in early diastole* (RVDC; Figure 11.7) correlates with obstruction to the *y* descent in the atrial pressure curve, i.e., obstruction to rapid filling; it tends to occur in *expiration* when RV volume is reduced. *Right atrial*

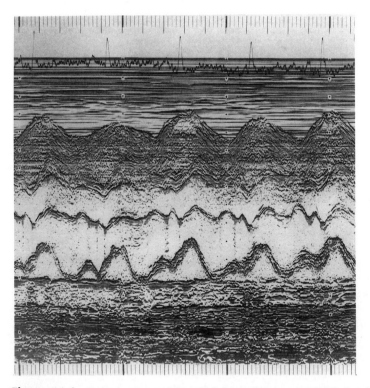

Figure 11.6 Swinging heart: M-mode echocardiogram and ECG showing 2:1 electric alternation due to alternate anterior and posterior swings, producing alternate larger and smaller QRS complexes in lead II (more leads would reveal directional vector alternation).

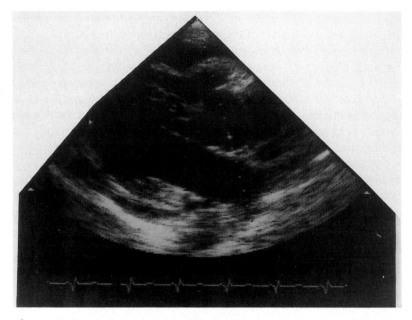

Figure 11.7 Cardiac tamponade: right ventricular diastolic collapse (indentation near top of two-dimensional echocardiogram).

wall collapse (RAC; Figure 11.8) occurs in very late diastole and early iso-volumic systole; in about 25% of cases, the *left atrial* wall also collapses (Figure 11.9). Each collapse marks transient increase of intrapericardial pressure over the collapsing chamber's cavity pressure—i.e., reversal of the chamber's transmural pressure (TMP) relations—yielding a negative TMP.

The *right ventricular diastolic collapse* occurs after a 15 to 25% drop in cardiac output and generally before a significant decrease in blood pressure in patients who are normovolemic or hypervolemic. Moreover, RVDC appears to be more specific than RAC and more sensitive and specific than pulsus para-doxus in detecting increased intrapericardial pressure, *particularly RVDC lasting at least one-third of the cardiac cycle*, which makes its specificity for tamponade approach 100%; duration of RVDC is quantitatively related to the elevation of pericardial pressure. (In hypovolemic patients the usefulness of RVDC paral-lels that of pulsus paradoxus.) Occasionally RVDC is seen when unilateral or bilateral *pleural effusion* causes increased pressure in an insignificant pericar-dial effusion; indeed, such RVDC, which occurs in *inspiration*, can be relieved by draining such pleural effusions. Rarely, acute left ventricular enlargement can also increase pericardial pressure sufficiently to cause right ventricular di-

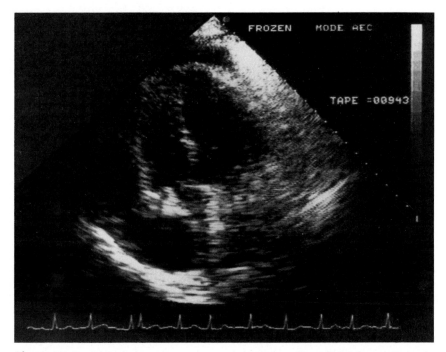

Figure 11.8 Cardiac tamponade: right atrial diastolic collapse (left bottom of two dimensional echocardiogram). The right atrium is almost obliterated by an "inverted L"-shaped collapse of its free wall.

astolic collapse, which disappears with treatment of the cause of the left ventricular enlargement. *Inferior vena cava (IVC) plethora* (diameter ≥ 20mm) with *absence of the normal IVC collapse* (≥ 50%; Figure 11.10A) is seen on subcostal echocardiography. When this accompanies right ventricular and/or atrial collapse, it markedly improves their diagnostic specificity for advanced tamponade, since chamber collapses can occur at relatively low intrapericardial (and therefore chamber) pressures while absence of normal inspiratory IVC collapse implies high right heart diastolic pressures (right atrial pressures ≥ 15 mm Hg). The *superior vena caval systolic flow* wave tends to be double-peaked, especially in patients with RA collapse, becoming single peaked after drainage. In "early" tamponade this occurs only in inspiration; later double-peaking occurs in both in- and expiration. In "early" tamponade this occurs only in inspiration; later, double peaking occurs in both in-and expiration. Finally, the most sensitive and specific indicator of right atrial pressure is hepatic vein Doppler: a difference between systolic and atrial reversal velocities < 0 cm/sec is inversely related (Table 10.3).

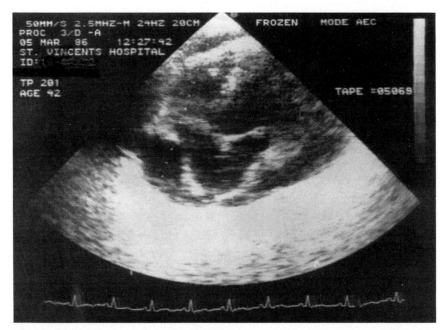

Figure 11.9 Cardiac tamponade: diastolic collapse of the left atrium as well as the right atrium (bottom of heart outline).

Respiratory effects parallel pulsus paradoxus (Chapter 13); thus, the right and left ventricular volumes vary reciprocally with respiration, as shown by *ventricular septal shift* from the right into the left ventricle in inspiration and its restoration in expiration (Figure 13.6). Doppler velocity recording permits gross estimation of the reduced stroke volume and also shows *markedly increased flow velocities across the right-sided valves in inspiration (Figure 11.10B), with a corresponding (but lesser) drop across the left-sided valves and their reversal during expiration; maximal changes are on the first beat after the onset of inspiration and the first beat after the onset of expiration;* thus, although

---

Figure 11.10 A. Cardiac tamponade: inferior vena cava diameter does not vary between inspiration (top) and expiration (bottom). This sign nonspecifically indicates right heart diastolic pressures of over 15 mm Hg and is also seen in constrictive pericarditis B. Cardiac tamponade: schemata of respiratory fluctuation in transtricuspid (right ventricular filling) and hepatic vein blood flow velocity. (Compare marked respiratory responses with their absence in the inferior vena cava in Figure 11.10A.) Above: right ventricular filling: E = early diastolic peak; A = active filling following atrial systole. During inspiration, flow velocities increase markedly and promptly fall with expiration. Middle: hepatic vein forward-flow velocities increase with inspiration and reverse promptly with expiration, reversing again at end expiration. Bottom: curve of breath-

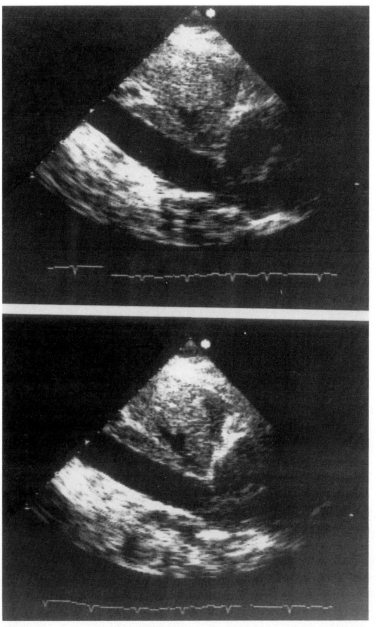

(A)

ing cycle. C. Inspiratory effects on transvalvular Doppler flows in patients with tamponade (striped bars) compared with normal subjects (solid bars). The degree (%) of changes between inspiration and expiration is normally small, but greatly exaggerated during tamponade. Inspiratory increases in right sided (tricuspid and pulmonic) flows are much larger than inspiratory decreases in left sided (mitral and aortic) transvalvular flows.

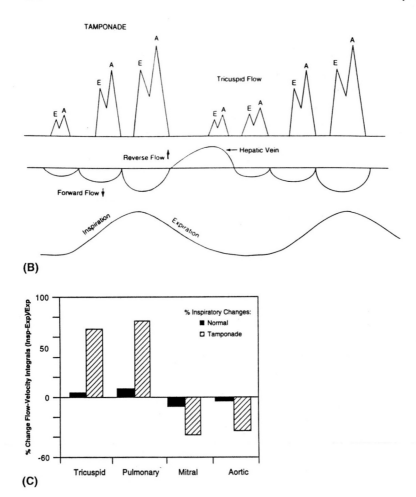

Figure 11.10 Continued

total transvalvular blood *volume* flows are reduced, right heart–left heart flow *velocity differences* are enormously magnified during these respiratory events. Figure 11.10C compares these with each other and with the much smaller normal respiratory changes. Concurrently, respiratory variations of *superior vena cava flow velocities* are exaggerated in tamponade. (Because volumetric venous flow changes parallel velocity changes, actual blood flow can be inferred.) Finally, all these striking changes disappear after successful pericardial drainage. *Hepatic vein flow velocities* increase during inspiration with retrograde flow in early expiration (Figure 11.10B).

DIAGNOSIS

In general, *cardiac tamponade should be suspected* in any patient with (1) unexplained shock and elevated systemic venous pressure; (2) unexplained low or falling blood pressure; (3) pulsus paradoxus; (4) unexplained tachycardia, dyspnea or tachypnea, especially if there are clear lung fields on physical examination and chest x-ray film (except occasional patients with severe myocardial failure or intrinsic lung lesions); (e) chest and abdominal wounds; (5) recent or concurrent evidence of pericarditis and unexplained "cardiac" enlargement or evidence on imaging (Figure 11.11) of pericardial effusion. Moreover, anticoagulant or thrombolytic therapy, certain drugs like cyclosporine, recent cardiac surgery, blunt chest trauma, malignancies, connective tissue disease, renal failure and septicemia all precipitate, aggravate, or predispose patients to cardiac tamponade. Patients with *indwelling instrumentation*, particularly of the thin right heart—like central venous lines, transvenous pacemakers, filtration catheters and hyperalimentation catheters—may have had subtle perforation of the right atrium or ventricle. Some of these provoke hemopericardium; those delivering parenteral fluids can rapidly fill and overload the pericardial cavity.

Certain conditions may inhibit chamber collapses and other respiratory phenomena, just as they limit pulsus paradoxus. These include left ventricular hypertrophy and dysfunction, aortic valve disease, hypertrophy and reduced

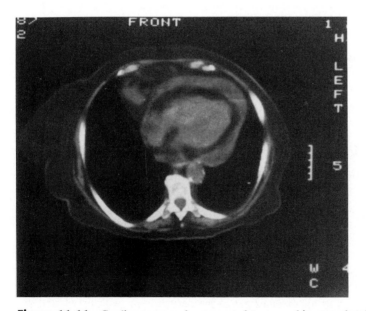

Figure 11.11 Cardiac tamponade: computed tomographic scan showing large pericardial effusion highlighted by underlying thick epicardial fat (black layer).

compliance of the right ventricle, and obstruction of right ventricular valves by intrinsic disease or masses. Moreover, the diagnostic sensitivities of chamber collapses and increased respiratory valve flows are decreased in postoperative cardiac patients. Finally, *left ventricular diastolic collapse* (LVDC) occurs with loculated, usually postsurgical, effusions over the left ventricle (page 388) and rarely in circumferential tamponade in patients with right ventricular hypertrophy.

VARIANT FORMS OF CARDIAC TAMPONADE

Low Pressure Tamponade

This usually occurs in hypovolemic patients with severe systemic diseases like tuberculosis and malignancies. They are weak, may seem normotensive and have dyspnea on exertion, with only mild if any jugular venous distension and no diagnostic pulsus paradoxus (Chapter 13); however, characteristic respiratory changes in diastolic inflow signals and isovolumic relaxation time are found. In low-pressure tamponade, the low-pressure pericardial effusion equilibrates with right ventricular diastolic pressure only, as in cases of early classic tamponade (Chapter 12). From this stage onward, diastolic pressure equilibration occurs first only in inspiration ("inspiratory tracking").

Hypertensive Cardiac Tamponade

This has all the features of cardiac tamponade except that these exceptional patients may have high and rarely very high—over 200 mm Hg—blood pressures. Moreover, pulsus paradoxus is demonstrable at high pressure. Typically, there is antecedent hypertension. Attempts to reduce the blood pressure may exacerbate the situation and precipitate or greatly exaggerate established pulsus paradoxus.

Tamponade with Ventricular Dysfunction

Right or left ventricular dysfunction can reduce or eliminate pulsus paradoxus. Left ventricular dysfunction, especially reduced compliance—notably in hypertensive or severe coronary artery disease, uremia, or aortic valve disease (especially aortic regurgitation)—may be associated with right atrial and right ventricular diastolic collapses at relatively small volumes of excess pericardial fluid. They essentially produce a right heart tamponade at lower intrapericardial pressures than with a normal left ventricle.

Tension pneumopericardium or pneumohydropericardium (Chapters 7 and 21). Accumulation of air or other gas in the pericardium, with or without excess pericardial fluid, blood, pus or chyle, can easily tamponade the heart, especially if the gas is relentlessly increasing. Examples include a check-valve mechanism admitting air from lung structures or gas-producing organisms multi-plying in the pericardium. Diagnostic and therapeutic principles are the same as in ordinary tamponade. However, there is a tympanitic precordial percussion note and frequently the "*mill-wheel sound*" of the heart splashing in a fluid-gas interface. The latter is also heard with *iatrogenic pneumohydropericardium* when air is injected after pericardial drainage to define the heart and pericardium on chest films, a procedure rendered unnecessary by modern imaging methods.

Regional Cardiac Tamponade

Compression of any part of the heart occurs from loculation of effusion over that part. Loculation is usually due to *localized pericardial adhesions*, especially postsurgical adhesions (pages 383–386), and presents hemodynamic abnormalities consistent with the chambers or zones that are compressed. For example, following *right ventricular infarction*, loculated effusion can cause selective right ventricular tamponade with right atrial pressure higher than left; absence of pulsus paradoxus make this difficult to recognize. Loculated effusions compressing the right atrium may act similarly and can also cause a *right-to-left shunt through a patent foramen ovale or atrial septal defect*, either by significantly increased right atrial pressure or by distorting the atrium so that blood entering from the inferior vena cava streams to and through the foramen ovale or defect. However, loculated effusion tamponading the right atrium can also reproduce all the hemodynamic findings of severe tamponade, including pulsus paradoxus (thus ventricular compression is not always necessary). Post-infarctional local tamponade and some postsurgical accumulations resolve spontaneously; others must be drained.

Effusive-Constrictive Pericarditis

This combination of effusion and constriction with mixed clinical, imaging, and hemodynamic signs can produce tamponade with relatively little fluid when there is a scarred, rigid, unyielding parietal pericardium or when a *constrictive epicarditis* underlies the tamponading fluid. (Discussed with constrictive pericarditis; Chapter 15.)

CARDIAC CATHETERIZATION (FIGURE 11.12)

It may be necessary to confirm the diagnosis of cardiac tamponade by either right heart or complete cardiac catheterization when an appropriate study of the heart and coronaries becomes desirable for any reason. Ideally, catheterization will show high pressures throughout ventricular diastole and *near-equilibration of atrial and ventricular diastolic pressures*. The tolerance limit for equilibration is within 5 mm Hg. A wider difference in an appropriate setting should

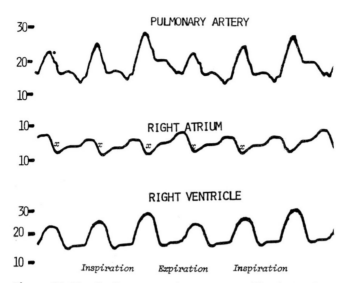

Figure 11.12   Cardiac tamponade; pressure equilibration: pulmonary artery diastolic, right atrial mean and right ventricular diastolic pressures each approximately 15 mm Hg. Respiratory fluctuation of right ventricular systolic pressure between 23 mm Hg in maximum expiration and 29 mm Hg at peak inspiration. Right atrial pressure has a single conspicuous drop, the *x* descent, there is no *y* descent. Pulmonary artery systolic pressure changes follow the right ventricular systolic pressures at approximately the same levels.

always raise a question of tamponade, especially if there are individual cardiac chamber abnormalities or the possibility of loculated fluid. Most tamponades equilibrate at pressures of 16 to 30 mm Hg. In *low-pressure tamponade*, levels may be as low as 5 to 10 mm Hg. Atrial traces will show partial amputation or absence of the *y* descent. Arterial and pericardial catheters disclose *exaggerated respiratory pressure fluctuations*. As pericardial pressure falls in inspiration, the arterial pressure pulse shows a systolic drop, which may be quite abrupt, depending on the patient's respiratory dynamics.

In the absence of preexisting coronary disease, compression of the epicardial coronary arteries and veins does not result in anaerobic metabolism, as measured by coronary sinus lactate level, demonstrating that the tamponaded and consequently underloaded myocardium has sufficient blood supply to avoid anoxia, despite the usual tachycardia and strong compensatory adrenergic response (pages 186–188).

Despite very high central circulatory pressures—indeed, pressures usually equal to those in left heart failure—*tamponade does not cause alveolar pulmonary edema*. Although there may be some interstitial lung edema, neither the alveoli nor the septa are affected, for incompletely understood reasons. In the systemic venous circulation, high pressure includes the hepatic veins and inferior vena cava. But unlike the respiratory effects in the heart and arteries, in tamponade, vena cava diameter does not change much with respiration (Figure 11-10). Subcostal echocardiography shows that *the intrahepatic inferior vena cava is plethoric*—i.e., wide—a more reliable sign than jugular venous distention. In fact, a highly sensitive sign of advanced cardiac tamponade (more specifically, right heart hypertension) *is a less than 50% decrease in IVC diameter with ordinary or deep inspiration.* This predicts elevated right atrial pressure (≥ 15 mm Hg) and, in tamponade, a relatively large pulsus paradoxus.

CHRONIC PERICARDIAL EFFUSION AND TAMPONADE (SEE ALSO CHAPTER 25)

Occasional patients present with vague complaints in the chest or during evaluation for other disease in which a large to massive, chronic pericardial effusion is discovered by accident. ("Chronic" arbitrarily indicates at least three months' documented duration.) In such patients, systemic complaints like fatigue, anorexia and weight loss may dominate the clinical picture. Progression is sometimes demonstrated by sequential chest films showing preceding chronic effusion. Occasionally the pathogenesis is demonstrable in conditions like cholesterol pericarditis or severe thyroid disease. However, the majority of cases prove to be of unknown origin, with pericardial fluid and tissue providing no clues. Unlike much pericardial disease, there is no male predominance. Some patients become symptomatic only after a long-standing effusion has been decompensated by an intercurrent event and some degree of overt tamponade appears. Tamponade, of course, dictates prompt intervention. However, the danger of eventual tamponade, especially after recent febrile illness, chest pain or with a pericardial rub, makes it prudent to drain the fluid and, if necessary, resect the pericardium. Cardiac catheterization may be desirable to evaluate the heart and coronary arteries. A pericardial catheter may show a surprising range of low to high pericardial pressures in patients with chronic effusions. Any tendency for constrictive pericarditis, especially constrictive epicarditis, indicates pericardectomy. Indeed, after drainage of chronic effusion with or without clinical tamponade, occasional patients go on to more or less rapid constriction.

TREATMENT OF CARDIAC TAMPONADE

Definitive treatment of cardiac tamponade is prompt evacuation of the compressing pericardial contents. Only in a relatively few patients who have dehydration and hypovolemia has it been possible to demonstrate that cardiocirculatory support by medical measures may be effective. Volume infusion *in hypovolemic patients* may indeed also be diagnostically useful, at least temporarily, by revealing the typical hemodynamics of cardiac tamponade, which is otherwise well concealed in some hypovolemic patients (*occult tamponade*; see low-pressure tamponade, page 168).

Medical Treatment

Even the experimental evidence for the usefulness of a wide variety of medical agents is conflicting and has been investigated in models that do not necessarily apply to human clinical tamponade. Medical treatment may indeed appear to be temporarily effective, partly because tamponade occasionally remits spontaneously. However, there is no evidence for its permanent or even satisfactory temporary effectiveness. Medical therapy has been aimed at supporting the wide-ranging compensatory mechanisms and physiologic responses to tamponade (Chapter 12), specifically by expanding intravascular volume, increasing or decreasing systemic vascular resistance and supporting inotropy. The latter, of course, is almost predictably useless because *most tamponaded hearts without preexisting cardiac disease are under effective endogenous inotropic stimulation*; this typically produces an excellent ejection fraction—but at critically low stroke volume. Supporting filling with various intravenous fluids can help hypovolemic patients, but otherwise tends to increase heart volume with a subsequent countervailing increase in pericardial pressure, leaving the patient no better and perhaps worse. Agents increasing peripheral resistance to support blood pressure have not been demonstrably effective, again because tamponade evokes maximal endogenous sympathetic stimulation and perhaps also because of untoward cardiac effects. Finally, *atropine* can be given or kept in reserve for depressive vagal reflexes during early and late tamponade.

If drainage equipment is not immediately available, of course, medical measures may be used in the hope that a transiently favorable effect may tide the patient over, perhaps permitting additional pericardial stretch. These include isoproterenol, norepinephrine, dobutamine and similar agents. Although respiratory alkalosis occurs in tamponade (page 188), correction of any *metabolic acidosis* avoids the myocardial depressant effect of that condition and increases responses to endogenous and exogenous catecholamines. Temporary results may also accrue from vasodilators. Nitroprusside plus blood transfusion in experimental animals produces some improvement in cardiac output. Hydralazine plus volume infusion appears to raise arterial pressure and cardiac output and improve blood flow to myocardium, central nervous system and kidney—all locations where slightly improving blood flow has not been critical, due in part to autoregulation. *Positive-pressure breathing of any kind should be avoided* at any stage of tamponade because it will further reduce venous return, right ventricular transmural pressure and cardiac output. On the other hand, maintenance of normal pH and avoidance of hypercarbia help protect the myocardium from chemical depression. Only after the pericardium is incised or the fluid drained, may positive-pressure breathing be used.

PERICARDIAL DRAINAGE

Whenever possible, limited or open *surgical drainage is the treatment of choice* for both safety and effectiveness.

Drainage of pericardial fluid, particularly tamponading fluid, has several objectives: (1) to definitively treat tamponade, (2) to treat the cause of tamponade, (3) to prevent recurrence of effusion and tamponade, and (4) for diagnosis. Several methods are available (Table 10.6); *all may be hazardous*, especially in patients with a bleeding diathesis or in the postirradiated chest of patients who have had radiotherapy for malignancy and other conditions. Choice of procedure usually depends on urgency. For example, when death appears to be impending, the quickest method, percutaneous needle paracentesis, can be the procedure of choice. On the other hand, with brisk pericardial bleeding—as in wounds, ruptured ventricular aneurysm or dissecting hematoma of the aorta—the thrombotic process can overwhelm pericardial antithrombotic defenses, so that clotting makes it impossible for needle evacuation. Moreover, bleeding may be slowed by the tamponade pressure, so that *open surgical drainage and treatment of the bleeding source is safer and surer*.

The extent of the drainage procedure chosen is related to the adequacy of drainage, the need for tissue samples and the patient's prognosis. In the latter respect, patients with advanced malignancy may require only palliation (e.g., by dependent tube drainage or by balloon or surgical pleuropericardial window; page 309). The choice must be individualized, but a *pericardiostomy* with suction drainage for at least 3 or 4 days appears to be optimal. Drainage should be as complete and prolonged as necessary, whether by catheter, tube or window, into a neighboring cavity. *Preventing recurrence* is important in disorders prone to reaccumulation. Treatment of underlying disease processes with specific agents may suppress reaccumulation. However, some resistant processes like malignancies and stubborn infections may ultimately require pericardiectomy or suppression of effusion by obliteration of the pericardial cavity, using tetracycline, bleomycin (instilled with a local anesthetic) or other agents (page 309). In some patients prolonged tube drainage stimulates obliterative adhesions.

Traditional percutaneous *needle paracentesis (pericardiocentesis)* is usually effective and relatively safe with fluids of at least 1 cm depth anteriorly by echocardiogram. Moreover, although imperfect, *echocardiographic guidance* has improved its safety. Pericardiocentesis is essentially blind and sometimes the needle may not be visualized, so that an injection of saline must be utilized to locate it. *Fluoroscopic* and even *computed tomographic* monitoring are also feasible. [*Electrocardiographic monitoring* via the needle, long advocated, impairs the sense of touch, and the needle or catheter can contact or enter any cardiac chamber even before registration on the electrocardiogram (Figure 11.13).] The main danger is not cavity puncture, except the unusual puncture of a vital structure; it is *laceration* either of the right heart chambers or a coronary vein, resulting in brisk bleeding and frequent clotting, further decompensating tamponade and a high risk of death. Whenever a needle must be used, *a catheter should be placed via the needle or over a J-tipped wire as soon as possible*; after maximum complete drainage, it should be left in place as long as further drainage proceeds; aseptic conditions are maintained along with a heparin lock and frequent flushing. Contraindications to thoracotomy—like pleuropulmonary diseases, which make intolerable even temporary compromise of lung tissue, or extensive pleural adhesions—may necessitate prolonged tube drainage or even a *pericardioperitoneal shunt* via special equipment (Table 10.6).

Pericardiocentesis can be initiated from almost any reasonable place on the precordium over the distended pericardium except over the internal mammary arteries, 2.5 cm on each side of the sternum. Apical and especially subxiphoid approaches are preferred. A *balloon-equipped catheter* may be used through the subxiphoid approach to produce a large opening in the pericardium for drainage into the peritoneum or pleura.

SURGICAL DRAINAGE; ANESTHETIC IMPORTANCE

Modern cardiothoracic surgery, including thoracoscopic drainage, has greatly reduced the justification for needle pericardiocentesis. The *subxiphoid surgical incision* or *thoracoscopic drainage* produce little morbidity and can be done in emergencies with only local anesthesia. They permit direct inspection, biopsy

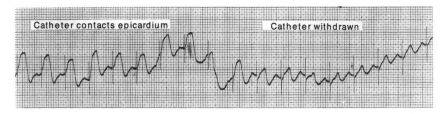

Figure 11.13 An ECG monitor attached to needle during drainage of tamponading pericardial effusion. Epicardial contact by catheter causes J (ST) segment elevation.

of both visceral and parietal pericardium, and resection. When extensive pericardial resection is an option, perhaps the optimal technique is *video-assisted thoracoscopy*, which gives the operator a wide field of view (although a lung must be collapsed, depending on which side this is approached from—usually the left). Through the thoracoscope, much pericardial tissue can be removed if necessary, permitting both extensive inspection and generous biopsies, always taking care to preserve the phrenic nerves.

Open Operation

Other chest conditions or failure of thoracoscopic drainage may mandate an open surgical approach through a sternum-splitting or anterolateral chest incision. However, the strong desirability of surgical over needle drainage may impose a "catch 22." In the operating room, attempts must be made to *drain the pericardium under local anesthesia before induction of general anesthesia.* This is because most general anesthetics tend to worsen tamponade by provoking tachycardias and bradycardias, including junctional rhythms, and hypotension, especially during induction, that will further reduce cardiac output. However, if clotting or other factors defeat attempts to initially reduce tamponade, operative treatment must proceed. Ketamine is currently a preferred anesthetic because its sympathomimetic effects augment myocardial performance.

EFFECTS OF PERICARDIAL DRAINAGE

As pericardial fluid is withdrawn, hemodynamic or echo-Doppler monitoring should be maintained. *Postpericardicentesis cardiac pressure and volume changes reflect the presence and degree of cardiac compression and are not predictable from the amount of fluid removed.* However, because critically tamponaded hearts operate on the steep portion of the pericardial pressure-volume curve (Figure 3.1), *the initial fluid decrement will produce the greatest improvement in stroke volume.* Drainage in severe tamponade may eliminate pulsus paradoxus, but the Doppler may still show respiratory fluctuation of aortic and pulmonary flows resembling low-pressure tamponade.

   In general, after drainage, right ventricular (RV) volume increases more than left because the more compliant RV is more compressed. Indeed, the RV occasionally dilates after pericardiocentesis, and echocardiography shows abnormal ventricular septal motion characteristic of RV volume overload. Especially if there is *myocardial disease*, RV dilation may initiate congestive failure, as may left ventricular dilation with occasional pulmonary edema (*"pericardial shock"*). (Although pulmonary artery pressure usually falls after drainage, it may rise with a temporary mismatch of ventricular outputs.) Such acute right, and particularly left, heart failure occurs with ventricles unable to accommodate posttamponade increase in venous return exacerbated by continuing high afterload due to increased peripheral resistance induced by compensatory adrenergic responses during tamponade (page 187). Occational patients

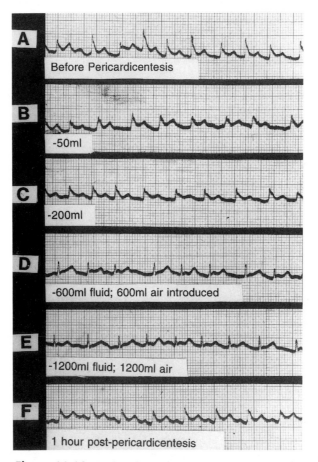

Figure 11.14 Pericardial drainage in cardiac tamponade: prompt resolution of electric alternation. Unusual case: 64-year-old man with strict 2:1 electric alternation despite atrial fibrillation. (A): baseline trace. (B): with removal of 50 mL (out of a total of 1200 mL), alternation disappears. (C): essentially the same after 200 mL. (D): after 600 mL fluid and introduction of 600 mL air (see Figure 11.15); slurred R-ST disappears (E); essentially the same after 1200 mL fluid removed and a total of 1200 mL air introduced; (F) 1 hr after drainage, patient is in sinus rhythm but RST slurring has returned.

develop transient systolic dysfunction after drainage of large effusions, possibly due to myocardial "disuse atrophy" analogous to the effects of chronic constriction.

On average, RV and LV ejection fractions do not change significantly after pericardial drainage. Hemodynamic improvement, and consequently clinical improvement, is related to increased stroke volume. This can be small, with drainage of even large but slowly developing effusions, since pericardial stretch modulates the degree of cardiac chamber compression by maintaining a gentle or relatively flat pericardial pressure-volume (P-V) curve. In contrast, drainage of even small aliquots of rapidly developing effusions can significantly relieve cardiac compression with significantly increased chamber volumes and consequently increased stroke volume.

Effective drainage is characterized by (1) disappearance of pulsus paradoxus, (2) frequent relief of dyspnea, (3) disappearance of signs of venous engorgement paralleling falling right atrial pressure, (4) reappearance of *y* descents, (5) loss of vena cava plethora, (6) loss of diastolic pressure equilibration and (7) prompt loss of electric alternation (Figures 11.14 and 11.15). A pericardial catheter (rarely necessary) documents normalization of pericar-

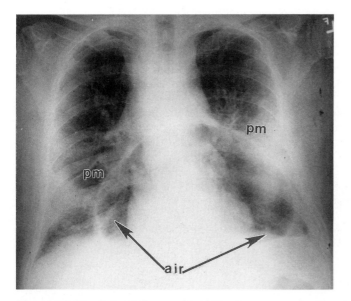

Figure 11.15 Induced (iatrogenic) 1200 mL pneumopericardium in patient in Figure 11.14. Air floats on residual fluid, outlines pericardium and reveals lung lesions (neoplastic and inflammatory). *Pm* = pericardium.

dial pressure. Exceptional patients improve their cardiac index (probably due to increased transmural pressure) while maintaining a high LV end-diastolic pressure in spite of reduced pericardial and right atrial pressures.

If atrial pressure shows an enlarged y descent, especially if with a third heart sound, epicardial constriction (effusive-constrictive pericarditis) should be suspected.

KEY POINTS

1. Cardiac tamponade is a broad pathophysiologic continuum from the clinically insignificant respiratory effects of almost any pericardial effusion to the symptomatically florid, life-threatening state of critical cardiac compression.
2. Symptoms of tamponade are nonspecific, ranging from weakness or faintness to breathlessness or tachypnea. Any symptoms of acute pericarditis or systemic disease may accompany or dominate the picture.
3. The picture of hemodynamically critical tamponade is one combining shock, usually with venous distention, absence of pulmonary edema and frequent pulsus paradoxus.
4. State of hydration can be a key factor in the rate of hemodynamic and clinical progression of tamponade. In hypovolemia, compensation breaks down earlier than in normovolemia. Hypervolemia contributes to later decompensation. Hypovolemic individuals account for most cases of low-pressure tamponade and for many cases improved by intravenous fluids.
5. Catheterization typically shows equilibration of central circulatory diastolic pressures.
6. Electric alternation of the QRS is a strong sign of tamponade in the presence of clinical signs and symptoms; P-QRS-T ("total") alternation is virtually pathognomonic. Electro-mechanical dissociation typifies end-stage, especially hemorrhagic, tamponade.
7. Echo-Doppler signs of tamponade of varying sensitivity and specificity include diastolic chamber collapses, especially of the right atrium and/or ventricle, and exaggerated reciprocal left-right respiratory variations in transvalvular flows, with plethora and less than 50% inspiratory collapse of the inferior vena cava. Inspiratory shift of the ventricular septum into the left ventricle is typical.
8. Variant forms of tamponade, often diagnostically confusing, include low-pressure, hypertensive and regional cardiac tamponade as well as effusive-constrictive pericarditis.
9. Definitive treatment is pericardial drainage. Medical therapy at best temporizes and at worst is ineffective.

BIBLIOGRAPHY

Cogswell, T.L., Bernath, G.A., Keelan, M.H., et al. Laboratory Investigation — cardiac tamponade: The shift in the relationship between intrapericardial fluid pressure and volume induced by acute left ventricular pressure overload during cardiac tamponade. Circulation 1986; 74:173–180.

Cooper, J.P., Oliver, R.M., Currie, P., et al. How do the clinical findings in patients with pericardial effusions influence the success of aspiration? Br.Heart J. 1995; 73:351–354.

Fowler, N.O. Cardiac tamponade. In: Fowler, N.O. (ed.). The Pericardium in Health and Disease. Mount Kisco, New York: Futura, 1985, pp. 247–280.

Friedman, H.S., Gomes, J.A., Tardio, A.R., Haft, J.I.: The electro-cardiographic features of acute cardiac tamponade. Circulation 1974; 50:260–265.

Karatay, C.M., Fruehan, C.T., Lighty, G.W., et al. Acute pericardial distension in pigs: Effect of fluid conductance on body surface electrocardiogram QRS size. Cardiovasc. Res. 1993; 27:1033–1038.

Plotnick, G.D., Rubin, D.C., Feliciano, Z., Ziskind, A.A. Pulmonary hypertension decreases the predictive accuracy of echocardiographic clues for cardiac tamponade. Chest 1995, 107:919–924.

Shenoy, M.M., Dhar, S., Gittin, R., et al. Pulmonary edema following pericardiotomy for cardiac tamponade. Chest 1984; 86:647–648.

Spodick, D.H. Cardiac tamponade: A physiologic approach to diagnosis and treatment. J. Cardiovasc. Med. 1983; 8:1085–1097. 1983.

Spodick, D.H. The technique of pericardiocentesis. J. Crit. Illness 1987; 2:91–96.

Spodick, D.H. Critical care of pericardial disease. In: Rippe, J.M., Irwin, R.S., Alpert, J.S., Fink, M.P. (eds.). Intensive Care Medicine, 2d ed. Boston: Little, Brown, 1991, pp. 282–295.

Venkatesh, G., Tomlinson, C.W., O'Sullivan, T. McKelvie, R.S. Right ventricular diastolic collapse without hemodynamic compromise in a patient with large, bilateral pleural effusions. J. Am. Soc. Echocardiogr. 1995; 8:551–553.

Hurrell DG, Symanski JD Chaliki HP, Klarick KW, Pascoe RD, Nishimura RD. Assessment of right atrial pressure by hepatioc vein doppler echocardiography. J Am Coll Cardiol 1996; 27:212A.

12

Physiology of Cardiac Tamponade

INTERACTION BETWEEN THE PERICARDIUM AND ITS CONTENTS

To compress the heart significantly, the pericardial contents must (1) fill the pericardial reserve volume (Figure 3.1), (2) increase thereafter at a rate exceeding the rate of stretch of the parietal pericardium, and (3) exceed the rate at which venous blood volume expands to support the small normal pressure gradient for filling the right heart. Pericardial volume increases at the expense of cardiac chamber volume (unless the pericardial contents increase very slowly), ultimately equalizing reduced diastolic compliance in all chambers. The key operational defect is *restriction of cardiac inflows due to compression of all cardiac chambers.*

Interaction between the rate of fluid accumulation and parietal pericardial stretch determines pericardial stiffness and consequently the character (shape) of the pericardial pressure-volume (P-V) curve (Figure 3.1). Thus, *pericardial stiffness determines fluid increments causing tamponade.* Patients with critical tamponade function on the steep portion of the pericardial P-V curve, so that small fluid increments provoke large pressure increments (Figure 12.1, left). In contrast, with slow fluid accumulation and a yielding pericardium, the initial portion of the P-V curve remains "flat" longer than with rapid effusions, so that relatively large fluid volume increases cause relatively little pressure rise (Figure 12.1, right).

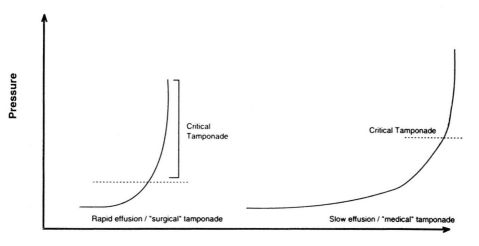

Figure 12.1 Cardiac tamponade: schema of pericardial pressure-volume curves (volume increases over time). Left: rapidly increasing pericardial fluid first fills the pericardial reserve volume (initial flat segment) then rises steeply to exceed the limit of parietal pericardial stretch, causing even steeper rise as smaller fluid increments disproportionately increase the pericardial pressure. Right: slower rate of pericardial filling takes longer to exceed pericardial stretch limit because of time available for "give."

Clinically, cardiac tamponade is defined as the decompensated phase of cardiac compression resulting from increased intrapercardial pressure. *Physiologically, tamponade is a continuum*, since even small increases in pericardial contents couple the pericardium to the heart, producing *significantly increased ventricular interaction with exaggeration of the normal reciprocal respiratory effects on the right and left heart*. These small increases need not be clinically significant. However, rising pericardial contents—serous effusions, blood, pus, gas and combinations of them—if unchecked by compensatory mechanisms, ultimately produce *critical cardiac compression*: severe cardiac tamponade. Fundamentally this depends on two *time-dependent pericardial factors*: the rate of pericardial fluid accumulation and the ability of the parietal pericardium to stretch. Their exact effect on intrapericardial pressure depends on the extent to which cardiac volume is maintained. If cardiac volume is reduced the pericardial pressure rise is less.

CARDIAC TAMPONADE: A PATHOPHYSIOLOGIC CONTINUUM (FIGURE 12.2; TABLE 12.1)

Rate of Fluid Accumulation

A cardiac wound, intrapericardial rupture of a dissecting aortic hematoma, or other such hemorrhagic catastrophe produces rapid tamponade ("surgical tamponade"; Figure 12.1, left) in minutes to hours, whereas a low-intensity inflammatory process may require days to weeks to critically compress the heart ("medical tamponade"; Figure 12.1, right). Apart from frank hemorrhage, the precise rate of accumulation is unpredictable but always prone to cause more or less sudden breakdown of compensation.

Pericardial Stretch

The other basic pericardial factor, capacity to stretch, is determined by rate of increase of its contents and two pericardial "springs": (1) wavy collagen, which tends to be smoothed by the burgeoning pericardial contents, and (2) elastic tissue (pages 9–11). Rapid accumulation of pericardial contents quickly exhausts these and the limit of stretch is quickly attained due to the pericardium's J-shaped P-V curve (Figures 3.1 and 12.1). The ensuing phase, *decompensated tamponade* tends to be a "last straw" (last drop) phenomenon, the last bit of fluid putting the pericardium, and consequently the cardiac chambers, on the steep portion of their P-V curves. Cardiac filling is resisted by compression of

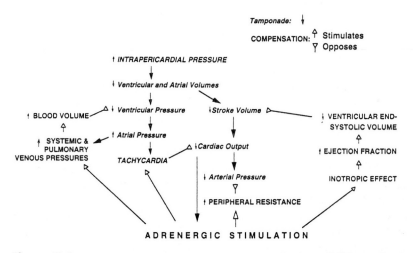

Figure 12.2 Cardiac tamponade and compensatory mechanisms. Solid arrowheads and italic print = tamponade. Open arrowheads and block letters = compensation; pointed open arrowheads = stimulatory compensatory mechanisms; blunted open arrowheads = opposing compensatory mechanisms.

Table 12.1 Cardiac Tamponade: Hemodynamic Progression

Phase	Pericardial pressure		Effects of pericardial drainage				
	vs. right ventricular diastolic pressure	vs. left atrial/pulmonary wedge pressure	Pericardial pressure	right atrial pressure	Inspiratory blood pressure fall	Cardiac output	Left atrial/pulmonary wedge pressure
I	Equal	Less	Reduced	Reduced	Variable	None	Variable
II	Equal	Less	Reduced	Reduced	Reduced	Increased	Variable
III	Equal	Equal	Reduced	Reduced	Usually Normal	Increased	Reduced

Source: Adapted from investigations by P. S. Reddy and colleagues.

all heart chambers, a form of diastolic dysfunction where, at any diastolic volume, there is necessarily excessive intracardiac pressure. The "last straw" phenomenon is mirrored by the reciprocal effect of draining pericardial fluid: *the first decrement produces the largest relative hemodynamic improvement* by shifting the stretched pericardium back toward the "flat" portion of its P-V curve, consequently tending to normalize myocardial P-V relations.

Although the key chambers in maintaining cardiac output are the ventricles, the earliest point of attack is on the right atrium and ventricle. These thinner chambers' pressures equilibrate with rising pericardial pressure before the left atrial and ventricular pressures do. (Interestingly, regional anatomic pericardial configurations normally change reciprocally with P-V changes in the subjacent right atrium and ventricle, but they vary synchronously with them during tamponade.) Table 12.1 shows the hemodynamic progression.

Normal right atrial and ventricular pressures are somewhat lower than in the corresponding left chambers, and the right ventricular wall is much thinner than the left. Thus, *in tamponade*, rising pericardial pressure due to increasing pericardial contents imposes a parallel rise in diastolic pressures, first in the right heart and later in the left heart. *Intrapericardial pressure* is normally lower than right atrial pressure, so that *right atrial transmural pressure* (right atrial pressure minus pericardial pressure) is normally higher than its cavitary pressure. In contrast, during tamponade, rising pericardial pressure progressively reduces—and ultimately makes phasically negative—the transmural pressure of the right, followed by the left, cardiac chambers. Like most tamponade-induced abnormalities, these are reciprocally exacerbated during expiration and inspiration (Chapters 10 and 12).

Cardiac filling is maintained by a parallel *rise in systemic and pulmonary venous pressures*; i.e., the venous beds must generate enough pressure to keep both sides of the heart filled—a pressure primarily determined by pericardial rather than myocardial compliance. While the rate of pericardial filling is one key factor affecting the ability to tolerate or resist cardiac tamponade, another is the *rate of venous volume expansion*. This occurs by fluid transfer from the tissues and the arterial side to the venous side of the cardiovascular system, which requires time and is inoperative in very rapid ("surgical") tamponade. Finally, *diastolic suction* may augment filling at very low ventricular volumes.

As this form of diastolic dysfunction proceeds, *pericardial pressure first equilibrates with right ventricular diastolic pressure* because of the factors mentioned: thinner myocardium and lower right heart pressures but also pericardial stiffness that is inherently greater than right but not left ventricular stiffness (Table 12.1). Concomitantly, despite multiple *compensatory mechanisms* (Figure 12.2), cardiac filling progressively decreases. Sooner or later, pericardial pressure equilibrates with left ventricular diastolic pressure and cardiac output decreases critically. Eventually, diastolic pressures in both ventricles and the pulmonary artery all equilibrate with mean right and left atrial pressures at approximately intrapericardial pressure—the characteristic hemodynamics of "pure" cardiac tamponade. (*"Equilibrate"* means diastolic pressures measure within a few millimeters of each other—conventionally 5 mm Hg or less.) Even the left ventricle ultimately equilibrates owing to drastic reduction in volume (Figure 10.9) such that its transmural pressure is very low.

During inspiration, left heart pressure differences are least or nil and commonly reversed; circulation is assisted by reciprocal flow changes in inspiration and expiration. During *pulsus paradoxus* (Chapter 13; Figures 11.2 and 13.2), the breathing phases have comparable but exaggerated differential effects; with inspiration, pulmonary wedge pressure falls below pericardial pressure. In contrast, right atrial pressure also falls, but not below pericardial pressure, enhancing inspiratory filling of the right ventricle.

The true "filling" (distending) cardiac pressures are the *myocardial transmural pressures*, i.e., cavitary pressures minus the normally nearly zero intrapericardial pressure. (Put differently, cavitary pressures are always the sum of transmural and pericardial pressures.) In severe tamponade, transmural cardiac pressures are drastically reduced, so that cardiac filling is drasticallly reduced. In fact, transient reversal of the transmural pressure gradient causes *right ventricular collapse early in diastole* (especially the RV outflow tract), and *right*, and sometimes left, *atrial collapse in late diastole* (Figures 11.7 through 11.9). That the RV inflow tract can continue to fill while the outflow tract collapses suggests a possible element of *diastolic suction* in the right heart. The thick left ventricle does not collapse unless there is either loculated high-pressure fluid on its free border or considerable right ventricular hypertrophy. The onset of chamber collapses coincides with a 20 to 25% decrease in cardiac output, while compensatory mechanisms still tend to maintain arterial pressures, mainly due to increased peripheral resistance (see below and Figure 12.2). Indeed, at least in euvolemic and hypervolemic patients, *right ventricular diastolic collapse tends to occur earlier than pulsus paradoxus.*

In tamponade, blood mainly enters the heart when blood is leaving it; pericardial volume and pressure vary continuously during the cardiac cycle, reflecting the variations in cardiac chamber volumes, although the high-pressure pericardial fluid compresses the heart throughout diastole. In *early diastole* the *peak filling rate* of the ventricles becomes radically reduced along with the *filling fraction*, emphasizing the importance of the atrial contributions. By *end-diastole or earlier, the ventricles are filled* and therefore maximally expanded within the pericardial sac, raising intrapericardial pressure to its maximum. Although atrial expansion due to filling would also tend to raise pericardial pressure at *end-systole*, ventricular ejection (emptying) is then complete, so that the ventricles are at minimal volume, permitting intrapericardial pressure to fall. Within these complex dynamics, the ventricles remain underfilled and therefore operate at the low end of their Frank-Starling curves while ejecting reduced stroke volumes. *Complexity of cardiac chamber responses is implicit in their simultaneous variations with the respiratory cycle as well as the cardiac cycle.* For example, right and left ventricular filling are reciprocal during inspiration and expiration and close to 180° out of phase with each other. Their outputs may not be; maximal flow and pressure in the pulmonary artery can precede minimal aortic flow and pressure by one to three beats. Atrial filling also varies with respiratory phase in severe tamponade.

Ventricular filling may occur only during differential pressure fluctuations. When the ventricles contract to eject blood, the pericardial "space" is increased and the atrial "floors" are pulled downward. Pericardial pressure falls somewhat, enhancing the atrial filling, since atrial cavitary pressure falls at the same time, producing the *x* descent in atrial pressure curves.

High pericardial pressure levels throughout the cardiac cycle prevent rapid ventricular filling in early diastole; there is no rush of blood through the atrioventricular (A-V) valves. Moreover, the A-V valves tend to close early. These key factors in tamponade progressively amputate the *y* descent of the atrial and venous pressure curves (Figure 11.1), reflecting curtailed and ultimately absent rapid ventricular filling (with a comparable effect on the Doppler E wave). Moreover, atrial reservoir function has increased importance: *in severe tamponade, the left atrium may fill only during expiration and the ventricles may fill only during atrial systole*, the mitral and tricuspid valves otherwise remaining closed. Decreased filling due to premature A-V valve closure exacerbates the reduced ventricular preload (shorter fiber length), further contributing to lower stroke volume and decreased ventricular ejection rate. Ultimately, the aortic valve opens only during expiration. During inspiration, leftward septal shift (Figure 13.6) may further reduce left ventricular chamber compliance and obstruct left ventricular filling. Correspondingly, the ventricular pressure curves show an immediate, shallow (relatively flat to invisible) diastolic rise from a slight lowering just after A-V valve opening, rising to the high diastolic levels seen with pressure equilibration—typically between 15 and 30 mm Hg in euvolemic patients.

With normal coronary arteries, *coronary blood flow is reduced, but remains adequate to support aerobic metabolism* because there is proportionate reduction in cardiac work—the ventricles are underloaded. Even coronary vasodilator reserve, capacitance and resistance are not significantly impaired. (Renal blood flow during tamponade is reduced, though partly supported by auto-regulation.)

Despite decreased cardiac output, *arterial blood pressure* is maintained until relatively late in slowly developing tamponade, partly by *alpha* adrenergic mechanisms (page 182), but thereafter it may decline precipitously due to fur-ther drops in stroke volume and cardiac output. Thus, tamponade is a form of severe diastolic dysfunction; in otherwise normal hearts, gross systolic function remains intact.

The *myocardium* itself is also important, so that previously diseased or injured hearts may not maintain circulatory pressure as well as normal hearts. Good myocardial function permits the ventricles to increase the amount of blood ejected per beat by an increased ejection fraction. With poor myocardial func-tion, hemodynamic decompensation occurs earlier.

COMPENSATORY RESPONSES; DECOMPENSATED TAMPONADE

Compensatory mechanisms for tamponade (Figure 12.2) include time-dependent pericardial stretch and blood volume expansion accompanied by tachycardia, increased ejection fraction, and peripheral vasoconstriction due to intense adr-energic stimulation stimulated by falling cardiac output. Rising pressure in the right atrium induces *tachycardia* to defend the minute cardiac output in the face of falling stroke volume. A neurogenic antinatriuresis reflexly increases renal *sodium and fluid retention* which, teleologically, defends cardiac filling by in-creasing blood volume and venous pressure. Concomitant *adrenergic stimula-tion*, including increased serum catecholamines, has four main effects: (1) al-pha-adrenergically *increased peripheral resistance* to maintain central blood pressure and support the gradient for coronary flow, (2) a beta-adrenergic contribution to *heart rate increase*, (3) beta-adrenergic–dependent *augmenta-tion of diastolic relaxation*, and (4) *increased inotropy* to minimize ventricu-lar end-systolic volume and improve ejection fraction, which is normal to high in tamponade.

In *decompensated tamponade*, the eventual drop in blood pressure is in-fluenced by an *opioid-dependent mechanism*—demonstrated by naloxone-induced blood pressure increase during tamponade without increasing cardiac output—a mechanism responsible for a large additional increase in systemic vascular resistance. (Additional evidence that systolic function does not limit cardiac output in tamponade.) On the other hand, while the increased peripheral vas-cular resistance is not affected by *beta* blockade, it is decreased by *alpha* block-ade, which can decompensate tamponade.

Due to arterial and atrial baroreceptor unloading, blood pressure is augmented by *neurohormonal activation*, including a limited late contribution by the *renin-angiotensin-aldosterone system*, via renin, angiotensin II, arginine vasopressin and aldosterone, with decreased urine flow and renal sodium and potassium excretion. These appear during decompensated tamponade after mean blood pressure decreases by about 30% and are followed by increased production of adrenocorticotropic hormone (ACTH). Unlike cardiac failure at comparable central pressures, atrial natriuretic factor (ANF) does *not* increase because tamponade prevents myocardial stretch. Thus tamponade prevents this mechanism for increasing renal sodium elimination.

Cardiac tamponade can produce a profound *arterial respiratory alkalosis*, even early on, with the cardiac output still maintained at 60 to 80% of normal and blood pressure still intact. In contrast, mixed *venous* (pulmonary artery) blood pH, Pco_2 and serum bicarbonate are relatively unchanged. With increasing tamponade, as the cardiac output falls critically, there is an increasing difference between arterial and mixed venous Pco_2.

ATYPICAL FORMS OF CARDIAC TAMPONADE: LOW PRESSURE; OCCULT; RIGHT-SIDED; HYPERTENSIVE

Hypovolemia attenuates compensatory increase in venous blood volume and pressure, permitting cardiac output to fall at lower ventricular pressures. In volume-depleted patients, *low pressure tamponade* may occur at mean atrial and diastolic pressures as low as 6 mm Hg, with few symptoms at rest, and with or without significant systemic hypotension. Despite this, both right ventricular diastolic collapse and pulsus paradoxus may be present. Pulse contours tend to be abnormal, although it may be necessary to expand blood volume by administering saline intravenously to produce diagnostic pulse morphology (*occult cardiac tamponade*). In these patients, pericardial pressure has equilibrated with right, and often left, ventricular diastolic pressure without a detectable compensatory increase in venous pressure. *Right-sided cardiac tamponade*, with right-sided diastolic pressures exceeding left, can occur when the left ventricular compliance is very low (e.g., left ventricular hypertrophy or fibrosis), or more commonly when, usually after cardiac surgery, fluid is loculated over the right side of the heart (page 389). Of course, early classic tamponade begins as right-sided tamponade (pages 183–184). In *hypertensive tamponade*, patients with significantly low cardiac output due to tamponade maintain an unusually high (i.e., normal to even hypertensive) systolic arterial pressure, probably due to excessive adrenergic drive. Individuals with preexisting hypertension are frequent in this group, and for these patients, even "normal" blood pressures may be low.

KEY POINTS

1. Cardiac tamponade, a pathophysiologic continuum, progresses at a rate determined by interactions among the rates of pericardial filling and stretch and a variety of compensatory responses.
2. The tamponade, pericardial and cardiac pressure and flow changes vary phasically with both the cardiac and respiratory cycles. This is made even more complex by right heart–left heart reciprocation during inspiration and expiration.
3. With progressive tamponade, rising intrapericardial pressure equilibrates with right heart diastolic pressures before equilibrating with left heart pressures and ultimately converts myocardial transmural pressures from slightly positive to phasically negative, significantly diminishing cardiac filling.
4. In severe tamponade, rapid early ventricular filling is abolished, along with the atrial y descents. Filling depends partly on reciprocal respiratory effects, inspiration favoring the right and expiration the left heart. Ultimately, A-V valves may be opened mainly by atrial systole.
5. Complex, time-dependent compensatory mechanisms respond to the physiologic handicaps of tamponade. These include tachycardia, blood volume expansion and adrenergic stimulation. An opioid-dependent mechanism associated with *alpha*-adrenergic activation ultimately supports blood pressure via increased systemic vascular resistance. Neurohormonal responses include activation of the renin-angiotensin-aldosterone system. Atrial natriuretic factor does not increase.

BIBLIOGRAPHY

Boltwood, C.M. Ventricular performance related to transmural filling pressure in clinical cardiac tamponade. Circulation 1987; 75:941.

Brown, J., MacKinnon, D., King, A., Vanderbush, E. Elevated arterial blood pressure in cardiac tamponade. N. Engl. J. Med. 1992; 327:463–466.

Cogswell, T.L., Bernath, G.A., Raff, H., et al. Total peripheral resistance during cardiac tamponade: Adrenergic and angiotensin roles. Am. J. Physiol. 1986; 251:R916–R922.

Fowler, N.O. Physiology of cardiac tamponade and pulsus paradoxus: II. Physiological, circulatory, and pharmacological responses in cardiac tamponade. Mod. Concepts Cardiovasc. Dis. 1978; 47:115–118.

Hynynen, M., Salmenpera, M., Harjula, A.L.J., et al. Atrial pressure and hormonal renal responses to acute cardiac tamponade. Ann. Thorac. Surg. 1990; 49:632–637.

Lader, A.S., Mihailescu, L.S., Abel, F.L. Effect of pericardial pressure on determinants of coronary flow. FASEB J. 1993; 7:A319.

Reddy, P.S., Curtiss, E.I., O'Toole, J.D., Shaver, J.A. Cardiac tamponade: Hemodynamic observations in man. Circulation 1978; 58:265–272.

Shabetai, R. Pericardial and cardiac pressure. Circulation 1988; 77:1–5.

Spodick, D.H. Low atrial natriuretic factor levels and absent pulmonary edema in pericardial compression of the heart. Am. J. Cardiol. 1989; 63:1271–1272.

Spodick, D.H. The normal and diseased pericardium: Current concepts of pericardial physiology, diagnosis and treatment. J. Am. Coll. Cardiol. 1983; 1:240–251.

Spodick, D.H. Threshold of pericardial constraint: The pericardial reserve volume and auxiliary pericardial functions. J. Am. Coll. Cardiol. 1985; 6:296–297.

13

Pulsus Paradoxus

CHARACTERIZATION

Normal breathing causes cyclic cardiocirculatory changes alternately favoring left heart and right heart filling and ventricular performance (stroke volume, for example), with corresponding aortic and pulmonary artery pressures and flows. Pulsus paradoxus, as Kussmaul described it, was a change in a pulse (*pulsus*), not a pressure. Indeed, he had no blood pressure cuff or catheter, and it *was* "paradoxic" to him, since the radial pulse disappeared intermittently (during inspiration) while the heart continued to beat without interruption. Pulsus paradoxus is an exaggeration of the normal phenomenon of an inspiratory fall in systolic arterial pressure (Figure 13.1). Arbitrarily, "normal" means up to 10 mm Hg; usually it is much less. "Pulsus," a fall of over 10 mm Hg, is thus not paradoxic, and it is *characteristic of uncomplicated cardiac tamponade*. A small pulsus (< 15 mm Hg) occurs occasionally in constrictive pericarditis (pages 228–229), in which it may be unexplained, but it is often due to residual pericardial fluid or accompanying pulmonary disease. Indeed, *transmission of pleural pressure variations* to the cardiac chambers via the pericardium explains pulsus paradoxus in tamponade, while their *insulation from transmission by constrictive scar* tends to prevent pulsus. Moreover, although inspiration increases right ventricular filling *velocity* in constriction, any filling *volume* increase is minimal. Since *increased inspiratory right ventricular filling volume is indis-*

(See also Chapters 12 and 15)

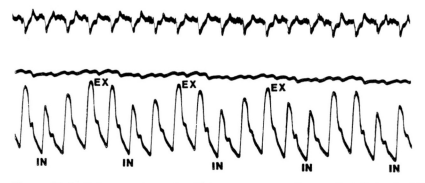

Figure 13.1 Pulsus paradoxus: brachial artery pressure. From a diastolic level of 72 mm Hg, systolic pressure fluctuates between a peak expiratory (EX) 114 mm Hg and a minimum inspiratory (IN) 96 mm Hg. "Size" of the pulsus is thereafter 18 mm Hg (114 to 96 mm Hg), which is 43% of the maximum expiratory pulse pressure (42 mm Hg).

pensable for pulsus (page 186), it should not occur with a pure, generalized constricting pericardium, unless with radical septal shifts..

Although usually elicited by blood pressure cuff, pulsus paradoxus is more sensitively found by catheter in some patients in early tamponade, when pericardial pressures are approaching equilibration with right heart pressure but not yet with left heart pressure (page 183) and in low-pressure tamponade (page 188). Many patients at these times have an exaggerated inspiratory fall in arterial pressure which is under 10 mm Hg—not quite conventionally "diagnostic." Moreover, the right heart is the crux of tamponade dynamics, and pulsus can occur in isolated right heart tamponade. This chapter primarily considers classic cardiac tamponade.

Along with increasing venous pressure, patients increasingly develop a full pulsus paradoxus as tamponade proceeds, with decreasing cardiac filling progressively decreasing cardiac output. Finally, *in florid tamponade, almost all patients develop pulsus paradoxus* when pericardial pressure equilibrates with left ventricular diastolic pressure and cardiac output falls critically. The amount of inspiratory systolic pressure decrease and its proportion of the maximum pulse pressure ("size" of pulsus; Figure 13.1) are broadly but imprecisely related to the hemodynamic severity of the tamponade.

PATHOPHYSIOLOGY (FIGURE 13.2)

The appearance of pulsus paradoxus usually signals both very large reductions in ventricular volumes and equilibration of mean pericardial pressure with all

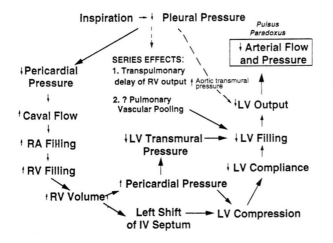

Figure 13.2   Physiology of pulsus paradoxus: complex sequential and simultaneous responses to inspiratory reduction of pleural pressure produce the inspiratory fall in arterial flow and pressure (see text).

cardiac diastolic pressures. Breathing now transiently causes this "razor's edge" equilibration pressure level to alternate: *expiration* favors left heart filling; *inspiration* decreases pericardial pressure and favors right heart filling. Indeed, pulsus occurs as inspiration depresses pulmonary venous pressure below systemic venous pressure so that pulmonary wedge and left atrial pressures fall below pericardial pressure, while right atrial pressure falls, but not below pericardial pressure. Inspiration may also transiently reverse pulmonary venous flow in severe tamponade and reduce left atrial volume. Indeed, inspiratory decrease in transmitral flow velocity significantly exceeds the normal decrease of $<15\%$.

While pulsus paradoxus is multifactorial and still incompletely understood, it clearly depends on *alternate reciprocal exaggeration of ventricular interaction by the respiratory cycle*. The "size" of the pulsus—the amount of inspiratory pressure fall—is *additionally related to the pattern and depth of breathing* and hence to the degree of pleural pressure fluctuation. Normally, intrapericardial and pleural pressures vary almost equally during breathing, but in tamponade, intrapericardial pressure during inspiration decreases somewhat less than pleural pressure; it increases as the right side of the heart fills, partly because the right heart expands into the pericardial fluid (Figure 13.2), thereby increasing its already high pressure. The increased pericardial pressure further compresses the left heart in inspiration, along with a sharp leftward shift of the ventricular septum (see below), tending to impede left ventricular filling (which is volumetrically decreased by reduced inflow from the compressed left atrium). The comparable *expiratory* decreases in right heart filling and cavitary pressures are dramatically seen on echocardiography: RA and RV diastolic collapses are maximal during expiration.

Directional respiratory changes in transmural pressures (Figure 13.2), flow and filling remain normal and approximately 180° out of phase, i.e., almost perfectly reciprocal for maximal changes (Figure 13.3). At the low chamber volumes of tamponade, *proportional* inspiratory pressure increases are very much greater than normal on the right; corresponding left-side inspiratory pressure decreases are relatively less than on the right, although much greater than normal (Figure 13.3). This is dramatically evident in the markedly fluctuating Doppler transvalvular and intravascular flow velocities during the respiratory cycle (Figures 13.4, 13.5, and 11.10C). Thus, because systemic venous return to the heart, and consequently cardiac output, are reduced in tamponade, inspiration accelerates systemic venous blood flow but augments the low right heart input more than normally only relative to left heart input. With the reciprocal changes in the left heart, this contributes to much greater than normal respiratory *variation* in the already low output of the ventricles. This is also reflected in the exaggerated fluctuation of the low ventricular ejection time, which reflects stroke volume (Figure 13.5).

A parallel effect due to inspiratory increase in right ventricular transmural pressure and filling is *displacement of the ventricular septum* into the underfilled left ventricle, enlarging the right ventricle at the expense of the left (Figure 13.6). The septal shift further impedes left ventricular filling (Figure 13.2),

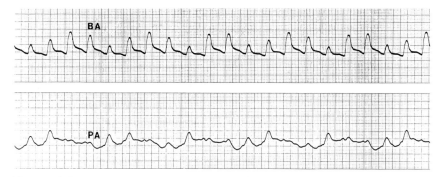

Figure 13.3 Pulsus paradoxus: brachial artery (BA) and pulmonary artery (PA) pressures 180° out of phase. Maximal BA pressures coincide with minimal PA pressures and vice versa. Changes are relatively much greater on PA, with little inspiratory systolic increase over the diastolic level. This reflects the proportionally much larger respiratory fluctuations in right ventricular performance.

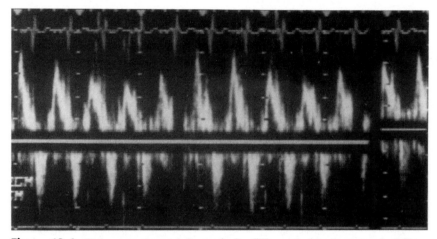

Figure 13.4 Pulsus paradoxus: left ventricular filling velocities by transmitral Doppler. Maximum (expiratory) flow velocity is almost 50% greater than minimum (inspiratory) flow velocity.

augmenting *inspiratory decrease in left ventricular transmural pressure* as well as reduced chamber compliance. This septal component of ventricular interaction becomes maximal when rising pericardial pressure finally equilibrates with left as well as right ventricular diastolic pressure. Left ventricular ejection is

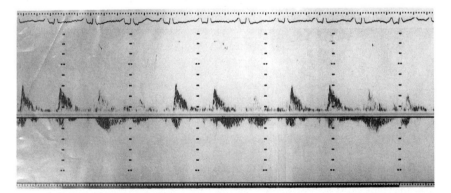

Figure 13.5 Pulsus paradoxus: Left ventricular ejection velocities by Doppler measurement in the ascending aorta. Marked respiratory fluctuation with peak (expiratory) flow velocity approximately 50% greater than minimum (inspiratory) flow velocity. Darker recording during inspiration suggests greater volume flow due to more "targets" (red blood cells) in the ejection volume. *Left ventricular ejection time* varies between approximately 210 msec and 160 msec, reflecting small stroke volume in expiration and very small stroke volume in inspiration. At a heart rate of 107 beats per minute, ejection time would be expected to be approximately 260 msec.

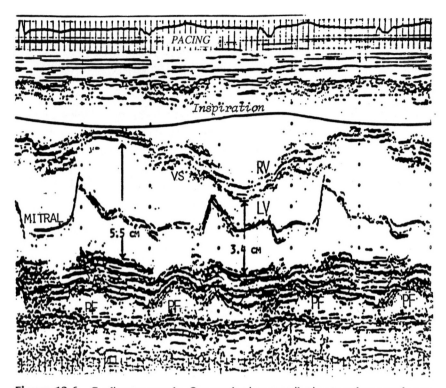

Figure 13.6 Cardiac tamponade. One mechanism contributing to pulsus paradoxus: with inspiration the ventricular septum (VS) plunges into the left ventricle (LV) enlarging the right ventricle (RV) at the expense of the left. In this example, LV diameter decreased by almost 40%: 5.5 cm maximum expiratory diameter to 3.4 cm minimum inspiratory diameter (these measurements will be different at papillary muscle level). The right ventricle measurement appears to fluctuate by approximately 100%. Although the patient was not specially positioned for right ventricular measurement, this is consistent with much greater respiratory fluctuations in the right heart.

also opposed by *inspiratory reduction of aortic transmural pressure*, causing the LV to contract against increased aortic impedance.

Finally, the left atrium is normally tightly clasped by the locally specialized parietal pericardium, often preventing penetration of fluid behind it. Thus, the left atrium sometimes continues to abut lung tissue and is variably subject to negative pulmonary inspiratory pressure. Moreover, with inspiration, pulmonary wedge, pulmonary vein and left atrial pressures fall below pericardial pressure and therefore below right atrial and systemic venous pressures, which do not fall below pericardial pressure. (This is the mechanism favoring inspiratory right-to-left shunting through an atrial septal defect or a patent foramen ovale during tamponade; page 169.) Consequently, in inspiration, some blood in the left ventricle may actually be "sucked" back toward the atrium and pulmonary veins contributing to transient reversal of pulmonary vein flow. All the foregoing factors combine to sharply decrease left ventricular filling in inspiration, while the left ventricle operates on a steeper-than-normal pressure-volume (P-V) curve because the pericardium is on the steep slope of its P-V curve (page 181). Thus, pulsus paradoxus, the exaggerated inspiratory decrease in systemic arterial flow and pressure, reflects a complex chain of events that reduce left ventricular stroke output in inspiration. Other factors may augment the respiratory differences:

1.   The *series effect of right ventricular activity*, which requires time—partly a function of heart rate—for the inspiratory increase in right ventricular output to cross the lungs and appear on the left, with the lungs acting to some degree as a capacitor, "pooling" the right ventricular output during inspiration. Two to four beats later, this further reduces the reduced left heart inflow by decreasing or even reversing the pulmonary artery, and ultimately the pulmonary vein, to left atrium gradient.

2.   However, *within one beat of the onset of inspiration, aortic flow and systolic pressure decrease*—immediately following inspiratory merging of pulmonary wedge and intrapericardial pressure. Thus, a large component of the change must be left-sided, *occurring before the series effect of inspiratory increase in right ventricular output can reach the left atrium*. This may also be a function of immediate transmission of negative inspiratory pleural pressure to the aorta and systemic arteries. This increases these vessels' own transmural pressures, which increases impedance to left ventricular ejection.

Pulsus paradoxus usually disappears with adequate pericardial drainage. In occasional patients with hyperpnea, pulsus may appear to persist despite relief of tamponade.

"NONPERICARDIAL" PULSUS PARADOXUS

Pulsus paradoxus occurs frequently in chronic obstructive airway disease and acute asthma but is distinguished by diastolic as well as systolic pressure fall. Pulsus occurs occasionally in hemorrhagic shock, tension pneumothorax, tracheal compression, right ventricular infarction (possibly due to pericardial constraint), severe pulmonary embolism, restrictive cardiomyopathy, and mediastinal and cardiac compression by tumors and other masses.

ABSENCE OF PULSUS PARADOXUS

Tamponade without pulsus paradoxus occurs under several circumstances.

1. The effect of respiration on right heart filling and the pulmonary vein–left atrial pressure gradient are essential for pulsus paradoxus. When left ventricular diastolic pressures and left ventricular stiffness significantly exceed those of the right ventricle (e..g, *marked left ventricular hypertrophy or severe left-sided heart failure*), pericardial pressure may effectively equilibrate only with right heart pressures, a form of right ventricular tamponade, with the much less compliant left ventricle resisting the phasically changing pericardial pressure. Here, respiratory changes cannot alternately favor both right- and left-sided filling. (Moreover, with left ventricular dysfunction, on echocardiography, cardiac chambers may collapse with hemodynamically insignificant effusions.)
2. *Severe aortic regurgitation*, even without severe left ventricular dysfunction, can produce sufficient regurgitant flow to damp respiratory fluctuations.
3. *Atrial septal defects*, with increased inspiratory venous return balanced by shunting to the left atrium.
4. *Extreme hypotension*, as in shock, and even severe tamponade, may make respiration-induced pressure changes unmeasurable.
5. *Acute left ventricular myocardial infarction* with tamponading effusion (occasionally) for uncertain reasons.
6. *Local* (usually postsurgical) *cardiac compression*.
7. *Pericardial adhesions*, especially over the right heart.

KEY POINTS

1. Pulsus paradoxus (PP), an exaggeration of the normal (<10 mm Hg) inspiratory drop in arterial pressure, is characteristic of manifest, uncomplicated cardiac tamponade but can precede the full hemodynamic picture. Volumes of the compressed, underfilled ventricles are significantly reduced so that respiratory changes, while absolutely small, are relatively far greater than normal.
2. The pathophysiology of PP is complex, multifactorial and only party understood, including differential intra- and extrapericardial respiratory effects, essentiality of right heart involvement, respirophasic exaggeration of the decreased myocardial transmural pressures due to tamponade, and phasic ventricular septal shifts.
3. With pulsus paradoxus, inspiration improves right heart hemodynamics at the expense of left, reversing on expiration. While changes of flow in the aorta reflect the series effect of those in the pulmonary artery after two to four beats, due to additional mechanisms, maximal reciprocal changes in filling occur almost simultaneously, i.e., about 180° out of phase.

BIBLIOGRAPHY

Curtiss, E.I., Reddy, P.S., Uretsky, B.F., Cecchetti, A.A. Pulsus paradoxus: Definition and relation to the severity of cardiac tamponade. Am. Heart J. 1988; 115:391–398.

Hoit, B.D., Ramrakhayan, K. Pulmonary venous flow in cardiac tamponade: Influence of left ventricular dysfunction and relation to pulsus paradoxus. J. Am. Soc. Echocardiog. 1991; 4:559–570.

Reddy, P.S., Curtiss, E.I., Uretsky, B.F. Spectrum of hemodynamic changes in tamponade. Am. J. Cardiol. 1990; 66:1487–1491.

Settle, H.P., Adolph, R.J., Fowler, N.O., et al. Echocardiographic study of cardiac tamponade. Circulation 1982; 66:887.

Shabetai, R., Grossman, W. Profiles in constrictive pericarditis, restrictive cardiomyopathy and cardiac tamponade. In: Grossman, W. (ed.). Cardiac Catheterization and Angiography, 2d ed. Philadelphia: Lea & Febiger, 1980, pp. 358–376.

Spodick, D. Pathophysiology of disorders of the pericardium. In: Levine, H.J. (ed.). Clinical Cardiovascular Physiology. New York: Grune & Stratton, 1976, pp. 621–634.

Spodick, D.H., Paladino, D., Flessas, A.P. Respiratory effects on systolic time intervals during pericardial effusion. Am. J. Cardiol. 1983; 51:1033.

Wayne, V.S., Bishop, R.L., Spodick, D.H. Dynamic effects of nontamponading pericardial effusion: Respiratory responses in the absence of pulsus paradoxus. Br. Heart J. 1984; 51:202–204.

14

Noneffusive Sequelae of Pericardial Inflammation: Pericardial Fibrin, Adhesions, Scarring, Calcification

PERICARDIAL ADHESIONS AND FIBROSIS (CICATRICIAL PERICARDITIS)

Structural Perspectives

Table 14.1 summarizes the noneffusive sequelae of pericardial inflammation.

Pericarditis often heals without detectable residua or with some degree of scarring of one or both pericardial layers. The plastic fibrinous exudate of acute and subacute pericarditis can be adhesive, but its fate is either fibrinolysis and reabsorption or organization with newly formed collagen fibrils, as a matrix for invasion by new blood and lymphatic vessels and later fibrous or fibrogranulomatous adhesion. A common denominator for the most intense scarring may be bleeding. Following drainage of bloody effusions, instillation of urokinase may eliminate this factor. Cicatrization is also probably intensified by local production of the interleukins and the tumor necrosis factors found in abnormal pericardial fluids.

Most pericardial scarring is usually clinically and physiologically unimportant—as, for example, following rheumatic pericarditis, many cases of infectious pericarditis and particularly rheumatoid arthritis, in which approximately 40 to 50 percent of patients are found at autopsy with incidental pericardial fibrosis and adhesions. Local thickenings are not rare on computed tomography in patients with healed myocardial infarctions, rheumatic heart disease, sar-

Table 14.1 Noneffusive Sequelae of Pericardial Inflammation

Cicatricial pericarditis: pericardial adhesions and fibrosis, constriction
Pericardial calcification, local and general
Inflammatory cysts (pseudocysts, loculated effusions)
Inflammatory diverticula
Granulomatous pericarditis
  Of unknown origin
  Due to systemic diseases
  Infectious
  Foreign-matter reactions

---

coidosis and other conditions. This contrasts with more destructive inflammation in severe infectious, especially tuberculous, pericarditis, which may heal without further consequences but frequently provokes constrictive scarring involving the heart, any portion of the heart or of the great vessels, producing illness by compressing or distorting structures it entraps. Such compressive syndromes arise from lesions that are primarily pericardial, differing from primarily myocardial lesions (rheumatic heart disease, myocardial infarction, etc.), which are often associated with conspicuous pericardial adhesions and fibrosis of little or no dynamic significance. Some pericardial adhesions may buttress a myocardial wound or infarct and, indeed, contribute mural and microvascular support. Some contain an otherwise fatal myocardial rupture (*pseudoaneurysms*; page 346).

Metabolic Activity in Healing Pericardium

Fibroblasts, other constituents of scarring, and granuloma cells are metabolically active. This property of fibrotic and granulomatous tissues and inflammatory cells requires further investigation for local, and perhaps systemic, effects favorable or pathophysiologic. These include high angiotensin II (AT2) receptor binding in pericardial fibrosis; marked angiotensin converting enzyme (ACE) binding at sites of high collagen turnover; ACE production by macrophages and AT2 by leukocytes. Tissue repair may involve regulation of local AT2 by macrophage and granuloma ACE. Indeed, ACE-inhibiting medications should limit pericardial fibrosis but as yet have no such clinical role.

Finally, inflamed pericardial mesothelium produces plasminogen activator inhibitors that check mesothelial plasminogen activating activity, impairing the normally strong serosal fibrinolytic activity (also directly impaired by tissue trauma; page 24), prolonging fibrin production and consequently the matrix for collagenization.

Clinical Considerations (Table 14.1)

Adhesions on the *external* surface of the parietal pericardium, even when combined with internal adhesions, may well be due to inflammatory disease of the mediastinum and pleura; they seem to be extremely rare in modern times. They have a potential effect on the appearance of the cardiac silhouette and may permit systolic tugging on adjacent organs as well as *exopericardial friction sounds* (Chapter 4), including *pleuropericardial rubs*, in patients who have had pleuritis and mediastinitis abutting the pericardium.

All forms of pericarditis can cause adhesions (Figure 14.1A and B) and fibrotic thickening (Figures 14.2 and 14.3A through C). *Blood and thrombi in the pericardial sac* (Figure 14.4), particularly blood lipids, especially when combined with pericardial injury and exudate, contribute to fibrosis and adhesions. However, even following cardiac surgery, apart from the occasional case of postsurgical constrictive pericarditis (much less common since irritating irrigations of the pericardium have been avoided), it is remarkable how rarely significant problems arise from pericardial healing. Thus, *pericardial adhesions are nearly always clinically silent*, although often easily detected by echocardiography (Figures 14.2 and 14.3).

Distortion by simple adhesions of the cardiopericardial silhouette on the chest x-ray is quite rare; any unusual configurations can be resolved by imaging methods like computed tomography (CT) and magnetic resonance imaging (MRI). In the past, it was thought that auscultatory clicks and electrocardiographic (ECG) voltage reduction were related to pericardial adhesions and fibrosis, but these appear to be related to pericardial compression or disease of the heart itself. However, dense pericardial scarring, like pericardial effusion, may abolish the ECG response to ingestion of a standard swallow of ice water—normally, orientation of the T vector away from the cooled area, best noted in leads II, III, aVF, V1 and V2.

PERICARDIAL CALCIFICATION

Calcification (rarely ossification), also known as *Panzerherz* or "armor heart," may be taken as "concrete evidence" of antecedent pericardial injury of greater destructiveness than conditions that result in healing without calcification. Although young children have developed pericardial calcification, the usual chronicity of the process makes it rare early in life. Neither its occurrence nor its extent directly correlates with abnormal cardiocirculatory function; even extensive calcification, often of almost the entire pericardium, can be well tolerated and asymptomatic even with widespread chronic Stage III T-wave inversions. However, any degree of calcification—microscopic to rigid armor plating—can be found in constrictive pericarditis. So many of the cases, especially those with ECG abnormalities, are associated with constriction that *constrictive pericarditis should always be ruled in or out when any pericardial calcification is discov-*

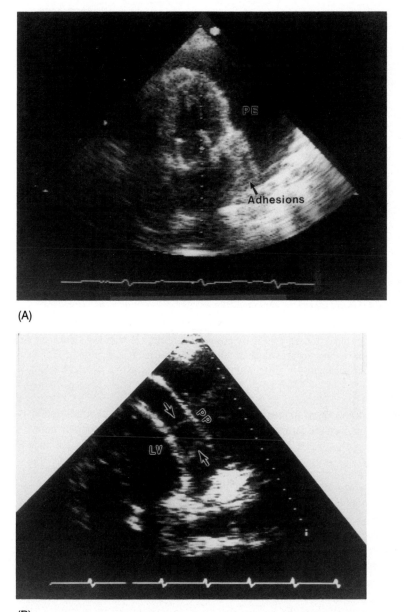

(A)

(B)

Figure 14.1   A. Linear pericardial adhesions on two-dimensional echocardiogram, made visible by a pericardial effusion (PE). B. Two-dimensional echocardiogram revealing linear, strutlike pericardial adhesions (arrows) between the visceral pericardium of the left ventricle (LV) and the parietal pericardium (PP), made visible by a pericardial effusion.

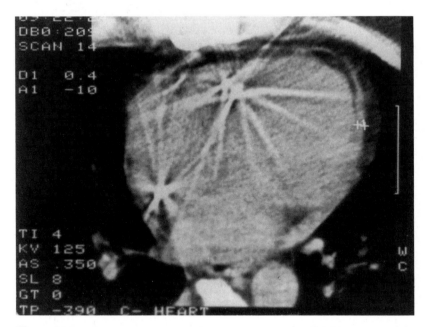

Figure 14.2 Computed tomograms showing variable pericardial thickening highlighted by epicardial fat (black zones), especially posteriorly. Compare with less thickened lateral pericardium (caliper marks) and virtually normal anterior pericardium. (On two-dimensional echocardiography, there was no fluid.)

ered. Movie-mode *rapid acquisition computed tomography* can simultaneously identify and map calcifications and identify any hemodynamic impairment.

Distribution

In asymptomatic patients and those with constriction-related or unrelated abdominal symptoms (page 343), pericardial calcification may be discovered in gastrointestinal x-ray series, because the pericardial-diaphragmatic interface is often heavily involved (possibly because gravity causes inflammatory pericardial contents to sediment inferiorly). Calcification inferiorly, over the apex of the left ventricle, and particularly its relative frequency over the right atrium, the sternal aspect of the right ventricle and in the atrioventricular grooves— seems related to *involvement of these areas of least heart movement and of greatest friction* between the epicardium and the parietal pericardium.

  Microscopic calcific foci may first be detected by careful tissue examination and may begin only weeks after pericardial injury. Resected, well-calci-

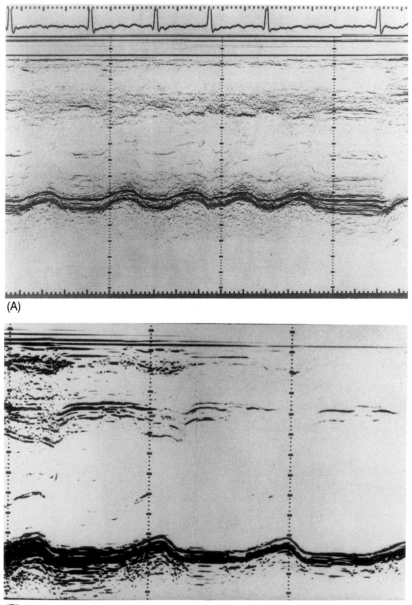

(A)

(B)

Figure 14.3 (See following page for legend.)

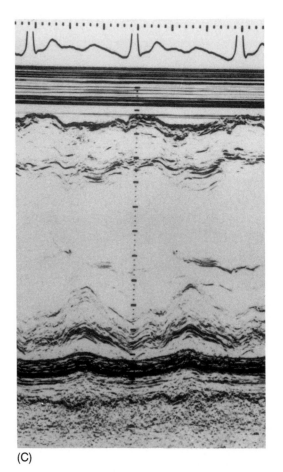

(C)

Figure 14.3 A. M-mode echocardiogram showing a dense double band—separate thickening of the visceral and parietal pericardia separated by material that may be fibrinous or fibrous adhesions. Strictly parallel movement of each band with the left ventricular wall indicates adhesion. B. Pericardial thickening and adhesion of both layers. M-mode echocardiogram showing marked pericardial density that remains intensely echogenic during a damping maneuver (left half of illustration). C. M-mode echocardiogram showing small posterior and anterior pericardial effusion, posteriorly highlighting marked thickening (echogenicity) of the parietal pericardium.

fied pericardial tissue is often associated with hypocellular scar tissue but also frequently shows chronic, subacute and even acute inflammatory changes. *X-ray detectability* of pericardial calcification probably takes at least a year and often many years to discover. In occasional individuals operated for constric-

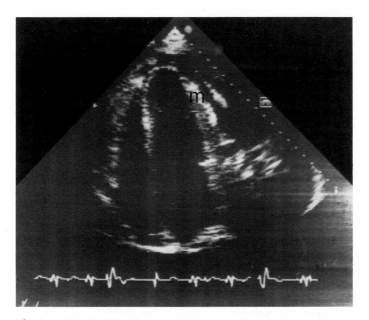

Figure 14.4 Small pericardial effusion. Two-dimensional echocardiogram shows elongated fibrinous or thrombotic mass (m) on the left ventricular epicardium.

tive pericarditis, calcium first appears or reappears in pericardial remnants several years later.

Clinical Impact

The clinical importance of asymptomatic pericardial calcification, particularly if local, rather than a completely armored heart, lies in its confusion on x-rays with calcium in cardiac structures like the coronary arteries, the myocardium and in the walls of aneurysms, particularly at the apex. Deposits appear in a vast array of shapes: granules, streaks, needles, strands, bands, plaques, disks, plates, buckles and sheets, any of which may be smooth or irregular. Odd configurations may result, including those resembling the letters C, U, J, Y, or O (rings) and may completely or partially clasp portions of the heart (Chapter 15). Calcifications increase the technical difficulties of pericardial resection by requiring instruments for removing them, and, where pericardial calcification invades the myocardium, the procedure is particularly difficult and dangerous (pages 255–256). Concomitant pericardial constriction can make calcific material spring apart when cut. Sharp-edged plaques must be removed with extreme care to avoid myocardial injury. Ultrasonic instruments may be needed.

The location of pericardial calcific deposits should be demonstrated before surgery; this may be possible with ordinary roentgenography (lateral films are best: Figures 14.5 through 14.7A and B). However, more sensitive and accurate imaging methods (CT; MRI) are desirable, especially to differentiate any other calcified structures and to help surgeons prepare operative approaches.

INFLAMMATORY CYSTS OF THE PERICARDIUM

These include pseudocysts as well as encapsulated and loculated pericardial effusions. Pericardial scarring may trap portions of an intrapericardial exudate or hemorrhage, producing a pocket or cystlike structure with or without symptoms and signs of its presence. Previously, these were due largely to rheumatic pericarditis, bacterial infection, particularly tuberculosis (cold abscess), or traumatic hemopericardium; today they are more frequent following cardiac surgery. Their capsules are scarred parietal and visceral pericardium in which low-grade inflammatory activity persists. Dense and constrictive scarring can form inflammatory cysts which may calcify individually or along with the adhesions. Rarely, encapsulation by intact serosa resembles a congenital cyst (Chapter 6). The contents are sometimes under pressure and, with chronicity, calcification is common both in the walls and contents. While frequently asymptomatic,

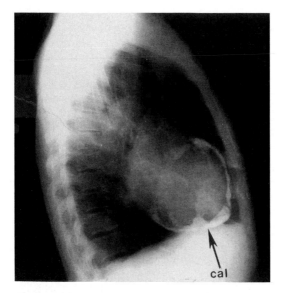

Figure 14.5 Pericardial calcification (cal): circumcardiac dense irregular distribution in lateral chest film.

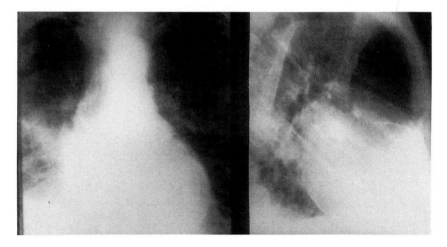

Figure 14.6 Constrictive pericarditis with enlarged cardiopericardial silhouette. Posteroanterior (PA) chest film shows no definite calcification; light calcification on lateral film.

postsurgical loculations can cause localized tamponade and individual diastolic chamber collapse on echocardiography (page XX). The importance of the more chronic inflammatory cysts lies in their differentiation from ventricular pseudoaneurysms and true (congenital) cysts of the pericardium, which tend to be smooth, with a predilection for the low right cardiac border and sometimes the left. In contrast, the inflammatory pseudocysts, like parasitic cysts, have variable contours and can occur anywhere.

INFLAMMATORY DIVERTICULA

Inflammatory pericardial diverticula are related to encapsulated pericardial effusion in that they follow exudative pericarditis, especially tuberculous, but acute idiopathic (presumably viral) pericarditis can be a precursor. Unlike the case with inflammatory cysts, only parietal pericardium is primarily involved, so that communication with the pericardial cavity is maintained. The walls of pericardial diverticula are usually serosa and fibrosa with variable amounts of scar tissue. Rarely, scarred serosa can herniate through a defect in the fibrosa (*false diverticulum*); this is more characteristic of congenital than inflammatory diverticula. Diverticular contents resemble those of inflammatory cysts. These diverticula, for some reason, tend to be right-sided, perhaps because the fibrosa over the right ventricle is particularly thin. They may result from the effect of elevated intrapericardial pressure on a weakened portion of the stretched pari-

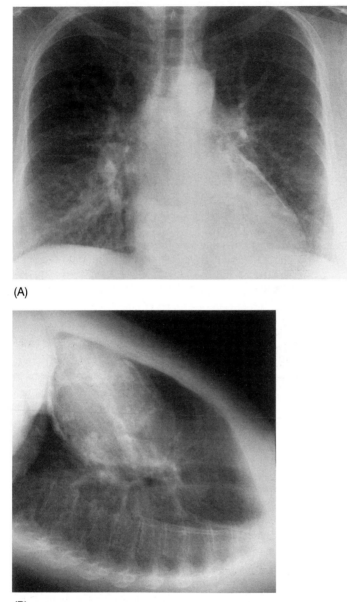

(A)

(B)

Figure 14.7   A. Nonconstrictive calcified pericardium appears confined to the left heart border in PA view. B. Lateral view of Figure 14.7A; dense circumcardiac calcific deposits.

etal pericardium, creating a *pulsion diverticulum*. The occasional diverticulum with external adhesions about its sac may represent *traction diverticulum*. Inflammatory diverticula are usually asymptomatic and the differential diagnosis resembles that of inflammatory pericardial cysts (page 208). Rarely, an aneurysm of the root of the aorta may be confusing, but abnormalities elsewhere in the aorta should suggest that diagnosis. Omental hernia through the foramen of Morgagni at the right cardiophrenic angle may be distinguished by imaging procedures. Like cysts, inflammatory diverticula may be resected if they become symptomatic or if thoracoscopy makes the diagnosis.

GRANULOMATOUS PERICARDITIS

A variety of agents incite granuloma formation, characterized by simultaneous inflammation and repair, a process well suited to produce subacute and chronic pericardial disease. Granulomas, basically focal nodules or masses, are composed mainly of granulation tissue and fibrous tissue with a variable degree of leukocytic infiltration (Figure 14.8). Yet they can spread throughout the pericardium, with larger granulomas tending to coalesce; accompanying fibrotic processes ultimately bridge and overgrow them. The tendency to form a static, avascular scar usually makes etiologic diagnosis progressively more difficult because, during the progress of the granuloma, important clues may disappear. Infection may be liquidated by treatment or by the patient's humoral and tissue defenses. Telltale necrotic and foreign matter can be dispersed or removed

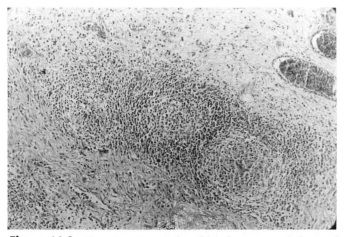

Figure 14.8 Granulomatous pericarditis: simultaneous inflammation and repair with leukocytic infiltration, fibrosis and nodular cellular aggregations.

piecemeal by phagocytes and the fibrosis itself distorts or overwhelms formerly characteristic histologic patterns.

Severity and chronicity vary widely among the granulomatous pericarditides. In many, particularly the infectious forms (notably tuberculous pericarditis), the clinical picture is of acute pericardial disease, irrespective of whether the inflammatory process is truly acute and recent or whether the granuloma has advanced silently and for some reason is provoked into a dramatic flare. In many cases, the borderline between an advanced but active inflammatory process and constrictive pericarditis due to scarring is indistinct, either because of great clinical similarity or because both processes are in fact present. *Tuberculous pericarditis* epitomizes all of the foregoing possibilities and is by far the most important member of this group.

In general, the etiology of granulomatous pericarditis includes four main groups:

1. *Of unknown origin*, including "idiopathic."
2. Due to *systemic disease* like rheumatoid arthritis and other connective tissue diseases and to sarcoidosis.
3. *Infections*, particularly tuberculosis, histoplasmosis, coccidioidomycosis, actinomycosis and tularemia (also, rarely, syphilis).
4. *Foreign-matter reaction*, particularly silicosis and asbestosis; however, if sterile, each has few acute clinical repercussions.

Many granulomas of multiple etiologies are rich in cholesterol and represent one source of *cholesterol pericarditis* (Chapter 7), in which cholesterol crystal deposition in the pericardium tends to provoke a strong reaction, including copious effusion, secondary granuloma formation and constriction.

While *rheumatoid arthritis* causes a great number of pericardial adhesions and *rheumatoid nodules* have been recognized in the pericardium (sometimes with acute or subacute fibrinous pericarditis), the prevalence of rheumatoid arthritis is so great that a chance coincidence with many other pericardial lesions is highly probable. Thus, the presence of rheumatoid arthritis may make it difficult to prove etiology in a given patient with clinically important pericardial disease, although some rheumatoid granulomas have the histologic structure of rheumatoid nodules.

Pulmonary *silicosis* and *asbestosis* may be associated with pericardial granulomas and widespread pericardial and pleuro-pericardial adhesions. Granulomatous lesions have been induced by poudrage with asbestos and magnesium silicate, a discarded operative treatment for ischemic heart disease. Talc-containing powders used on surgeons' gloves may affect the pericardium during cardiac surgery, as in the peritoneum, where granulomatous inflammation can occur. In general, many such *foreign-matter reactions* tend to form static scars with uncertain (usually low) constrictive potential.

KEY POINTS

1. Postinflammatory pericardial scarring is a complex process with a range of effects from clinically silent (most common) through distortions of diagnostic imaging to compression (constriction) of the heart and vessels.
2. Pericardial calcification, often innocent, indicates a search for general or local constrictive scarring.
3. Inflammatory pericardial cysts and diverticula are uncommon; main importance is identification in chest x-ray films and the range of imaging studies.
4. Granulomatous pericarditides involve a wide range of inflammatory lesions, notably rheumatoid pericarditis (only occasionally clinically important) and tuberculous pericarditis (usually serious).
5. Fibrotic and granulomatous cells and tissues are metabolically active, with important local and perhaps general effects, including ACE and AT2 production and inhibition.

BIBLIOGRAPHY

Leak, L.V., Ferrans, V.J., Cohen, S.R., et al. Animal model of acute pericarditis and its progression to pericardial fibrosis and adhesions: Ultrastructural studies. Am. J. Anat. 1987; 373–390.

Mitchell, J.D., Lee, R., Hodakowski, G.T., et al. Prevention of postoperative pericardial adhesions with a hyaluronic acid coating solution. J. Thorac. Cardiovasc. Surg. 1994; 107:1481–1488.

Spodick, D.H. Chronic and Constrictive Pericarditis. New York: Grune & Stratton, 1994, pp. 19–100.

Sun, Y., Weber, K.T. Angiotensin II receptor binding following myocardial infarction in the rat. Cardiovas. Res. 1994; 28:1623–1628.

Chello M, Mastroberto P, Romano R, Perticone F, Marchese AR. Collagen network remodelling and left ventricular function in constrictive pericarditis. Heart 1996; 75:184–189.

15

Constrictive Pericarditis

Constrictive pericarditis is a form of cardiac compression with important similarities to and differences from cardiac tamponade (Tables 15.1 through 15.4). Like almost every type of "traditional" disease, constrictive pericarditis, which makes the heart the prisoner of a diseased, usually scarred, pericardium (Figure 15.1), has changed its dominant etiologic spectrum and its clinical manifestations over the years. The latter relate mainly to the tempo of the disease—i.e., the aggressiveness of the inciting processes and the point in its development where it becomes significantly compressive or symptomatic—and, perhaps even more important, where it becomes diagnosable. With progress in understanding constrictive (restrictive) hemodynamics and other features related to the constrictive clinical syndromes and in diagnostic testing (particularly imaging of the heart and pericardium), diagnosis is now rarely greatly delayed. There remains variably difficult differential diagnosis from restrictive cardiomyopathy, other causes of systemic congestion, particularly right ventricular failure, and cirrhosis of the liver. Moreover, the presentation may be subtle and may mimic other conditions clinically and hemodynamically, including constrictive compression of coronary vessels, causing ischemic syndromes. Sometimes direct inspection and biopsy of the pericardium are required to rule in or out constriction or one of its variants, especially in the presence of more generalized diseases that may or may not be related to it. Indeed, constrictive scarring may follow pericardial resection or pericardiotomy for any condition, *including constrictive pericarditis*. (Fortunately, while obliterative adhesions regularly follow cardiac

Table 15.1 **Etiology of Constrictive Pericarditis** (Western/advanced countries).
Great Majority: Unknown or uncertain etiology/"Idiopathic pericarditis"

Relatively Common
  Infectious
    Viral or probable viral
    Tuberculosis
    Pyogenic
  Therapeutic Irradiation
  Cardiopericardial surgery
Relatively uncommon; increased incidence in special populations
  Neoplasia
    Metastatic
    Mesothelioma
        Pericardial
        Pleural
  Uremia (on dialysis)
  Vasculitus - connective tissue disease group
    Esp.: rheumatoid arthritis; lupus; scleroderma (including CREST syndrome)
  Infectious
    Fungal
    Parasitic
  Myocardial infarct-related
    Post hemopericardium (from thrombolysis)
    Postmyocardial infarction (Dressler's) syndrome
  Trauma
    Blunt
    Penetrating
  Drugs
    Procaineamide (lupus)
    Methysergide
    Practolol
    Hydralazine (lupus)
  Hemopericardium/encapsulated hemopericardium in hemorrhagic disorders
Rare
  Cholesterol pericarditis
  Chylopericardium
  Intrapericardial instrumentation
    AICD patches
    Epicardial pacemaker
    Whipple's disease
    Wegener's granulomatosis

(*continued*)

Table 15.1   Continued

Hypereosinophilic syndromes
Cardiac transplant
Hereditary: Mulibrey nanism
Sarcoidosis
Asbestosis
Pericardial amyloidosis
Dermatomyositis
Lassa fever
Chemical trauma: sclerotherapy of esophageal varices

---

surgery, constrictive scarring is uncommon.) Finally, atrial septal defects seem unusually frequent with constriction (possibly due to ascertainment bias); they modify the clinical and hemodynamic signs and are identified during catheterization or color Doppler study.

Pathogenesis

A striking variety of conditions produce acute pericarditis, and nearly all are capable of inducing constriction, some more frequently than others. The notable

Table 15.2   Cardiac Compression; Tamponade and Constriction: Features Common to Both [a]

Decreased stroke volume due to:
  Decreased preload
  Decreased diastolic compliance
  Decreased ventricular volumes, *esp.* diastolic
  Increased ventricular diastolic pressures
Diastolic pressure equilibration [b]
Increased venous pressure
Neurohormonal activation, *esp.* renin-angiotensin-aldosterone system
  Increased adrenergic activation/sympathetic tone producing:
    Increased heart rate [c]
    Increased systemic vascular resistance
After relief of compression, sharply increased plasma antinatriuretic peptides (ANF)

---

[a]Any systolic impairment is very late or due to associated or unassociated cardiac disease or myocardial collagenization.
[b]Includes pulmonary artery (PA) diastolic pressure; cardiac compression rarely causes significant reactive PA hypertension.
[c]*Rate increase* may be restricted or absent in uremic pericarditis; *bradycardia* in some cases of critical acute tamponade with ultimate electromechanical dissociation (*esp.* acute hemopericardium).

Table 15.3 Cardiac Compression: Clinical Comparison

	Tamponade	Constriction	
		Subacute	Chronic
Pericardial effusion	+	Often[a,b]	0/+[c]
Pericardial calcification	0	Usually 0	Often
Abnormal P or atrial fibrillation	0[c]	Usually 0	Often
Jugular pulse	X or Xy	Xy or XY	XY or xY
Paradoxic pulse (>10 mm Hg)	+	+[a,d]	Rare[d]
Kussmaul's sign	0	Usually 0	Occasional
Abnormal S3	0	0/+	Nearly always

[a]In effusive-constrictive pericarditis.
[b]Often loculated.
[c]In absence of cardiac disease (related or unrelated).
[d]Usually explained by additional lesions (see text) and respiratory shifts of atrial and ventricular septa.

exception is acute rheumatic fever, which can produce extremely dense pericardial adhesions that mysteriously appear rarely if ever to constrict. The majority of cases are of undetermined etiology—"idiopathic"(see Chapter 23).

The responsible attack of acute pericarditis may be silent, though it is more often clinically apparent irrespective of whether it had been correctly diagnosed as a pericardial inflammation. The essential pathologic process is *healing resulting in a thick or thin scar that restricts cardiac filling*, particularly of the ventricles. The pattern of healing is usually one of total obliteration of the pericardial space or near-total obliteration, with remaining lacunae of fluid, pus or blood. On the other hand, *loculated* larger collections of fluid may compress individual cardiac chambers and *bandlike* constriction can involve any portion of the heart, including the valve rings and the great vessels, mimicking disease in those structures. Traditionally, constriction has been chronic, sometimes with surprising pericardial thickness (Figure 15.1); recently relatively thin and very thin constricting pericardia are increasingly evident. However, early diagnosis and some shift of the majority of recognizable etiologies, from processes like tuberculosis to viral infections, have resulted in most contemporary cases being *subacute constriction* (arbitrarily occurring 3 to 12 months after the original acute pericardial insult). *Acute constriction* occurs hard on the heels of an episode of acute pericarditis, often with cardiac tamponade; indeed, the healing process occasionally causes constrictive cicatrization within days after drainage of tamponading fluid, the cardiopericardial silhouette remaining small, with the central diastolic and systemic venous pressures reascending progressively. More recently, *transient acute constriction* in patients soon after acute peri-

Table 15.4 Cardiac Compression; Tamponade vs. Constriction: Differential Features

	Tamponade[a]	Constriction
Pericardial pressure	Pressure increased; acts throughout cardiac cycle	Not measurable; acts at limit of ventricular expansion
Limit of ventricular expansion	Reduced throughout cardiac cycle	Set by scar[b]; maximum heart volume in early diastole
Ventricular septum	Inspiratory bulge into left ventricle	Respiratory variations less
Ventricular pressure curve	No dip	Dip and plateau
Venous pressure curves	x only	x and y (usually $y > x$)
Venous return	Unimodal: during x only, i.e., during ventricular ejection; inspiratory increase	Bimodal: during x and y; insignificant respiratory effects on volume
Ventricular filling in severe cases	Early and late diastole; most severe only with atrial systole	Early diastole only (extremely rapid);[b] atrial systole usually ineffective[c]
Peak filling rate	Greatly reduced	Increased
Rapid filling period	Absent	Brief; may be only filling period[b]
Inspiratory decrease in intrathoracic (pleural) pressure	Transmitted to fluid in pericardial space; reduces transmural pressure by 1–2 mm Hg	Not transmitted into pericardium; space obliterated[d]
Special respiratory phenomena	Pulsus paradoxus	Kussmaul's sign
Diastolic suction	Possibly	Probably
Blood pressure	Supported mainly via increased systemic vascular resistance	Supported largely by blood volume expansion

[a]In classic tamponade, filling is reduced to absent throughout diastole; decreased left ventricular volume stems mainly from decreased pulmonary venous return due to greater compression of the thin-walled right ventricle.
[b]Blood rushes into ventricles until abruptly halted at limit imposed by scar.
[c]Variable in local and unequal constriction; atrial systole may be effective in elastic constriction (with corresponding S4).
[d]Except when with fluid: effusive-constrictive pericarditis or sufficiently large fluid locules entrapped by scar tissue.

Table 15.5 Current Etiology of Constrictive Pericarditis

Principal Etiologies
  Unknown
  Idiopathic/"nonspecific" pericarditis
  Infectious pericarditis
    Viral
    Suppurative (pyogenic organisms)
    Tuberculous
    Other
  Trauma (usually with hemopericardium; generalized or loculated)
    Cardiopericardial surgery
    Penetrating wounds
    Indirect/blunt trauma
  Therapeutic/accidental irradiation
  Neoplasia, primary and secondary
  Vasculitis/connective tissue diseases
  Uremia
  Other
Unusual Etiologies
  Congenital
    Mulibrey nanism
    Afibrinogenemia (hemopericardium, spontaneous or traumatic)
  Trauma
    Intrapericardial electrodes
      Pacing
      Cardioverter-defibrillator (AICD)
    Endoscopic sclerosis of esophageal varices
  Drugs
    Methysergide
    Procainamide (SLE)
    Mitomycin-C Hydralazine (pericardial sclerosant)
  Myocardial infarction
    Postinfarction (Dressler's) pericarditis
    Clotted hemopericardium
  Asbestos
    Inhaled
    Intrapericardial
  Exotic organisms
    Parasites
    Nocardia
    Lassa virus
    Whipple's disease
  Sarcoidosis
  Amyloidosis of pericardium
  Degos disease
  Campylobacter: arthropathy-pericarditis syndrome
  Coccidioidomycosis

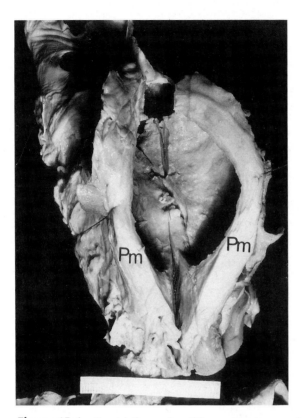

Figure 15.1 Constrictive pericarditis: postmortem specimen of unusually thickened pericardium (Pm). The heart has been removed.

carditis, usually with tamponade, has been observed by echocardiography, inspection of the jugular venous pulse and auscultation (transient abnormal third heart sound) with or without symptoms, and resolving in days to weeks. In *chronic constriction*, pericardial tissue usually shows nonspecific fibrosis with few inflammatory cells (Figure 15-2) and frequent myocardial atrophy. Both subacute and acute constriction show many more inflammatory cells and lighter connective tissue (Figures 15.3 and 15.4). Depending on etiology, there may be giant cells and granulomas.

Pathophysiology

A constricting pericardial scar sharply accentuates the ventricular pressure–volume relation (Figure 15.5) and increases ventricular coupling (ventricular interaction; page 20) while restricting filling of the ventricles progressively ear-

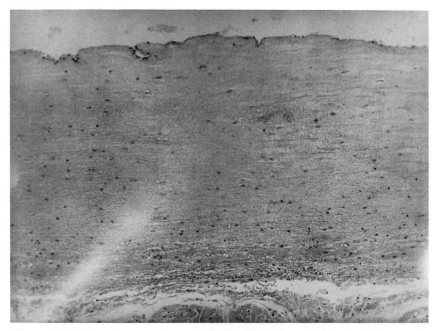

Figure 15.2 Chronic constrictive pericarditis: microscopic section of densely scarred, avascular pericardium with few inflammatory cells.

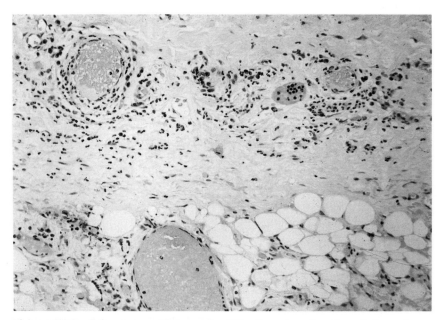

Figure 15.3 Subacute constrictive pericarditis. Scar tissue is quite cellular and vascular with active leukocytic infiltration.

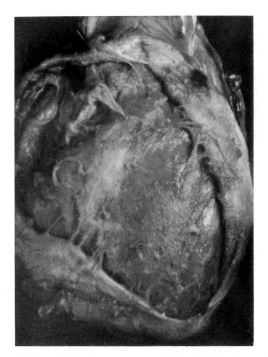

Figure 15.4 Subacute constriction: thickened pericardium with abundant adhesions. The heart bulges through the incised, relatively elastic pericardium.

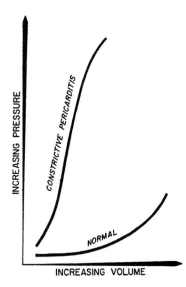

Figure 15.5 Ventricular pressure–volume relation in constrictive pericarditis. Increasing ventricular volume (filling) imposes markedly greater than normal pressure increase for every increment. This is seen in diastole when volume rise due to ventricular filling raises pressure so rapidly that filling is abruptly halted early in diastole. (From Spodick, Chronic and Constrictive Pericarditis, 1994; author's copyright.)

lier during diastole until *70 to 80% of the reduced filling occurs in the first 25 to 30% of diastole.* (In contrast, cardiac tamponade *continuously* restricts filling from the beginning of diastole as filling progressively decreases.) Elevated atrial pressures reflect the elevated ventricular diastolic pressures. Moreover, early diastolic filling is at high velocity due to (1) high atrial pressure as the atrioventricular valves open and (2) *diastolic suction*, augmented by the *"rubber bulb" effect*: springing back of the pericardial scar sheathing the ventricles, which had been contracted like a spring by ventricular systole. (Interestingly, despite the constricting carapace, if ventricular systole causes the cardiac volume to fall below pericardial volume, the ventricles may briefly behave as if they were more compliant.) Such factors produce the "square root" configuration of ventricular diastolic pressure curves (Figure 15.6) and other findings (detailed under "Cardiac Catheterization"; page 241). *All cardiac diastolic pressures are nearly equilibrated*, similar to cardiac tamponade, and often at com-

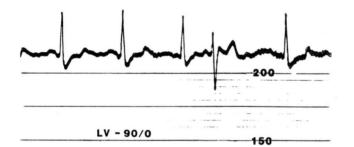

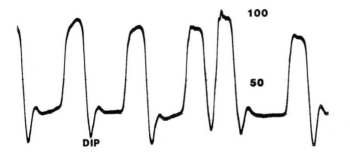

Figure 15.6 Constrictive pericarditis: left ventricular pressure curve showing typical diastolic "square root" configuration composed of an early dip rising rapidly to high plateau of pressure (left ventricular end-diastolic pressure, LVEDP, 25 mm Hg). Almost all filling occurs during the dip. A ventricular premature beat shows increased peak pressure. Wide P waves (interatrial block) are common in constrictive pericarditis.

parable levels. (NB Equilibration may be "unbalanced" by vigorous diuretic therapy). Unlike tamponade, the venous and atrial pressure wave forms resemble the normal; that is, the *y* descent is preserved—it is deep and usually larger than a more or less deep *x* descent (Figure 15.7). (In tamponade, the *y* descent is sharply truncated or amputated.) Venous *flow* toward the heart occurs with the *x* and *y* descents of venous pressure, with the major acceleration during the *y* descent (normally during the *x* descent).

There are no systolic abnormalities except with coexistent myocardial lesions due to ischemia, myocardial atrophy or myocardial damage, including antecedent myocarditis. *Ischemia* includes both underlying coronary disease and when the constricting scar compresses coronary arteries, veins or bypass grafts. Systolic dysfunction may also be due to severe antecedent *myopericarditis* (Chapter 9), with local or generalized myocardial injury and scarring. With chronic constriction, *myocardial atrophy, fibrosis and calcification* can also produce systolic abnormality, generally related to the degree of chronicity. Thus, constriction can differ from uncomplicated tamponade by a variable element of systolic impairment and the occasional significant compression of the coronary arteries and veins, especially in patients with intrinsic coronary disease (even producing angina). In contrast, in uncomplicated constriction, as in tamponade, coronary blood flow is adequate for aerobic metabolism.

Compensation for constriction resembles compensation in cardiac tamponade (Figure 12.2). The *heart rate* is the major mechanism defending cardiac output, as stroke volume is nearly fixed by the rigid halt to filling in early

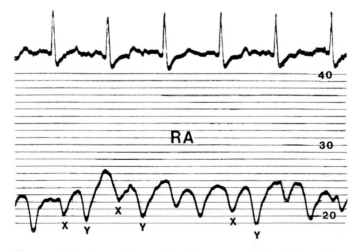

Figure 15.7 Constrictive pericarditis: characteristic right atrial pressure curve with well-formed *x* and *y* descents and *y* > *x*. Mean atrial pressure approximately 22 mm Hg. Electrocardiogram shows interatrial block.

diastole. Thus, increasing the number of beats tends to increase cardiac output. (Yet a truly maximal effect on cardiac output is rarely attained, since there is an untapped "rate reserve." This is disclosed during modest heart rate increases by pacing, e.g., to 140 beats per minute, and also by an inadequate heart rate response to exercise, both relieved by successfully pericardiectomy.) *Increased heart rate mainly amputates the diastolic pressure plateau following the abbreviated filling period.* This is why tachycardia and atrial fibrillation are relatively less important in constriction than in some other conditions where the more rapid beats severely encroach on filling. However, heart rate control is essential to find the optimal rate for a given patient. This may be critical in older patients and those with ischemia or other heart disease, since rapid rates can shorten diastole sufficiently to reduce coronary blood flow. Moreover, increasing the number of beats per minute may raise minute cardiac output, but it also raises cardiac energy expenditure and oxygen demand—potentially critical in patients with coronary artery disease.

Humoral, hormonal and renal responses are similar to those of cardiac failure and tamponade (page 188) with *electrolyte and water retention.* Yet, as in tamponade, restricted atrial distensibility prevents a significant rise in atrial natriuretic factors (ANF) until relief of cardiac compression. Sodium and water retention contributes, with high hepatic vein pressure, to *ascites,* and with high systemic venous pressure, to *edema.* The attendant *blood volume expansion* is more important than the simultaneously *elevated systemic vascular resistance* in maintaining arterial pressure.

Respiratory Changes

(See also echo-Doppler findings; pages 234–241; Table 15.6.)

The heart and pulmonary vessels are intrathoracic. Normally, they are simultaneously affected by respiratory pressure changes, so that pulmonary venous flow to the left atrium is not significantly changed by respiration. But in classic constrictive pericarditis, the heart is totally encased and thus insulated from thoracic pressure changes, so that when inspiration decreases intrathoracic pressure, cardiac pressures remain high. Consequently, pulmonary venous blood cannot easily enter the high-pressure left atrium; therefore, *total pulmonary venous flow and flow velocity are decreased in inspiration, decreasing left ventricular filling* and time to peak filling rate. Respiration does not change the superior vena cava pressure or flow velocity. Although the inferior vena cava is affected by diaphragmatic movements and abdominal pressure fluctuations, there is *diminished (<50%) to undetectable respiratory change in inferior vena cava diameter* (Figure 15.12).

Inspiration does not greatly increase right ventricular filling (*volume*), although filling *velocities* definitely increase. *Inspiration increases pulmonary*

Table 15.6 **Constrictive Pericarditis: Echo-Doppler Findings** (None Obligatory—Varying Sensitivities and Specificities)

Generalities
1. Respiratory observations require a precise respirometer/thermistor recording accompanying echo-Doppler recordings.
2. For accurate Doppler observations during irregular rapid heart rates, convert the rhythm or make long-duration tracings.
3. Central venous and right atrial observations assume no significant tricuspid regurgitation.
4. Most patients have reciprocal right-left sided respiratory variations. (Respiratory variations in mitral inflow velocity with hepatic vein flow velocity quasidiagnostic.)
5. When mitral Doppler is difficult to obtain, respiratory variation >25% in pulmonary vein diastolic forward flow (by transesophageal echocardiography; TEE) represents respiratory variation in LV filling.

M-Mode Echocardiograms
Pericardium appears thick and may show two or more parallel "lines."
Left ventricle: Flat posterior wall throughout diastole; shortening fraction normal or increased.
Ventricular septal abnormalities (components of "septal bounce")
    Abnormal systolic motion: involves proximal or entire septum
        Paradoxic: Left side of septum
            Anterior (type A); begins at end of P wave
            Flat (type B)
        Right side of septum
            Parallels left side, *or* moves slightly more anteriorly
    Decreased systolic thickening
    Abnormal early diastolic motion
      Abrupt posterior motion
      Abrupt anterior motion
      Abrupt posterior, then anterior motion, or the reverse; varies with respiration
    Sharp notch following P wave of ECG ("atrial notch").
Septum to left in inspiration; to right in expiration (Note: generally less than in tamponade).
Atrial septum: Brisk inspiratory displacement to left
Aortic root and valve
    Reduced motion
    Abrupt early diastolic posterior motion
    Gradual systolic closure of aortic valve; reduced ejection time (open time of "aortic box") for any heart rate

Table 15.6 Continued

Pulmonic valve
  Premature opening
  Exaggerated respiratory variation of A wave
Mitral valve
  Later opening in inspiration: LV isovolumic relaxation time short but longer in
    inspiration
Inferior vena cava
  Dilated, with reduced ($<50\%$) to absent respiratory diameter change
Two-Dimensional Echocardiograms (TEE optimal)
  Pericardium thick, bright (well seen next to lung)
  Septal "bounce" (best seen in SAX plane)
    = *composite of septal motions detailed in M-mode tracings* (p. 226)
  Ventricles may be narrow, tube-like
  Atria
    Normal, *or*
    One or both slightly enlarged
    TEE: RA wall excursion reduced
  Atrial septum: Brisk inspiratory displacement toward LA
  LV: Quantitative measurements
    Ejection fraction normal or increased
    Filling restricted to early diastole
    Wide angle between LV and LA posterior walls (P-LAX plane: $>150°$)
  Inferior vena cava and hepatic veins dilated with small ($<50\%$) to absent respiratory
    variations

Doppler Flows
Generalities
1. Most *directional* changes in constriction are similar to those of tamponade because
   the tight pericardium similarly increases ventricular interaction.
2. *Absolute* changes smaller than normal; *phasic* respiratory (inspiratory/expiratory)
   and cardiac (systolic/diastolic) changes much greater than normal and usually with
   the first beat of inspiration or expiration after first inspiratory/expiratory diastole.
3. Inspiration decreases *extracardiac* thoracic pressure, decreasing velocity of cardiac
   input while the tight pericardium insulates the heart from thoracic pressure changes.
4. Generally, *intracardiac* inspiratory and expiratory changes are reciprocal, inspiration
   increasing right-sided and expiration left-sided velocities.
5. *Overall changes compared to normal*: Reduced ventricular filling (flow integrals);
   decreased peak E and A velocities; decreased E and A durations (filling periods);
   decreased pulmonic vein and systemic vein flow integrals (diastolic decrease
   proportional to atrial pressures); hepatic vein end-systolic flow reversal and early
   cessation of diastolic flow. Venae cavae: minimal variations.

(*continued*)

Table 15.6 Continued

Summary of Respiratory Variations

	Inspiration (vs. expiration)	Expiration (vs. inspiration)
Mitral valve flow velocity	Decreased	Increased
E wave		
Peak	Decreased	Increased
Deceleration time	Usually decreased (≤160 msec)	Usually increased (>160 msec)
Duration (rapid filling period)	Decreased	Increased
A wave		
Peak	Decreased	Increased
Duration	Decreased	Increased
Left ventricle		
Filling (flow integrals)	Decreased	Increased
Isovolumic relaxation time	Increased (e.g., 85–95 msec)	Decreased (e.g., 55–65 msec)
Rapid filling period	Decreased	Increased
Pulmonary vein velocities		
Overall	Decreased	Increased
Systolic	Decreased	Increased
Diastolic	Decreased[a]	
Tricuspid valve velocities		
A and E waves		
Peak	Increased	Decreased with first beat
Deceleration time	Decreased (E—usually ≤160 msec)	Increased (E—usually >160 msec)
Atria: flow reversals	Decreased	Increased
Hepatic veins; inferior vena cava		
Overall flow	Decreased	Increased
Diastolic flow reversal	Decreased	Increased
Diastolic forward flow	Increased	Decreased
Right ventricle		
Filling	Increased	Decreased
Rapid filling period	Decreased[b]	Increased

[a]Proportional to left atrial pressure.
[b]With decreased difference between right and left ventricular rapid filling periods.
NB: Hepatic vein systolic velocity *minus* atrial reversal velocity < 0 cm/s highly specified.

artery flow velocity but has minimal effects on the aortic pressure in pure con-striction. However, in some cases, inspiration does decrease systemic blood pressure over 10 mm Hg, strongly suggesting an element of concomitant tam-ponade (effusive-constrictive pericarditis) or other cause for pulsus paradoxus, such as pulmonary disease or marked respiratory shifts of the ventricular and atrial septa. Indeed, *the ventricular and atrial septa are free of constriction can respond to pressure differences across them and tend to move with respiration.*

Kussmaul's Sign

During classic constriction *Kussmaul's sign—inspiratory jugular venous distention*—replaces the normal inspiratory venous "collapse" that reflects the normal inspiratory fall of 3 to 7 mm Hg in right atrial pressure. (Note: Sometimes there is only absence of this normal "collapse.") The neck veins are extrathoracic and face an impediment to flow into the high-pressure right atrium (RA), which the constrictive scar insulates from respiratory changes; thus, the normal inspiratory acceleration of venous blood toward the heart is resisted, causing the neck veins to distend (Figure 15.13), while there is little or no respiratory variation in RA mean pressure (Figures 15.7 and 15.8). There may be an additional contribution to the atrial filling impediment from increased abdominal pressure on the inferior vena cava (IVC) caused by descent of the diaphragm. (Note: Kussmaul's sign does not occur in cardiac tamponade un-

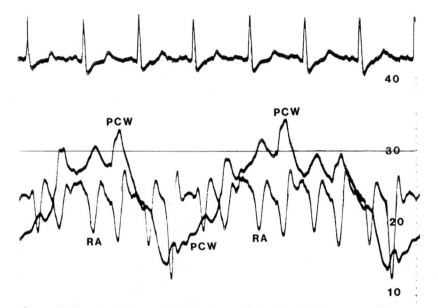

Figure 15.8 Constrictive pericarditis: right atrial (RA) and pulmonary capillary wedge (PCW) pressures in a patient with Kussmaul's sign. PCW pressure varies markedly with breathing, but RA pressure does not. The right atrium is insulated from respiratory changes. In contrast, the PCW is intrapulmonary and therefore sensitively reflects expiration (PCW peaks) and inspiration (PCW nadirs).

less complicated by effusive-constrictive disease due to a constricting epicarditis underneath the tamponading fluid.) Finally, other conditions with markedly increased right atrial and venous pressures may also produce the Kussmaul phenomenon, including right ventricular failure, right ventricular myocardial infarction (with hemodynamic similarities to constriction; page 241), restrictive cardiomyopathy (pages 250–251), chronic cor pulmonale and acute pulmonary embolism.

CLINICAL ASPECTS

Cardiovascular Graphics of Constriction

Various methods of demonstrating constriction essentially depend on two factors: pericardial thickening and abnormal ventricular filling. Imaging methods show greatly decreased ventricular diastolic volumes, abrupt transition from rapid to slower or no filling and dilated superior and inferior venae cavae and hepatic veins, with little or no respiratory variation.

Chest Roentgenogram (CXR)

The cardiopericardial silhouette is usually of normal size or only modestly enlarged (Figure 14.6), since pericardial thickening, rarely more than 1 cm, is usually much less. However, the shape depends on the configuration of the scar tissue and any fluid that remains; thus it is sometimes unusual. It can be triangular with some loss of the normal arcuate contours and angles (for example, filling in of the angle between the superior vena cava and the right atrium or of the right cardiophrenic angle). Irregularities along the diaphragm may be due to pleuropericardial adhesions, especially in patients with a background of pneumonia or tuberculosis. The superior vena cava and azygos vein are dilated. Pleural effusions are frequent and usually bilateral. Occasional concomitant *constrictive pleuritis* tends to be missed on CXR and discovered only by computed tomography or at operation or postmortem. The only chamber enlargement that can be recognized by CXR is occasional left atrial enlargement, particularly in cases with heavy scarring of the left ventricle or the left atrioventricular groove (functional mitral stenosis). Pulmonary blood flow often redistributes, with upper-zone vascular dilation and decreased lower-zone vessel caliber, particularly in patients with left atrial enlargement. Kerley B lines may be present. However, *alveolar edema is rare and implies either unequal chamber constriction or concomitant heart or lung disease*.

Previously, one-third to one-half of cases, mainly chronic, had obvious *pericardial calcification*; modern diagnostic efficiency has markedly reduced its incidence due to earlier surgery. Calcification is best seen on lateral films, appearing in sheets, hoops, bands and irregular shapes (Figure 15.9); it is

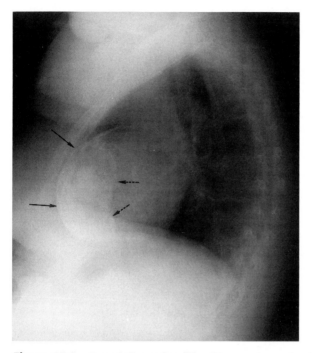

Figure 15.9   Constrictive pericarditis with extensive pericardial calcification (arrows).

heaviest over the right heart, the diaphragmatic surface directly under the left ventricle and the atrioventricular groove, especially on the left (Figure 15.10). With appropriate hemodynamics and other findings, the presence of calcium strongly favors the diagnosis of constriction. However, pericardial calcification per se is not specific, since it may occur without cardiac compression (Chapter 14).

   Blood pool radionuclide ventriculography shows time to peak filling rate to be shorter in inspiration, which may be unique to constriction.

Computed Tomography (CT) and Magnetic Resonance Imaging (MRI)

Pericardial thickening is best demonstrated by cine and gated MRI and CT, with and without contrast studies (Figure 15.11). Each technique has high time and spatial resolutions that are dependable for identifying and measuring pericardial thickening and geometric changes. Both CT and MRI are more specific than echocardiography in differentiating scarring from fluid or tumor. They dramatically demonstrate the dilated venae cavae and frequently deformed ventricles and atria. *The enlarged venae cavae contrast sharply with the aorta which their*

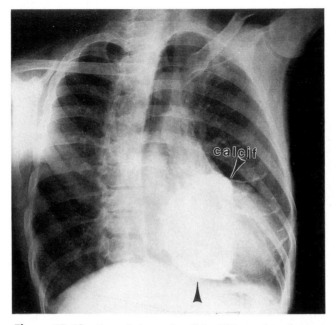

Figure 15.10 Constrictive pericarditis. Oblique view shows annular calcification involving the atrial ventricular groove.

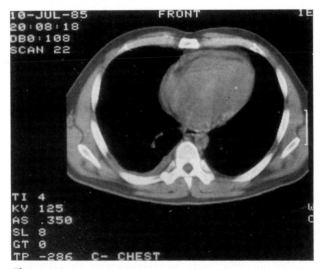

Figure 15.11 Constrictive pericarditis. Computed tomograms showing marked pericardial thickening highlighted by epicardial fat (black zones).

diameter normally matches. The atria, particularly the left atrium, may be enlarged and the ventricles narrowed and tubelike. The ventricular septum is frequently sinuous or bowed or angulated. *Pericardial thickness* by CT and MRI varies from subtle increase over the normal hairline pericardium seen by these techniques up to 10 to 15 mm (rarely more); *any* thickening over 4 mm helps differentiate constriction from restrictive cardiomyopathy; over 6 mm adds great specificity. However, *constricting pericardia may be so thin as not to be recognizable as abnormal by any contemporary imaging techniques*; direct, open inspection is required. Finally, *absence of myocardial signals* (especially absence of parts of the left ventricular wall) due to atrophy and fibrosis indicates a poor prognosis, including disastrous operative results, particularly irreversible decompensation after pericardectomy. On the other hand, CT and MRI permit detailed planning of the surgical approach in patients with adequate myocardium by revealing the distribution and varieties of pericardial thickenings and calcifications and any myocardial invasion.

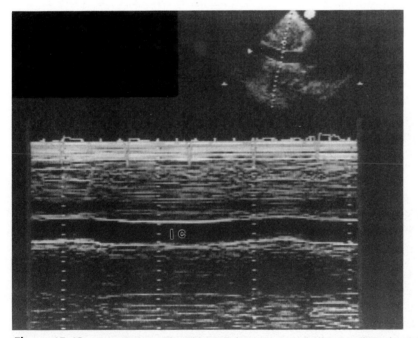

Figure 15.12 Constrictive pericarditis. Inferior vena cava (ic) by two-dimensional (inset) and M-mode echocardiography: little or no change in diameter during the respiratory cycle (indicating right heart diastolic pressure of at least 15 mm Hg).

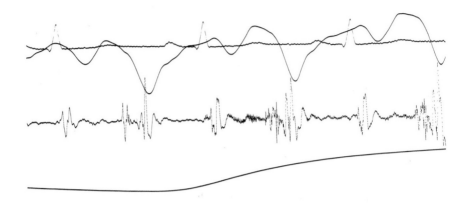

Figure 15.13 Constrictive pericarditis: jugular venous pulse with Kussmaul's sign. Traces top to bottom: electrocardiogram, jugular venous pulse, phonocardiogram, respiratory trace with inspiration registered upward. JVP shows characteristic *x* and larger *y* descents, the nadir of the *y* concurrent with the abnormal third heart sound, which is the largest heart sound. Inspiration causes respiratory curve to rise and with it the JVP level (Kussmaul's sign; compare with absence of respiratory effect on RA pulse in Figures 15.7 and 15.8).

Echocardiography

Echocardiography (Table 15.6) reflects constricting anatomic changes, the accelerated ventricular filling rate and restricted diastolic expansion and filling. Transesophageal echocardiography (TEE) can accurately display pericardial thickening comparably to CT. Transthoracic echocardiography (TTE) may not be as reliable for measuring pericardial thickness precisely, although it can disclose a very thick, highly echogenic pericardium acceptably (Figure 14.3A to C and Figure 15.14). Echocardiography with Doppler recording is excellent and probably optimal (on a cost-effectiveness basis) for dynamic changes. While there are many echo and Doppler signs (Table 15.6), no single one is pathognomonic for constriction. When pericardial thickening is identified, particularly on M-mode recording, it may be solid, may show two parallel lines separated by at least 1 mm, representing visceral and parietal pericardia (Figure 14.3A), or there may be multiple dense linear echoes (Figure 15.14). However, echocardiography can mistake fibrosis or tumor for effusion, necessitating CT or MRI. If a good trace is available, the *pulmonary valve may open prematurely* when the high right ventricular diastolic pressure exceeds pulmonary artery diastolic pressure, and there is extreme respiratory variation in the size of the pulmonic valve *A* wave (both nonspecific) (Figure 15.15). In contrast, the ventricular septum—pliant compared to the constricted walls (page 229)— tends to shift leftward with inspiration and rightward with expiration.

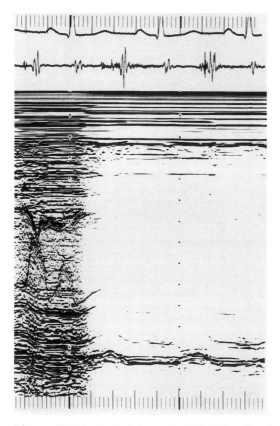

Figure 15.14 Constrictive pericarditis: M-mode echocardiogram at mitral valve level. Damping maneuver eliminates almost all structures except thick pericardium at bottom of trace. Before damping, one cardiac cycle shows mitral valve with rapid E-F slope concurrent with deep septal notch and large third heart sound on the phonocardiogram above.

The ventricular septum often shows *paradoxic systolic motion*: anterior (type A; Figure 15.16) or flat (type B). Unlike such motion with right ventricular volume overload, in constriction it begins at the end of the P waves (Figure 15.16). It is accompanied by reduced to absent diastolic ventricular expansion with a *"flat" left ventricular posterior wall* almost (within 1 to 2 mm) equally distant from the chest wall signal in early and late diastole (Figure 15.17). This is characteristic but not specific. Normal or paradoxic septal motion is bracketed by the components of septal "bounce" seen on two-dimensional echography. *Septal "bounce"* (at rapid heart rates, sometimes better named "septal dance") can be further analyzed in the M-mode tracings (Figure 15.18).

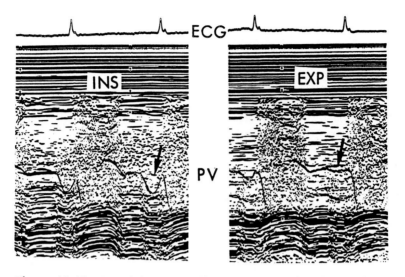

Figure 15.15 Constrictive pericarditis. M-mode recording of pulmonic valve (PV). Arrows indicate A wave that is markedly deeper in inspiration (INS) than in expiration (EXP).

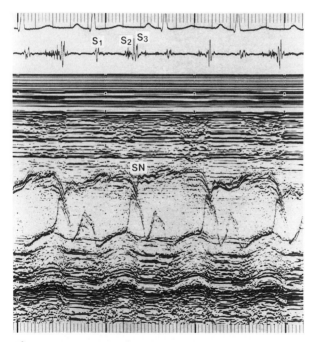

Figure 15.16 Constrictive pericarditis. M-mode recording of left ventricle at mitral valve level showing type A (anterior) paradoxic septal motion beginning at the end of the P wave (ECG, top line) and following a sharp septal notch (SN) coincident with the abnormal third heart sound and the accelerated mitral E-F slope.

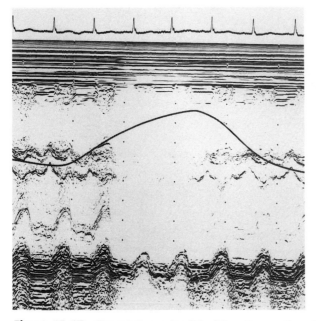

Figure 15.17 Constrictive pericarditis. M-mode recording of the right ventricle (top), ventricular septum (middle), and left ventricle (bottom), with respiratory curve and damping maneuver in center of recording. The posterior left ventricular wall and the pericardium are flat throughout diastole.

These may show an *"atrial" notch* beginning in the middle of the P wave: rapid posterior or anterior motion, or posterior then anterior motion following atrial systole, and a *"ventricular" notch*: often a more abrupt posterior (Figure 15.16), posterior-anterior or occasionally anterior-posterior sequence in early diastole. This "ventricular" septal notch coincides with the early diastolic abnormal third heart sound and the corresponding sudden halt to rapid filling. *The exact directional sequence of such ventricular septal movements depends on instantaneous pressure differences between the ventricles and their differing relative compliance* due to variations in the pericardial content of fibrous tissue and calcium. The *digitized M-mode echocardiogram* clearly shows the excessively rapid early diastolic motion (which in restrictive cardiomyopathy usually ends somewhat before the end of rapid filling).

The *aortic root* may show abrupt early diastolic posterior motion, best seen on two-dimensional TTE and TEE. These modalities also demonstrate enlargement of one or both atria with reduced wall excursion and dimensional change (particularly on the right). The superior and inferior venae cavae and hepatic veins are dilated with *restricted respiratory fluctuations*. In the inferior vena cava, these usually vary from well under the normal 50% of diameter to no

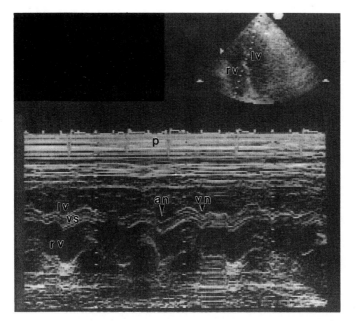

Figure 15.18 Constrictive pericarditis: "septal bounce." Two-dimensional (inset) and M-mode recording through the left ventricle (lv), ventricular septum (vs) and right ventricle (rv). The two-dimensional tracing shows a part of the sharp repetitive ventricular septal "bounce." In this patient, septal motion is normally posterior in systole (toward the left ventricle) and is bracketed by an atrial notch (an) beginning with the ECG P wave (P) and a ventricular notch (vn) at the beginning of diastole.

change, as in cardiac tamponade and other conditions with ≥ 15 mm Hg of elevated right atrial pressure (Figure 15.12). The *atrial septum*, like the ventricular septum, is compliant because it is free of the constricting pericardium; TEE shows its sharp leftward displacement during inspiration.

Echo-Doppler Cardiography

These modalities (Figure 15.19; Table 15.6) as well as transmitral (Figure 15.20) and transtricuspid (Figure 15.21) Doppler recordings show rapid forward flow in diastole and reverse flow in late systole. The *short total filling period* can be measured as *shortened individual and combined durations of the E (early filling) and A (late filling) waves.* (Indeed, with greatly reduced left ventricular compliance, the duration of normal phasic reversal of pulmonary vein flow during atrial systole may exceed the short mitral A wave duration.) The E and A waves show increased velocity of filling and abnormally rapid deceleration from their peaks (Figures 15.20 and 15.21). On the left, *these*

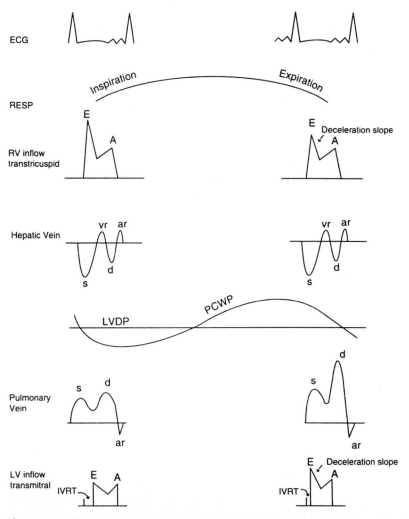

ECG

RESP

Inspiration   Expiration

RV inflow
transtricuspid

E   E
    A   Deceleration slope
                                           A

Hepatic Vein

vr   ar   vr   ar

    d   d
s   s

PCWP

LVDP

Pulmonary
Vein

s   d   d

                                     s

ar   ar

LV inflow   E   Deceleration slope
transmitral   E   A   A
          IVRT   IVRT

Figure 15.19 Constrictive pericarditis: schemata of Doppler flows (top to bottom) across tricuspid valve, in hepatic veins, in pulmonary veins and across mitral valve. Top: ECG and respiratory traces. Middle: LVDP = constant elevated level of left ventricular diastolic pressure; PCWP = respiratory variation of PCW pressure (as in Figure 15.8); s and d = systolic and diastolic waves of hepatic and pulmonary veins; ar = atrial reversal; vr = ventricular reversal; E = peak early filling velocity in right (RV) and left (LV) ventricles; A = peak presystolic filling velocities due to atrial contraction; IVRT = isovolumic relaxation time of left ventricle (sharply decreased in expiration indicating more rapid relaxation). (See text.)

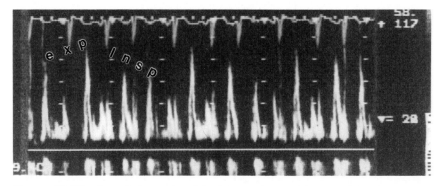

Figure 15.20 Constrictive pericarditis: *left ventricular filling velocities*. Transmitral flow velocities showing sharp inspiratory (insp) decreases and expiratory (exp) increases.

maximum velocities decrease on the first beat after the onset of inspiration. However, Doppler signals from the venae cavae and hepatic veins may lack the normal respiratory changes (Figure 15.19). (As in tamponade [Page 163] the difference [< 0 cm/sec] between hepatic vein systolic and atrial-reversal velocities correlates best with right atrial pressure. In contrast, although pulmonary venous forward flow *velocity* is reduced, pulmonary venous flow shows exaggerated respiratory variation of early diastolic peak velocity and time integral that is even more pronounced than across the mitral valve. *Reciprocal respiratory flow changes* resemble those in tamponade with decreased left-sided and increased right-sided transvalvular velocities at the very onset of inspiration and the reverse at the very onset of expiration. (Note: These are reliable, but their absence does not exclude constriction.)

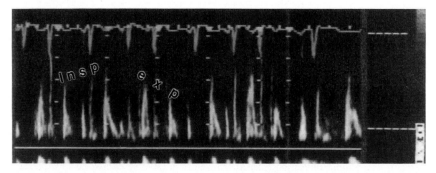

Figure 15.21 Constrictive pericarditis: *right ventricular filling velocities*. Transtricuspid flow velocities showing sharp inspiratory (insp) increases and expiratory (exp) decreases.

Doppler tissue imaging shows normal left ventricular expansion velocity (Ea) contrasting with greatly reduced velocity in restrictive cardiomyopathy. The slope of the color M-mode wave indicates a much more rapid flow from left atrium to left ventricle in constriction. Finally, rapid *mitral annular velocity* also reflects these conditions (Table 15.7)

Cardiac Catheterization

Catheterization is required if the sum of other findings only suggests constriction. It is desirable in any case, since it permits quantitation of pressures as well as helping to solidify the diagnosis and identify concomitant cardiac disease. Moreover, *coronary angiography should minimize operative accidents* with the vessels, especially if there is an unusual or anomalous distribution of the coronary arteries.

Constrictive hemodynamics are "restrictive" and therefore closely resemble those of restrictive cardiomyopathy—often the principal differential diagnosis (Table 15.7)—and right ventricular myocardial infarction, in which the right ventricle dilates, tightening a normal pericardium upon the heart in a constricting manner. The major finding, similar to tamponade, is *near equalization of all diastolic chamber pressures and venous pressures*. Both left and right ventricular traces have a dip and plateau, the *"square root" configuration* (Figures 15.6 and 15.22)—more pronounced in the RV—due to the sharp, short early diastolic fall toward zero pressure (*dip*), rising rapidly to a restrictive *plateau* as the relaxing ventricles rapidly reach the tight, limiting pericardium. Typically, right ventricular and pulmonary artery systolic pressures are 30 to 45 mm Hg (occasionally as high as 70 mm Hg) with the *right ventricular end-diastolic pressure at least one-third of the right ventricular systolic pressure* (Figure 15.22). Negative atrial waves, like negative venous waves, are preserved, with the y descent usually deeper than the x descent, although they are often equal (Figure 15.23); in contrast, $x > y$ suggests effusive-constrictive pericarditis (page 253). The nadir of the dip of the ventricular "square root" sign coincides with the atrial y nadir (Figure 15.23) and ranges from below 0 to over 20 mm Hg with fluid-filled catheters. (High-fidelity catheters show these to be exaggerated extremes; the nadir is usually between 4 and 12 mm Hg.) *Liver vein catheterization* identifies high hepatic venous pressure and, when wedged, any portal hypertension when the liver develops cardiac "cirrhosis" (page 246). *Cardioangiography* shows normal or decreased left ventricular end-systolic and end-diastolic volumes. The superior vena cava is dilated and continuous with a frequently flat right atrial border. *Coronary arteries* are usually seen well within the cardiopericardial silhouette, i.e., deep to their normal, more superficial location unless the constricting pericardium is thin (*which is not rare*). Occasionally, there is strategic coronary compression by inequalities in the scar

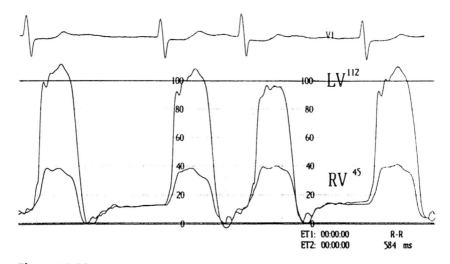

Figure 15.22 Constrictive pericarditis: simultaneous left (LV) and right (RV) ventricular pressure curves showing virtually superimposable early diastolic pressure dip rising rapidly to a plateau early in diastole; in the RV, pressure level reached is more than one-third of systolic pressure. The patient has atrial fibrillation; short diastole in middle beat shows that amputation of the plateau of rapid heart rates has little effect on ventricular filling, which virtually halts at the onset of the plateau.

tissue. Whereas these epicardial coronary arteries may display less than normal overall mobility, the septal coronary arteries may appear hypermobile.

CLINICAL CHARACTERISTICS

Symptoms, signs and clinical laboratory results, like the hemodynamic and graphic findings, are related to the pathogenesis and pathophysiology of constriction (pages 215–217). A *history* of antecedent pericarditis or pericarditis-inducing disease or drugs (e.g., procainamide; methysergide) or processes like thoracic irradiation may be strong clues to diagnosis. Aggressive organisms, like tubercle bacilli (pages 269–274), have figured prominently in the slow or rapid induction of constriction. However, today "idiopathic" (Chapter 23) or viral (Chapter 16) pericarditis is the major antecedent and absence of any history of a recognizable provocative disorder is common. Table 15.5 lists the principal etiologies of constrictive pericarditis. It is well to remember that constriction (especially if chronic) may have deceptive presentations, such as congestive heart failure, pleural effusions, right atrial thrombosis, and even hepatic coma.

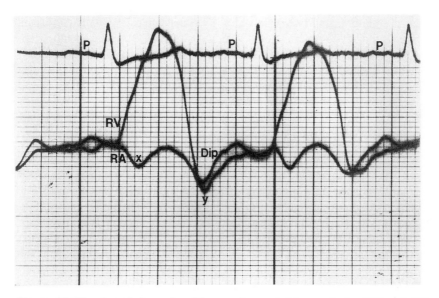

Figure 15.23 Constrictive pericarditis: superimposed right ventricular (RV) and right atrial (RA) pressure curves. Nadir of *y* descent of RA curve coincides with dip of RV curve and is deeper than the *x* descent. Patient in sinus rhythm with interatrial block— a wide bifid P wave, common in constrictive pericarditis. Following the P waves, relatively small a waves on RA curve.

Symptoms

Symptoms may be subtle or overt and are closely related to the degree of systemic and central venous congestion and fluid retention. Constrictive pericarditis resembles heart failure but is not "heart failure" in the ordinary sense; the heart has not failed—it has been prevented from "succeeding." Constriction features venous congestion resembling right heart failure with the appropriate compensatory systemic responses. Patients may have pedal edema, ascites and abdominal discomfort due to splanchnic engorgement. Ascites is often conspicuous and often occurs without peripheral edema, as in hepatic cirrhosis or tricuspid stenosis. (Ascitic fluid accumulation is initiated by liver lymph, which exudes due to high hepatic vein pressures.) Abdominal involvement can be prominent at early, lower cardiac diastolic pressures, and patients may have difficulty putting on belts and abdominal garments, which may leave a skin impression. Like a tight collar due to neck vein engorgement, this is an occasional early clue. Each may be reported by the patient.

At higher central diastolic pressures (arbitrarily over 15 mm Hg), "central" symptoms are more prominent, including dyspnea, easy fatigability, cough, occasional orthopnea and rarely platypnea. Detectable alveolar pulmonary edema is rare, and likely to be due to other conditions (page 230). Cardiac output cannot rise adequately with sufficient exercise, so that at any pressure level, *dyspnea on exertion* is characteristic; it is a nonspecific symptom related also to pleural effusions (usually bilateral) and a diaphragm limited by ascites as well as the reduced, relatively fixed stroke volume.

Physical Examination

In symptomatic patients, mild *tachycardia* is the rule, even with light exertion. More chronic or aggressive subacute constriction may be accompanied by *atrial fibrillation* (Figure 15.22) or other atrial arrhythmias. The blood pressure is normal or relatively low, although occasionally in the hypertensive range. Significant (> 10 mm Hg) pulsus paradoxus occurs only if there is effusive-constrictive disease or other extracardiac conditions like lung disease or if pliant ventricular and atrial septa have very exaggerated respiratory mobility. The *Valsalva maneuver produces a square-wave response*—detectable by sphygmomanometry but more precisely by catheter (Figure 15.24)— owing to central vascular congestion. *Pedal edema* may appear early, although at any stage there

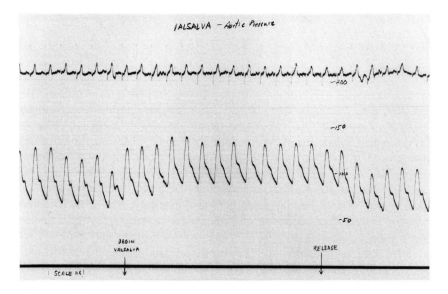

Figure 15.24 Constrictive pericarditis: Valsalva maneuver: "square wave" response of aortic pressure due to central circulatory engorgement. The entire curve shifts upward through the strain phase and promptly returns to baseline at release without the normal "overshoot."

may be *ascites* with or without pedal edema. Significantly diminishing cardiac output ultimately produces pale, *cool extremities* with *peripheral cyanosis* due to low blood flow and venous oxygen depletion. *Jaundice* in chronic constriction signals severe congestive or fibrotic liver impairment (Figure 15.25A and B).

Jugular venous distention is a hallmark, although peripheral venous distention is also easily detected in advanced cases. The patient should be sitting to determine if indeed a pressure level can be seen, measured as distance above right atrial level. Neck veins are better seen in constriction, as in tamponade, than in most other conditions because of the exceptionally high level of venous pressure with sharp x and y descents. These should be sought as *collapses from a high standing level.* (Positive a and especially c waves are often indistinct, even in venous pulse traces.) (However, despite high central venous pressure, jugular distention may not be visible due to overriding venoconstriction, enhanced by volume loss due to diuretic therapy.) *Retinal veins* are engorged. *Kussmaul's sign* (page 229; Figure 15.13) is the rule, although respiratory exaggeration of the amplitude of atrial and venous waves ("atrial pulse pressure") can mimic this but with no change in mean pressures.

Precordial palpation may be "quiet" with no point of maximal impulse or with paradoxic *systolic retraction* of the chest wall (Figure 15.26), well seen on precordial pulse recordings and sometimes partly due to pericardial adhesions. Frequent and characteristic is a sharp, early *diastolic thrust* (Figure 15.26), especially in chronic constriction. As shown in Figure 15.26, both can occur simultaneously. Such phenomena may be easily appreciated (and visible) with bodily wasting or cachexia. The early diastolic thrust corresponds to the ventricular rapid filling period and coincides with a loud *abnormal third heart sound (S3)* Figure 15.27) produced in both ventricles, which sometimes has a "knocking" quality; it is easily mistaken for the first heart sound, especially if the accompanying diastolic thrust is simultaneously mistaken for the apex beat (Chapter 4). Hemodynamic embarrassment can mute first (S1) and second (S2) heart sounds, although the pulmonic component of the second sound may be relatively or absolutely increased. The S2 may also show a fixed split or a peculiar sudden inspiratory widening if the aortic component (A2) occurs unusually early (demonstrable by phonocardiography). The fixed split is related to damping of normal respiratory changes in S2 by semifixation of right ventricular volume. The sudden early occurrence of A2 is related to reduced left ventricular filling due to sharp inspiratory diminution in left atrial filling from the pulmonary veins.

The *abnormal early diastolic sound* (EDS; S3), often palpable and tending to occur earlier than other abnormal third heart sounds, sometimes resembles the opening snaps of mitral and tricuspid stenosis. If equivocal or faint, it is enhanced by squatting or during contrast injection. *Bedside timing identi-*

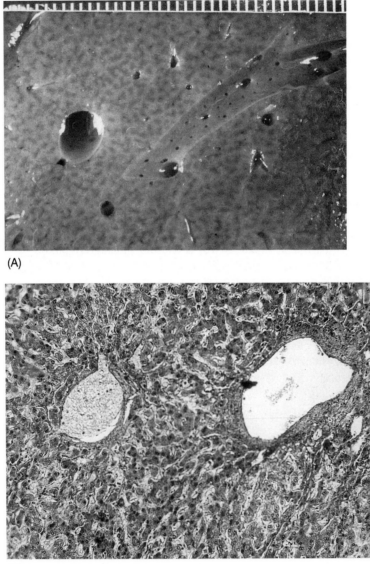

(A)

(B)

Figure 15.25   A. Constrictive pericarditis: grossly congested liver with typically difuse "mottled" appearance. B. Constrictive pericarditis: microscopic appearance of dilated hepatic central vein (left) and sinusoids with some atrophy of hepatocytes. (From Spodick, Chronic and Constrictive Pericarditis, 1994; author's copyright.)

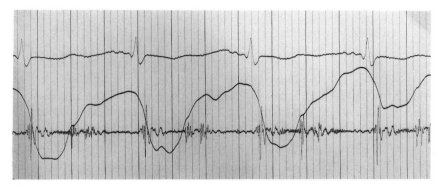

Figure 15.26 Constrictive pericarditis: paradoxic systolic retraction of precordium shown by "mirror image" apexcardiogram. Inward pulsation (downward) on precordial pulse curve during systole with sharp upward (outward) diastolic thrust initially peaking in early diastole but concurrently with a relatively small abnormal third heart sound (first heart sound is larger than usual for constriction). ECG shows interatrial block (notched wide P waves). Isovolumic relaxation time (from onset of S2 to onset of S3) is short, approximately 80 msec.

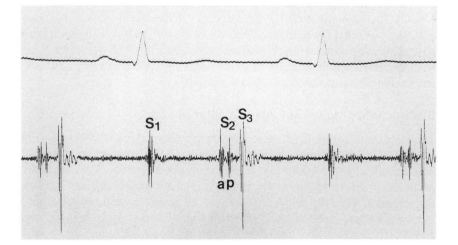

Figure 15.27 Constrictive pericarditis: phonocardiogram showing high-amplitude third heart sound (S3) larger than S1 and both components (a and p) of well split second heart sound (S2).

fies certain events: the abnormal third sound follows a usually well split second heart sound (Figure 15.27); when its loudness mimics a first heart sound (especially when S3 is palpable), it is identifiable because it follows the readily palpated peak of the carotid pulse, whereas S1 precedes the carotid peak. The jugular *x* descent occurs approximately with the carotid peak and the *y* descent coincides with the third heart sound and its concomitant diastolic precordial thrust (Figures 15.23 and 15.26). The *liver* is often palpable and may have a definite double pulsation. *Ascites* is recognized by abdominal protrusion and fluid wave; rarely it is chylous. The *spleen* may be palpable after portal hypertension is established.

Laboratory Abnormalities

The hemogram may be normal or reveal a normocytic normochromic anemia. Otherwise, especially in more acute constriction, blood counts may be normal or reflect etiologic agents or processes (Table 15.5). Rarely, congestive *hypersplenism* causes selective or pancytopenia. *Liver function tests* are likely to be abnormal due to hepatic congestion and particularly with chronicity and the late occurrence of *cardiac cirrhosis*, including increased conjugated and unconjugated bilirubin, which can rise to the point of cutaneous and conjunctival icterus. Ascitic fluid may be an exudate (typically >2.5 g/dL protein) or a transudate, but with chronicity may have a lower protein concentration and decreased specific gravity. The serum-ascites albumin gradient tends to exceed 10 g/dL, but is nonspecific for the diagnosis. *Hypoalbuminemia* is common, associated with liver impairment, *protein losing enteropathy* or the proteinuria of a *nephrotic syndrome*; each is related to chronically high venous pressure and more prominent in children, in whom each can be the presenting syndrome. An intestinal biopsy may show lymphangiectasis.

Electrocardiography (See Also Chapter 5)

The electrocardiogram (ECG) is nearly always *nonspecifically abnormal* (Figure 15.28), although rarely within normal limits. The T waves are almost always involved, either low to flat, or they show generalized or, less commonly, localized, T inversions; these are usually symmetric unless digitalis has been administered. The QRS and T voltage may be normal or reduced. *Interatrial block* is common, especially with chronicity, with P waves wider than 100 msec and usually notched; sometimes these resemble P mitrale, especially with A-V groove constriction and left atrial enlargement. Right atrial enlargement may accompany, with a large positive P wave or dominantly positive "+–" P in V1. Other local or unequal constriction (page 253) causes changes due to overload of "upstream" cardiac structures, so that some ECGs are consistent with right ventricular hypertrophy or "strain" and may show right axis deviation (Figure 15.28). In chronic constriction, myocardial atrophy probably contributes to low

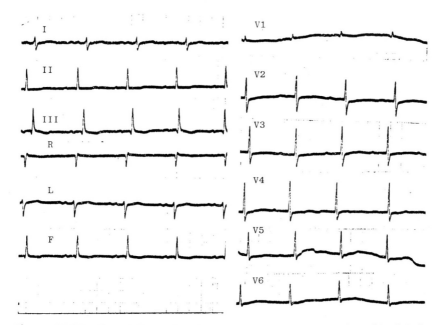

Figure 15.28 Constrictive pericarditis: nonspecific T-wave flattening with slight inversion in III and a VF. The patient has interatrial block resembling P mitrale in lead I, and right axis deviation ($+95°$) with simulation of right ventricular hypertrophy (dominant R wave in V1) probably due to unequal constriction or left AV groove constriction.

voltage, along with fluid retention and pleural effusions. Calcification and fibrosis involving the myocardium, especially with any impeded coronary flow, can produce atrioventricular blocks, intraventricular blocks and even abnormal Q waves. *Mixed ECG pictures* are particularly common in constriction following cardiac operations because of frequently localized or unequal postoperative constriction and also whatever heart disease necessitated surgery.

Constriction can compress even normal coronary arteries sufficiently to produce a positive ECG response to exercise. Subacute and especially chronic constriction is often accompanied by atrial arrhythmias, particularly atrial fibrillation (interatrial block is predictive). Ventricular ectopic beats occur occasionally and are usually followed by reduced left ventricular systolic pressure in the postextrasystolic beat (Figure 15.6).

Differential Diagnosis

Congestive failure due to myocardial, valvular or coronary heart disease is the principal differential diagnosis, usually easily recognized unless coexisting with innocent pericardial lesions. *Restrictive cardiomyopathy* (RCM), often due to myocardial amyloidosis or fibrosis, is particularly important because of virtually identical hemodynamics. The basic problem is to distinguish between abnormal chamber stiffness and abnormal muscle stiffness. *Table 15.7 analyzes its often complex differential diagnosis from constriction.* The principal differential points are the usual thickness of constricting pericardium on imaging and timing of the respiratory changes in Doppler flows. The latter occur within one beat of the onset of inspiration and expiration in constriction and occur later (if they occur at all) in restriction. The atrial and ventricular septa, free in constriction, are more often restricted by the cardiomyopathic process and therefore much less likely to show exaggerated respiratory mobility on echo and other imaging. More rapid early filling and shorter duration of filling characterize constriction, but such relative changes, while helpful, are not decisive. Fortunately, meticulous Doppler echocardiography, combined if necessary with CT, will nearly always make the diagnosis and Doppler tissue imaging, slope of the color M-mode wave and mitral annular velocity give clear separation (Table 15.7). However, occasional cases, particularly those critically constricted by a thin pericardium, will be sufficiently confusing to require endomyocardial and/or pericardial biopsy.

Venous obstructive syndromes, e.g., superior vena cava syndrome and the nephrotic syndrome, especially with gross edema and ascites, are usually easily differentiated by imaging, as is *abdominal disease with ascites*, such as ovarian carcinoma and Laennec's cirrhosis and other forms of hepatic failure. *Right atrial tumors*, especially myxomas, can mimic constriction by compressing the tricuspid valve; any ventricular involvement adds to the mimicry. The congested liver of chronic constriction may develop "reversal" of lobular architecture due to fibrosis extending from central vein to central vein, so that the portal triads appear "central" in these false lobules. In any unclear syndrome, *imaging, hemodynamic data and liver biopsy will often be decisive.* However, a few patients have *simultaneous restrictive cardiomyopathy and constrictive pericarditis*, usually due to radiation therapy of the thorax and mediastinum but also occurring in transplanted hearts. Here, operative intervention with biopsy may be necessary for identification and appropriate choice of management.

Quite suggestive for differentiation are a history of acute pericarditis, especially purulent or tuberculous, but of almost any etiology excepting acute rheumatic fever. A strong S3 and demonstrably rapid termination of early filling (typical of constrictive/restrictive syndromes) indicate the appropriate pathophysiology, whereas pericardial calcification and sufficiently thick pericardium on CT or MRI strongly support the dynamic findings as indicating constriction rather than other conditions.

Table 15.7 Constrictive Pericarditis vs. Restrictive Cardiomyopathy: Differential Features

Generalities
1. Positive diagnosis essential; negative test for one does not imply probability of the other.
2. Eventual endomyocardial and/or pericardial biopsy occasionally inescapable.
3. Both may coexist, *esp.* postirradiation.
4. Physical examination (unless residual pericardial rub) unhelpful.
5. Hemodynamics generally unhelpful.
6. Echo-Doppler + computed tomography nearly always make the diagnosis.

	Constrictive pericarditis	Restrictive cardiomyopathy
Significantly different diastolic pressures	Absent	Occasional
Septal myocardium	Normal	Stiff, may be thick
Systolic function	Normal	Reduced or normal
Ventricular filling	Very rapid in early diastole	Variable
Endomyocardial biopsy	Usually normal (except fibrosis postirradiation or vasculitides)	Abnormal: infiltration; fibrosis, inflammation; amyloidosis
ECG	Usually only ST~T and P wave abnormalities	May have QRS changes: abnormal Q wave conduction defects
Imaging		
Chest x-ray	Calcification sometimes	Absent
Gated MRI/CT	Parietal pericardium thick (may be localized)	Pericardium normal
Angiography	Pericardium thick (may be localized)	Pericardium normal
RA wall	Straight/slightly concave	Convex
Epicardial coronaries	Relatively deep; reduced motion	Normally superficial; normal motion
Echocardiogram		
Transthoracic (TTE)	Probable pericardial thickening	Absent
Transesophageal (TEE)	Pericardial thickening	Absent
Digitized M~mode	Early diastolic abnormal septal motion	Ends before end of rapid filling
	Absent	Reduced LV posterior wall thickening and thinning

(continued)

Table 15.7 Continued

Doppler		
Mitral regurgitation	Occasional	Common
Tricuspid regurgitation	Occasional	Common
Marked respiratory flow changes	Usual; with first beat of each respiratory phase	Occasional; after first beat of respiratory phase
Mitral flow		
E velocity	E velocity increased;	(E velocity usually increased)
	Inspiratory E < expiratory E	No respiratory phase variation
Isovolumic relaxation time	Moderate respiratory variation	Small respiratory variation
Mitral annular motion in early filling (Doppler tissue imaging)	Higher velocity (>8 cm/sec)	Lower velocity (<8 cm/sec)
Tricuspid flow		
E velocity	Inspiratory E > expiratory E	Small respiratory variability
Hepatic vein forward flows	Greatly decreased in diastole in expiration	Systolic > diastolic forward flow
	Increased diastolic reversal in expiration	Increased diastolic and systolic reversals in inspiration
Pulmonary vein flows		
Velocity	Expiratory increase during systole and diastole	Expiratory increase during diastole
x/y	Higher than restrictive cardiomyopathy (RCM)	Lower due to large y
Overall	Increased inspiratory systolic velocity; nearly equal expiratory systolic and diastolic velocities	Diastolic velocity much greater than systolic throughout respiratory cycle

VARIANTS OF CONSTRICTIVE PERICARDITIS

A variety of cases are not "typical" or "classic" due to the unpredictability of the pericardial scarring process (Chapter 14), particularly in contemporary patients following cardiac surgery, with variants that can resemble other conditions.

Unequal/Local Constriction

Chambers, valves and great vessels can be individually or unequally affected by pericardial scarring and calcification, producing murmurs due to locally turbulent blood flow (Chapter 4) and "local" ECG and hemodynamic changes. Echocardiography (TEE or TTE), MRI, or CT scanning may demonstrate thickened or calcified pericardium in the appropriate locations. Annular constriction may be striking, even on chest films (Figure 15.10).

Effusive-Constrictive Pericarditis (ECP)

This condition produces symptoms and objective findings due to variable mixtures of pericardial effusion or tamponade accompanied by constriction of the visceral pericardium (*constrictive epicarditis*) or constriction with local tamponade of one or more chambers due to loculated effusions. *Usually the physical and laboratory findings resemble tamponade more than constriction until after the fluid is drained, when a constrictive picture emerges.* (This includes electric alternation when the parietal pericardium is separately scarred without significant adhesions.) Occasionally tamponade is recognized, but often with an abnormal third heart sound, which is ruled out by pure, classic tamponade dynamics (i.e., no rapid filling period). Table 15.8 summarizes the clinical clues to ECP. In contrast to pure constriction, some degree of pulsus paradoxus is frequent. A large or dominant x descent ($x > y$) in the atrial and venous traces also suggests an element of tamponade. The usual finding of a constrictive epicarditis with an overlying high-pressure fluid layer accounts for such mixed

Table 15.8 **Clinical Clues to Effusive-Constrictive Pericarditis (ECP)**

ECP = epicardial constriction + compressive or noncompressive pericardial
  effusions with hemodynamics of variable constriction + variable tamponade
Abnormal third heart sound (S3) with
  Tamponading effusion
  Effusion without compression
  After drainage of pericardial fluid in absence of heart disease
Kussmaul's sign with
  Tamponade
  Effusion without compression
  After drainage of pericardial fluid
Constriction with
  Pulsus paradoxus > 10 mm Hg
  $x > y$ in jugular venous pulse (and atria)

pictures, although there must be some elasticity in the epicardial constriction to permit this. [Indeed, *elastic epicardial constriction* (see below) underlying an otherwise nontamponading fluid layer can produce classic tamponade dynamics.] After the fluid is drained, pericardial pressure drops to near zero, hemodynamic curves become more typical of constriction and any pulsus paradoxus usually disappears. Conversely, a Kussmaul's sign in what appears to be dominantly tamponade is a clue to effusive-constrictive pericarditis and may be accentuated after the fluid is tapped.

Elastic Constriction

Thick pericardial fluids, particularly rich in blood and fibrin, may organize and resemble tamponade, owing to continuous elastic compression, usually by clot, throughout diastole. The venous and atrial wave forms may show a predominant *x* descent like tamponade, yet there is nearly always no third heart sound because there is no early rapid filling; there may be a fourth heart sound. Variable respiratory responses occur. Occasionally, remarkable growth of malignancies will surround the ventricles, producing a similar picture.

Latent (Occult) Constriction

Patients with dyspnea, fatigue and mild edema with or without a history of acute pericarditis and no specific cardiac findings may show *excessive rises in heart rate and venous pressure with exercise, which may also induce a third heart sound*. Some such patients are volume-depleted due, for example, to diuretics. *Administration of fluids may bring out constrictive dynamics*. In this respect, the situation is analogous to that in low-pressure cardiac tamponade (page 165). Here, an intravenous volume load may be needed to demonstrate high levels of cardiac diastolic pressures as well as characteristic ventricular and atrial pressure curves.

Transient Constriction

Some patients with acute pericarditis appear to show a transient period of subclinical cardiac constriction for days or weeks following apparent recovery. Most have had an effusion, usually during idiopathic, viral or purulent pericarditis, followed by nonspecific symptoms with signs and echo-Doppler and catheterization features of mild constriction. These disappear spontaneously or during continued treatment of the original pericardial insult.

MANAGEMENT

Medical management does not relieve constriction unless there is a very dynamic inflammatory component responsive to anti-inflammatory agents. Of course, the underlying disease should be treated; if it is or is likely to be infection, especially tuberculous, specific therapeutic agents should be instituted before operation and continued afterwards. *Surgery is the definitive treatment and is technically easier early*, before calcification and myocardial abnormalities develop with chronicity (Figure 15.29). Indeed, ultrasonic dissection or a high-speed burr may be needed to safely sculpt and remove calcified pericardium. (Sometimes calcified islands must be left.) Good surgical results occur in patients in better cardiac and systemic condition as well as with less pericardial scarring, calcification and hepatic congestion.

In the modern era, the majority of patients respond well. Some have an immediate postoperative diuresis (often profuse), others a slower recovery in weeks or months following pericardiectomy. Removal of pericardium should be as extensive as possible, especially the diaphragmatic surfaces contacting the

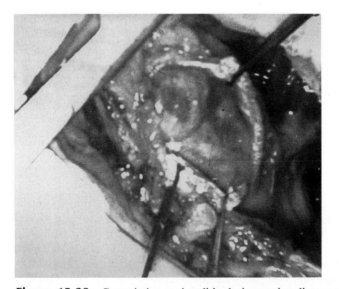

Figure 15.29 Constrictive pericarditis during pericardiectomy. The heart bulges through the incised, partly resected pericardium. (From Spodick, Chronic and Constrictive Pericarditis, 1964; author's copyright.)

ventricles, always taking care to spare the phrenic nerves, which descend in the anterior pericardium. *Appropriate depth is achieved when the coronary arteries are exposed and myocardium is visible between them.* Indeed, removal of an adherent pericardium may require a prolonged procedure complicated by frequent hypotension, decreases in cardiac output and arrhythmias. Venous inflow and cardiac outflow should not be subject to excessive tension from manipulation and blood replacement should be readily available for bleeding from raw surfaces. Of course, antiarrhythmic agents and a defibrillator must be available.

Poorer results are seen with (1) inadequate resection, (2) uncorrected coronary disease, (3) higher New York Heart Association classifications for "congestive failure," (4) older age, (5) after radiation pericarditis, (6) with chronicity—including peripheral organ failure (particularly renal and hepatic), ascites, edema, or both are ominous; (7) with severe myocardial atrophy and fibrosis (detectable by CT and MRI); and (8) with significant arrhythmias reflecting myocardial impairment. In high-risk patients, subtotal pericardiectomy through a median sternotomy may be effective. It may be necessary also to decorticate lungs affected by a constrictive pleuritis traceable to the original viral, tuberculous or other inflammation.

Preventive therapy (not always successful) depends on adequate treatment of acute pericarditis and drainage of significant collections of fluid and pus. *Corticosteroids frequently fail to prevent constriction.* Whether colchicine and nonsteroidal anti-inflammatory agents have a preventive effect is unknown. There is considerable promise for *intrapericardial urokinase* following drainage of bloody and purulent fluids, common harbingers of future constriction. However, before urokinase is used, the etiology of the pericardial disease should be clear and contraindications absent (neoplastic implants, for example, may tend to bleed).

KEY POINTS

1. Constrictive pericarditis can follow most etiologies of pericardial disease acutely (*acute constriction* and *transient constriction*). More often there is a delay of months (*subacute constriction*) to years (*chronic constriction*).
2. Pericardial constriction resembles tamponade hemodynamically, with some similar respiratory responses to cardiac flows and pressures. Kussmaul's sign is characteristic of constriction only. True pulsus paradoxus is rare and usually due to complicating disorders. *Effusive-constrictive pericarditis* has features of tamponade and constriction, one or the other usually predominant.
3. Constrictive (restrictive) hemodynamics are characterized by diastolic pressures equilibration and an early halt to ventricular filling expressed in ventricular pressure

curves with a dip-and-plateau ("square root") diastolic configuration. Atrial and venous curves have deep y and x descents (typically $y > x$).

4. Imaging methods can identify pericardial thickening and calcification which, because of virtually identical hemodynamics, may be decisive in differentiating constriction from restrictive cardiomyopathy and others of its mimics. However, improved diagnostic methods identify restrictive dynamics with an increasing number of thin pericardial constrictions.

5. Doppler flows in constriction show reciprocal respiratory changes beginning with the first beats of inspiration and expiration following the first respective respiratory diastoles.

6. A characteristic very early and loud abnormal S3 coincides with the ventricular diastolic dip and the nadir of the atrial and jugular y descents—an auscultatory marker of the sudden halt to ventricular filling—which is often palpable and may be mistaken for the first heart sound.

7. Symptoms mainly reflect systemic venous congestion and poor ventricular stroke volume. Fluid and electrolyte retention and venous hypertension contribute to ascites (along with exudation of liver lymph) and edema. Ascites frequently occurs without or out of proportion to edema, particularly in chronic cases.

8. Medical therapy may help symptomatically, but definitive treatment is pericardiectomy.

BIBLIOGRAPHY

Anand, I.S., Phil, D., Ferrari, R., et al. Pathogenesis of edema in constrictive pericarditis. Circulation 1991; 83:1880–1887.

Appleton, C.P. Editorial comment—Doppler assessment of left ventricular diastolic function: The refinements continue. J. Am. Coll. Cardiol. 1993; 21:1692–1700.

Bernardi, L., Saviolo, R., Spodick, D.H. Noninvasive assessment of central circulatory pressures by analysis of ear densitographic changes during the Valsalva maneuver. Am. J. Cardiol. 1989; 64:787–792.

Browing, C.A., Bishop, R.S., Heilpern, R.J., et al. Accelerate constrictive pericarditis in procainamide-induced systemic lupus erythematosus. Am. J. Cardiol. 1984; 53:376–377.

Byrd, B.F., Linden, R.W.: Superior vena cava Doppler flow velocity patterns in pericardial disease. Am. J. Cardiol. 1990; 65:1464–1470.

Candell-Riera, J., DelCastillo, H.G., Permanyer-Miralda, G., Soler-Soler, J. Echocardiographic features of the interventricular septum in chronic constrictive pericarditis. Circulation 1978; 57:1154–1158.

Doi, Y.L., Sugiura, T., Spodick, D.H. Motion of pulmonic valve and constrictive pericarditis. Chest 1981; 81:513–515.

Fowler, N.O. Clinical pathologic correlations: Constrictive pericarditis: Its history and current status. Clin. Cardiol. 1995; 18:341–350.

Garcia, M.J., Rodriguez, L., Ares, M., Griffin B.P., Thomas, J.D., Klein, A.L. Differentiation of constrictive pericarditis from restrictive cardiopathy: assessment of left ventricular diastolic velocities in longitudinal axis by Doppler tissue imaging. J. Am. Coll. Cardiol. 1996; 27:108-114.

Hancock, E.W. Subacute effusive constrictive pericarditis. Circulation 1971; 43:183-192.

Ling LH, Oh JK, Seward JB, Danielson GK, Tajik AJ. Clinical profile of constrictive pericarditis in the modern era: A survey of 135 cases. J Am Coll Cardiol 1996; 27:32A-33A.

McCaughan, B.C., Schaff, H.V., Piehler, J.M., et al. Early and late results of pericardiectomy for constrictive pericarditis. J. Thorac. Cardiovasc. Surg. 1985; 89:340-350.

Meijburg, H.W.J., Visser, C.A., Bredee, J.J., Westerhof, P.W. Clinical relevance of Doppler pulmonary venous flow characteristics in constrictive pericarditis. Eur. Heart J. 1995; 16:506-513.

Meyer, T.E., Sareli, P., Marcus, R.H., et al. Mechanism underlying Kussmaul's sign in chronic constrictive pericarditis. Am. J. Cardiol. 1989; 64:1069-1072.

Nakatani, S., Yoshitomi, H., Wada, K., et al. Noninvasive estimation of left ventricular end-diastolic pressure using transthoracic Doppler-determined pulmonary venous atrial flow reversal. Am. J. Cardiol. 1994; 73:1017-1018.

Rienmüller, R., Gürgan, M., Erdmann, E., Kemkes, B.M., Kreutzer, E., Weinhold, G. CT and MR evaluation of pericardial constriction. J. Thorac. Imag. 1993; 8:108-121.

Runyon, B.A., Montano, A.A., Akriviadis, A., et al. The serum-ascites albumin gradient is superior to the exudate-transudate concept in the differential diagnosis of ascites. Ann. Intern. Med. 1992; 117:215-220.

Sagrista-Sauleda, J., Permanyer-Miralda, G., Candell-Riera, J., et al. Transient cardiac constriction: An unrecognized pattern of evolution in effusive acute idiopathic pericarditis. Am. J. Cardiol. 1987; 59:961-966.

Santamore, W.P., Bartlett, R., VanBuren, S.J., et al. Ventricular coupling in constrictive pericarditis. Circulation 1986; 74:597-602.

Shabetai, R. The pericardium and its diseases. In: Hurst, J.W. (ed.). The Heart. New York: McGraw-Hill, 1986, pp. 1249-1275.

Spodick, D.H., Kumar, S. Subacute constrictive pericarditis with cardiac tamponade. Dis. Chest 1968; 54:62-66.

Spodick, D.H. Acoustic phenomena in pericardial disease. Am. Heart J. 1971; 81:114-124.

Spodick, D.H. Low atrial natriuretic factor levels and absent pulmonary edema in pericardial compression of the heart. Am. J. Cardiol. 1989; 63:1271-1272.

Spodick, D.H. Disease of the pericardium. In: Parmley, W.W., Chatterjee, J. (eds.). Cardiology. Vol. 2. Philadelphia: Lippincott, 1992, Chap. 43.

Spodick, D.H. Chronic and Constrictive Pericarditis. New York: Grune & Stratton, 1994.

Takata, M., Beloucif, S., Shimada, M., Robotham, J.L. Superior and inferior vena caval flows during respiration: Pathogenesis of Kussmaul's sign. Am. J. Physiol. 1992; 262:H763–H770.

Tei, C., Child, J.S., Tanaka, H., Shah, P.M. Diagnostic techniques: Atrial systolic notch on the interventricular septal echogram: An echocardiographic sign of constrictive pericarditis. J. Am. Coll. Cardiol. 1983; 1:907–912.

Tona, I.C., Danielson, G.K. Surgical management of pericardial diseases. Cardiol. Clin. 1990; 8:683–696.

Wilkinson, P., Pinto, B., Senior, J.R. Reversible protein-losing enteropathy with intestinal lymphangiectasia secondary to chronic constrictive pericarditis. N. Engl. J. Med. 1985; 273:1178–1181.

16

Infectious Pericarditis

Generalities

Virtually every infectious form of pericarditis presents a clinical picture conforming to some degree to the descriptions in Chapter 8, the differences being characteristic of particular etiologic types. For example, acute viral pericarditis is especially likely to provoke the entire range of subjective and objective acute findings. In contrast, tuberculous and fungal pericarditis can provide the classic acute tableau, but they are often quite insidious, overshadowed by manifestations of systemic disease and first recognizable by a complication like cardiac tamponade. Since any infectious agent that can reach the pericardium can inflame it directly or set up conditions for damage from a variety of immune responses, pericardial involvement occurs in every kind of infectious disease. Finally, whenever the common signs of an infectious process are muted or absent, it is important to rule out pericarditis as a complication of inapparent myocardial infarction (pages 349–356) or a postmyocardial injury syndrome (page 350) mimicking infectious, particularly viral, pericarditis. Table 16.1 presents the etiologic spectrum of the infectious pericarditides.

VIRAL PERICARDITIS

Pathogenesis

The most common form clinically encountered, viral pericarditis, has been provoked mainly by the same viruses that cause myocarditis (Table 16.1). The

Table 16.1 Etiology of Infectious Pericarditis

I. Viruses	II. Bacteria
Coxsackie B and A	*Staphylococcus*
Other enteroviruses	*Streptococcus* (aerobic and anaerobic)
Echovirus	*Meningococcus*; other Neisseria
Adenovirus	*Pneumococcus* (*S. pneumoniae*)
Epstein-Barr virus	*Salmonella*
Cytomegalovirus	Gram-negative organisms
AIDS/HIV	*Haemophilus*
Hepatitis A, B, (?C)	*Legionella*
Varicella	*Francisella tularensis*
Variola/vaccinia	*Escherichia coli*
Rubella	*Klebsiella*
(Infectious mononucleosis)	*Pseudomonas* (including melioidosis)
Herpes simplex	*E. coli*
Poliovirus	*Spirillum*
Lassa virus	*Serratia*
Parvovirus	*Yersinia*
(Kawasaki disease)	*Eikenella*
(Influenza)	*Vibrio*
	Brucellaceae Acti
	Actinobacillus
	Bacteroides
	Moraxella
	Listeria monocytogenes
	Campylobacter
	Mycobacterium
	M. tuberculosis
	M. avium
	M. kansasii
	M. chelonei
	Others
	Helicobacter
	Clostridium group
	Rhodococcus equi
	Peptostreptococcus
	Whipple's disease: *Tropheryma whippeli*; other
	Acinetobacter calcoaceticus
	Corynebacterium

(*continued*)

Table 16.1 Continued

III. Fungi	VII. Spirochetes
Histoplasma	*Borrelia burgdorferi*
Coccidioides	*Treponema pallidum*
Blastomyces	
Candida	VIII. Other
Aspergillus	*Actinomyces*
Cryptococcus	*Nocardia*
Pneumocystis	*Mycoplasma*
Zygomycetes (mucormycosis)	*Morganella morganii*

IV. Parasites
Echinococcus
Microfilaria
Trichinella
Protozoa
   Toxoplasma gondii
   Amoebae (esp. *Entamoeba histolytica*)
   Trypanosoma cruzi (Chagas' disease)
   Babesia microti
Necator americanus
Fasciola hepatica
Dracunculus (guinea worm)
Schistosoma
Trichuris

V. Rickettsiae
R. rickettsii (Rocky Mountain spotted fever)
Coxiella burnetii (Q fever)
R. mooseri (endemic typhus)
R. conorii (Mediterranean spotted fever; boutonneuse fever)

VI. Chlamydiaceae
C. trachomatis
Psittacosis–lymphopathia venereum group
C. psittaci
C. pneumonitidis

degree of involvement of either or both tissues depends on host susceptibility and the particular agent, with inflammatory abnormalities due to immune complexes, or direct viral attack, or both. Thus, early viral replication in pericardial tissue elicits cellular and humoral immune responses, which, if adequate, eliminate the virus. If inadequate, direct tissue damage continues or a destructive autoimmune reaction develops. Indeed, viral genomic fragments have been identified in pericardial tissue that may not be capable of replication, yet may serve as a constant source of antigen to stimulate immune responses.

Pericarditis is relatively common during *enterovirus* epidemics with characteristic spring and fall peak incidences, particularly *Coxsackie B* and *A* groups, *adenovirus, rhinoviruses, echovirus* type 8 and *influenza*. Familiar systemic infections like *hepatitis* (particularly type *B*), infectious mononucleosis (particularly *Epstein-Barr* virus) and *Mycoplasma pneumoniae* can involve the pericardium. These, *cytomegalovirus* (CMV) and *herpesvirus* particularly target immunocompromised patients. Other examples of the wide etiologic range include, fortunately uncommonly, *mumps, varicella, rubella, rubeola* and even *poliovirus* among others. *Variola* is extremely rare, although hypersensitivity pericarditis occasionally follows *vaccinia* (vaccination). *Parvovirus* has been implicated in some cases of Kawasaki's disease with pericardial effusion.

Virus-specific IgM, often with IgG and occasionally IgA, can be found in pericardium and myocardium even years after the original infection. Most cardiotropic viruses involve the pericardium and myocardium hematogenously, although cardiac and thoracic surgery afford opportunities for direct involvement (see "Postpericardiotomy Syndrome," page 403). A latent period between a recognized viral infection and the onset of acute pericarditis is compatible with both direct pericardial infection and immunopathic induction of pericardial inflammation.

Distinctive Clinical Features

Most cases of pericarditis of unknown origin—"idiopathic" or "nonspecific" pericarditis—are probably viral, and the majority of these, due mainly to enteroviruses, frequently produce the clinical epitome of acute pericarditis: pain, pericardial rub, more or less typical electrocardiographic (ECG) changes, elevated acute-phase reactants (e.g., sedimentation rate, C-reactive protein), varying degrees of fever, leukocytosis (with a relative or absolute lymphocytosis) and variably elevated myocardial enzymes. "Variably" ranges from normal levels to modest and occasionally very high elevations, reflecting, as does the ECG, variably intense myocardial inflammation (page 40). In common with most forms of acute pericarditis, there is a male preponderance of 3 or 4 to 1. Pericarditis may occur during the initial viral infection, but more often appears 1 to 3 weeks after an upper respiratory or gastrointestinal inflammatory syndrome—too late to recover the virus itself. Many patients will have pulmonary infiltrates and pleural effusions, often with cough. Any viral pericarditis may have smaller or larger pericardial effusions and develop tamponade, although most are "clinically dry," i.e., with no or clinically silent effusion (Chapter 8). Clinical illness lasts a few days to a few weeks; it most often resolves within 2 weeks and is self-limited.

Complications of viral pericarditis include unresolved inflammation, particularly recurrent pericarditis due to an immunopathy rather than reinfection and characterized mainly by pain but often recurrent pericardial effusion. One to three recurrences affect up to 50% of patients, mainly within 8 months of the initial attack. Typically, they are shorter and milder, characterized by pain and usually without ECG changes, which are nearly always present in the index attack. Sometimes they are provoked by some unrelated infection or physical (rarely mental) stress. (See Recurrent Pericarditis, Chapter 24). *Pleural effusions*, particularly on the left, are common; more so in those patients with pericardial effusions. Some patients, especially those with an initial pericardial effusion, develop *transient, usually asymptomatic pericardial constriction* detected by noninvasive or catheter follow-up over a period of weeks. Acute effusive viral pericarditis, particularly after tamponade, is also associated with ultimate *classic constriction* more often than "dry" pericarditis. (See "Constrictive Pericarditis," Chapter 15). In occasional patients with a significant element of myocarditis, heart muscle disease may proceed after the pericardial manifestations have become clinically silent; this is more common in children. *Any significant arrhythmias or conduction defects suggest independent heart disease or a significant element of myocarditis*; uncomplicated acute pericarditis appears not to provoke arrhythmias.

Differential and etiologic diagnosis includes acute myocardial infarction, particularly when there is an atypical ECG or when computer interpretation misdiagnoses acute pericarditis as "anterolateral infarction," for example. Pericarditis accompanying a true myocardial infarction may be identifiable by a rub or pleuritic pain (Chapter 20). These may be confusing when pericarditis follows a "silent" myocardial infarction (page 339). Other conditions to differentiate include traumatic pericarditis, systemic lupus erythematosus and nonviral, especially bacterial, pericardial infection. Preceding upper respiratory infections or gastrointestinal "flu"—rare in tuberculous and neoplastic pericarditis—and the presence of related systemic viral disorders (e.g., hepatitis) should suggest viral etiology. Those with infectious mononucleosis, especially younger patients, usually present with severe sore throat, adenopathy and positive heterophile antibody and Monospot tests. Even a fourfold increase in neutralizing antibody titer is only supporting evidence but helps in the etiologic diagnosis. However, newer techniques can identify minute amounts of viral nucleic acid; viral genomes can be demonstrated by the polymerase chain reaction (PCR), which amplifies viral DNA, along with in situ hybridization. Reverse immunoassay (RIA) can demonstrate virus-specific immunoglobulins like IgM, IgG, and IgA. However, it may not be necessary to use these procedures when the diagnosis seems clinically secure. In an otherwise healthy patient, a strong clinical suspicion of viral or idiopathic pericarditis should be adequate, especially since pericardiocentesis and other invasive procedures to obtain samples for diagnosis add little to the management and carry certain risks.

Management

Effective antiviral agents have not been available or even necessary for the management of most viral pericarditis. Perhaps those used in human immuno-deficiency virus (HIV) and allied infections have some impact. The vast majority of cases, being due to common viruses like the enterovirus group, are clinically recognized long after direct viral activity has ceased. Therefore, *treatment is for symptoms and complications*. Pain, usually pleuritic and usually limited to the first day or the first week, can usually be managed by giving nonsteroidal anti-inflammatory drugs (NSAID), notably aspirin and ibuprofen, at dose levels sufficient to suppress the symptoms as well as any accompanying fever. Cough, which sometimes exacerbates pericardial pain, should be suppressed by antitussive agents. Nontamponading pericardial effusions do not require drainage except in the rare event that they become very large and chronic. Tamponade, of course, requires prompt evacuation of fluid (page 173). Usually, acute management is quite successful. However, virus-specific immunoglobulins are found in many cases of chronic relapsing pericarditis (Chapter 24) and dilated cardiomyopathy.

BACTERIAL PERICARDITIS
(NONTUBERCULOUS SUPPURATIVE PERICARDITIS)

Acute suppurative pericarditis simultaneously threatens tamponade and septicemia. Pericarditis due to pus-producing organisms (*pyopericardium*) is often especially serious and severe in children and immunocompromised patients and when due to very destructive organisms like staphylococci. A surprising number, however, may be silent, presenting as cardiac tamponade or overshadowed by systemic disease and discovered at autopsy, particularly in the elderly. Although many forms due to gram-negative organism such as *Escherichia coli*, *Salmonella* and other nosocomially acquired infections and opportunistic organisms have appeared increasingly, *the most common forms remain streptococcal, pneumococcal* (*Streptococcus pneumoniae*) *and staphylococcal*. Rarely, gas-producing organisms like *Clostridia* cause *pneumopericardium*. Indeed, in adults, pneumopericardium and *pneumopyopericardium* of bacterial origin are most often due to a fistula between the pericardium and a hollow viscus (page 363).

Pathogenesis

Bacterial pericarditis (Table 16.1) is established by either intrapericardial implantation, with bacterial invasion breaching the pericardium, or by hematogenous (bacteremic) spread. Invasion from contiguous foci or traumatic implantation includes sources such as cardiothoracic surgery, mediastinitis, wound infection, myocardial abscesses (including infected myocardial infarction), infective endocarditis (particularly staphylococcal), subdiaphragmatic abscesses, wounds and perforation from neighboring viscera. The majority of pneumococcal cases occur during pneumococcal pneumonia, often with empyema. *Legionella* pericarditis also usually accompanies *Legionella* pneumonia, although sometimes isolated to the pericardium or accompanying a *Legionella* myocarditis.

Rarely, pericardial invasion proceeds from spread along fascial planes from oral cavity infections, particularly periodontal and peritonsillar abscesses, or via an esophagopericardial or other fistula. The latter may carry gas-producing organisms like *clostridia*, producing a *pyopneumopericardium*. Occasionally infected mediastinal nodes erode the pericardium.

Hematogenous dissemination includes bacteremia of any kind, though often from a distant infection involving skin, soft tissue wounds and, particularly in children, osteomyelitis. Children with staphylococcal bacteremias can develop staphylococcal pericarditis without endocarditis, although they can also develop endocarditis without cardiac disease. *Preexisting nonbacterial pericardial effusion, as in rheumatoid arthritis, sarcoid or uremia, can be infected hematogenously.* Indeed, this is probably the pathogenesis of various kinds of "primary" bacterial pericarditis in which only the pericardium seems to be the locus of disease. For example, *Neisseria* pericarditis, particularly involving *N. meningitidis* group C, occurs without or with meningitis, the latter circumstance producing "primary" meningococcal pericarditis. Other *Neisseria*, including the gonococcus, rarely do this. On the other hand, the *Neisseria* group and other organisms can evoke a sterile, immunopathic effusion, sometimes accompanied by immunopathic or infectious systemic reactions like arthritis and ophthalmitis. Finally, *Salmonella* pericarditis, usually due to *Salmonella* bacteremia, occurs with or without an enteritic syndrome.

While the success of antimicrobial therapy in recent decades has decreased the incidence of the common gram-positive infections, there is a definite (relative and absolute) increase, usually nosocomially acquired, of infection with *multiple organisms* and *gram-negative* organisms, especially in immunocompromised patients and after thoracotomy. These include an increasing number manifesting antibiotic resistance.

Although *Haemophilus influenzae* occurs sporadically in adults, children remain particularly susceptible to it. Such infection produces pericarditis during respiratory illness and even after, cellulitus of the skin. H. influenzae typically provokes a very thick, fibrinopurulent exudate similar to cottage cheese or scrambled eggs which can defeat attempts at percutaneous drainage. Moreover, all bacterial forms of pericarditis in children tend to produce tamponade and rapid constriction if not managed urgently.

Distinctive Characteristics

Suppurative pericarditis is most often acute and fulminant, particularly in younger patients, arising over several days with rapid development of tamponade or presenting as tamponade. In contrast, particularly in older patients, infections may have a reduced tempo and therefore be clinically silent or over-shadowed by other symptoms and signs of systemic disease. *Effusion is the rule*; the pericardial fluid is a turbid exudate characterized by polymorphonuclear leukocytes, increased lactic dehydrogenase and decreased glucose. Apart from the occasional slow, insidious infection, there is typically tachycardia, fever, toxicity, chills and night sweats. Chest pain is variable and a pericardial rub is audible in the majority of patients. Cough is common, especially when pleuropulmonary involvement produces pneumonia and empyema. Chest x-rays usually show an enlarged cardiopericardial silhouette With gas-producing or-ganisms, there are lucent "bubbles" or an "air"-fluid interface. *Leukocytosis* with a marked left shift is typical, although limited to absent in debilitated and immunosuppressed patients. Blood and pericardial fluid cultures should disclose the organism in the absence of effective antimicrobial treatment. The electro-cardiogram frequently shows stage I change (page XX), although it may be nonspecifically altered, particularly if the lesion is discovered late. The echo-cardiogram usually discloses an effusion. Inflammatory infiltration of the peri-cardium can be identified by scintigraphy with indium 111 or gallium 67, mod-alities that can also respond to leukemic infiltrations. With survival, there is a strong tendency to encapsulation and loculation, producing pericardial abscesses that may resemble cysts (page 73); these are identified by echocardiography, computed tomography or magnetic resonance imaging.

Etiology–specific diagnosis depends on smears, cultures and more sophis-ticated searching for the organism—for example, antigen detection by counter-immunoelectrophoresis of pericardial fluids (especially in patients in whom treatment appears to sterilize the fluid, producing negative cultures). The prin-cipal *differential diagnoses* include tuberculous pericarditis (page 269) and viral pericarditis (page 260).

Pericarditis Associated with Infective Endocarditis

Although pericarditis during endocarditis can produce a dramatic clinical pic-ture, it may be silent and is more often found at autopsy. *Acute endocarditis* may provoke an immunopathic pericardial effusion with immune complex depo-sition, while *subacute endocarditis* usually causes an infective pericardial ef-fusion. *Bacterial endocarditis* involves the pericardium most often by erosion of a valve-ring abscess, particularly aortic but also mitral, or by rupture of a mycotic aortic sinus abscess. Less often, myocardial abscesses due to septic coronary emboli penetrate the pericardium. Rarely, penetration produces a false ventricular aneurysm (page 346). The most common organisms are *Streptococ-cus viridans* and particularly *Staphylococcus aureus*, because of its great tissue destructiveness. Another mode of infection is hematogenous: the same bact-eremia infecting the endocardium simultaneously infects the pericardium. More-over, a sterile "sympathetic" effusion is not rare and congestive heart failure may produce an uninfected hydropericardium (page 130). The sterile, presumably immunopathic effusions resemble those of the postmyocardial infarction syndrome. Generalized immunopathic phenomena, as in any kind of endocarditis, include rheumatoid factor production and circulating immune complexes with decreased serum complement and increased gamma globulin. Hemorrhagic effusions in endocarditis follow direct pericardial irritation or bleeding from rupture of a mycotic abscess. Clues to accompanying myocardial and valve-ring invasion from bacterial endocarditis include degrees of atrioventricular block, particularly prolonged PR interval, and bundle branch block, each most common with staphylococcal endocarditis.

Management

The basis of management is effective systemic antimicrobial agents and pericardial drainage, preferably with exploration of the pericardium. *Systemically administered antibiotics appear to achieve excellent levels in pericardial fluid.* Exploration is needed, because these infections tend to loculate and form adhesions and to constrict. In critical tamponade, simple drainage may first be used to relieve the emergency, with exploration postponed. However, pericardial fluid and tissue should be obtained for Gram, acid-fast and fungal stains along with appropriate culturing, including cultures for aerobes and anaerobes, as well as antimicrobial susceptibility tests. (If initial treatment based on recognition of a systemic or bacteremic infection appears to be definitely successful, these studies become much less urgent.)

Mortality, due principally to cardiac tamponade, toxicity and rapid or slow constriction, traditionally approaching 100%, has been reduced to less than 50% by timely surgical drainage alone and further reduced by effective antibiotics.

Surgical drainage is always preferable, and particularly when etiologic diagnosis is uncertain; it also permits pericardiectomy when adhesions and loculations predict constriction (page 217). With or without definitive surgical intervention, urokinase may be used within the pericardial cavity to destroy fibrinous adhesions. Iodine-containing irrigation fluids should be avoided because they may provoke constriction. If, because of a patient's generally precarious condition, *catheter drainage* is elected, this must be prolonged, using large catheters with frequent irrigation including streptokinase or urokinase. Very thick purulent and sanguinopurulent exudates resisting free drainage may require repeated intrapericardial instillation of streptokinase (to activate the fibrinolytic system) combined with streptodornase (to liquify viscous nucleoproteins in pus) alternated with appropriate antibiotics. A clue to loculation and potential constriction is failure to improve after appropriate treatment.

TUBERCULOUS PERICARDITIS

Since the middle of the 20th century, the incidence of pericarditis due to *Mycobacterium tuberculosis* has fallen steadily due to improved public health measures and effective antimycobacterial treatments; more recently, *atypical forms of mycobacteria*, along with classic tubercle bacilli, have increasingly appeared in immunocompromised patients, particularly those with acquired immunodeficiency syndrome (AIDS) due to HIV, lymphocytotropic and other viruses, and some of those with impaired immune systems of other etiologies (e.g., antineoplastic therapies). High incidence continues, as with all tuberculosis, in the poorer nations; it is the commonest cause of pericarditis in Transkei and India, for example.

Tuberculous pericarditis is the classic main etiology of constrictive pericarditis; indeed, *the majority of books, series and case reports describing its symptoms, signs and laboratory findings are seriously confounded by those cases due to elements of constriction and tamponade* rather than tuberculous *pericarditis per se.* (For example, hepatosplenomegaly, pulsus paradoxus or an abnormal S3 are due to compressive sequelae.) On the other hand, although pleural effusions are common, a relatively small proportion of patients with tuberculous pericarditis have active pulmonary tuberculosis. In the United States, its principal importance has been differential diagnosis from a variety of pericarditic syndromes and the classic difficulty of isolating tubercle bacilli.

Pathogenesis

The pericardium may be infected by hematogenous, lymphatic, peribronchial or contiguous spread of tuberculous infection. *Hematogenous dissemination* occurs during all primary pericardial infections, and this may include acute pericarditis, particularly in children and immunocompromised hosts. Later, established tuberculosis and tuberculous abscesses, particularly in the genitourinary and skeletal systems, may spread hematogenously to the pericardium; only occasionally is the pericardium infected during miliary tuberculosis. *Lymphatic spread* occurs from lung, bronchi and peribronchial and other mediastinal lymph nodes. *Contiguous infection* may be most important and involves intrapericardial inoculation from mediastinal nodal, pleural and, rarely, myocardial tuberculosis. Some of the material penetrating into the pericardial cavity undergoes proteolytic degradation and antigen processing into individual peptides. *Immune responses to such components of the tubercle bacillus* cause much of the morbidity of the active tuberculous process. These include *antimyolemmal antibodies*, a subtype of antisarcolemmal antibody, which are very common in tuberculous pericarditis and probably play a role in its pathogenesis. The bacillus' protein antigens induce delayed hypersensitivity responses that stimulate lymphocytes to release *lymphokines*; these activate macrophages and influence granuloma formation. Moreover, tuberculous effusions are provoked by hypersensitivity to surprisingly small amounts of tuberculoprotein.

There are *three classic pathologic stages of tuberculous pericarditis* (with or without effective antituberculous therapy, constriction remains common enough that it may be considered a *fourth stage*): (1) Diffuse fibrinous exudation with initially a polymorphonuclear leukocytic response, relatively abundant mycobacteria and beginning granuloma due to loose organization of T cells and macrophages. (2) Serous, usually serosanguineous, effusion—usually slow and asymptomatic—with mainly a lymphocytic exudate including monocytes and foam cells. (3) Absorption of the effusion with dense organization of granulomas, caseation and pericardial thickening due to fibrin masses, collagenosis, and ultimately fibrosis; mycobacteria are now particularly difficult to find. (4) *Constrictive scarring*: survival with progressive replacement of the fibrinous and granulomatous matter by fibrous tissue, which progressively contracts on the cardiac chambers; this can develop despite effective antituberculous therapy for lesions in the pericardium and elsewhere. *Calcification* may occur at any stage, at first microscopically and, depending on the tempo and duration of the process, with a tendency to form hoops, bands and above all, irregular sheets of calcium salts over any part of or the entire cardiac surface. Although *the pericardium may be extensively calcified without clinical constriction*, gross calcification is a hallmark of classic chronic constrictive pericarditis and is much less common in subacute and more acute constriction, the forms more often seen in the United States and western populations. Most active infections are due to reactivation of a dormant remote infection, but recently growing numbers appear to represent initial (primary) infection.

Tuberculous pericarditis may surface in the clinical form of acute or chronic pericardial effusion and occasionally as a variant of cholesterol pericarditis (page 85) with or without overt cardiac tamponade and usually with considerable fibrin, adhesions and loculations demonstrable by imaging or by deliberate introduction of air into the pericardium after drainage of effusions (now rare). That "clinically dry" or noneffusive acute tuberculous pericarditis can heal without treatment is suggested by the de novo appearance of constriction without a recognizable acute stage.

Distinctive Clinical Features

The clinical expression of tuberculous pericarditis depends on the tempo of inflammation, which is usually relatively slow and indolent following an insidious onset and often accidental discovery (especially in those cases surfacing as rather large effusions). Occasionally, an aggressive course with acute tamponade, often mixed with constrictive components, discloses the lesion. Children and immunocompromised patients more often present with classic acute pericarditis. Indeed, most patients have no history of an acute phase of pericarditis and often no history of tuberculosis; *evidence of pulmonary tuberculosis is quite the exception*. On the other hand, like tuberculous meningitis, tuberculous pericarditis may even erupt during appropriate antimicrobial treatment for tuberculosis elsewhere. By the time it is clinically apparent, patients tend to have *lymphocytosis* both in the blood and in the pericardial fluid (over 50% small lymphocytes) with an increased proportion of T-lymphocytes. *Lymphopenia* is associated with decreased immunologic responsiveness. At any stage, tuberculosis may also invade the myocardium, usually without distinctive symptoms unless myocardial involvement is extensive.

There are eight general modes of presentation covering almost any "pericardial" syndrome:

1. *Typical, painful acute pericarditis* with or without minimal to large effusion; with or without fever, cough and malaise
2. *Silent pericardial effusion*, often large and chronic
3. *Tamponade* without other symptoms except perhaps fever
4. *Acute constrictive pericarditis* (i.e., constriction appearing over a period of days to a month), usually after drainage of an effusion or disappearance of fluid under therapy
5. *Subacute constriction* (a course of weeks or months) with varying amounts of fluid, i.e., *effusive-constrictive pericarditis*
6. *Chronic constrictive pericarditis*
7. *Pericardial calcification* with or without hemodynamic consequences
8. *Fever of unknown origin*, usually with constitutional symptoms like anorexia and weight loss

Tuberculous effusions typically increase slowly, with few or no signs and symptoms, ultimately producing tamponade or, after reabsorption or drainage, effusive-constrictive or constrictive pericarditis. This behavior, plus the general modes of presentation enumerated, ensures that tuberculous pericarditis may be first recognized at any stage, though more often with tamponade, constriction or combinations of the two. Yet, these may be misleading, especially when clinically silent constriction causes hepatic congestion and ascites simulating cirrhosis of the liver (page 246). On the other hand, those presenting as recognizable constrictive pericarditis may have few constitutional signs and symptoms if the inflammatory process has burned itself out. Moreover, the tuberculous etiology may not be clear, since so many forms of pericarditis are capable of causing constriction (Chapter 15).

Except in children and in the immunocompromised host, clinically typical acute pericarditis is uncommon, probably because of the usual insidious, slow tempo of the infection. Yet a few patients will have a pericardial rub and precordial pain; more often there is precordial discomfort which the patient may find difficult to describe. Dyspnea, particularly dyspnea on exertion, may follow pulmonary restriction due to a very large pericardial effusion, with unilateral or more often bilateral pleural effusions. Tuberculous pericarditis must be kept in mind as a cause of *fever of unknown origin* and suspicion should be increased if the cardiopericardial silhouette on chest film is increased, irrespective of any pulmonary lesions. Suspicion is heightened if the increased silhouette is demonstrated by imaging to be due to more or less chronic pericardial effusion that proves to be hemorrhagic. Indeed, *tuberculous pericarditis must be ruled in or out when any pericarditis does not rapidly resolve on nonsteroidal anti-flammatory drug (NSAID) treatment and in any tamponade of obscure origin.* This is particularly the case in immigrants from third-world countries; in elderly patients, in whom viral pericarditis is rare and cancer can be ruled out; and in immunocompromised patients, especially those with AIDS, in whom miliary or pericardial tuberculosis may be the first manifestation.

Diagnosis

Identification of *M. tuberculosis* in pericardial fluid or tissue is specific for the diagnosis, but *a negative result does not rule out tuberculous pericarditis.* Organisms are so difficult to find by smear that *all* fluid obtained from drainage should be centrifuged and studied by smear, culture, and, if necessary, DNA amplification. Demonstration of extrapericardial tuberculosis—including lung, pleura and lymph nodes—is only indirect support for the diagnosis, so that pericardial tissue should be biopsied either by subxiphoid incision (also excellent for drainage and inspection of the pericardium) or, better, by pericardioscopy. *Like negative smear and culture, negative biopsy does not rule out tuberculosis*, so that if the pericardial contents and tissue appear to be "sterile," differentiation from other granulomatous pericarditis, like that in rheumatoid arthritis and sarcoid (pages 330), is required.

   A positive tuberculin skin test (PPD) can support but not confirm pericardial tuberculosis, since it may reflect antecedent extrapericardial tuberculosis, as may positive sputum and gastric aspiration, none of which is specific. (In general if there is 10% tuberculin positivity in the general population, a positive test is worthless.) *Negative skin tests are quite common and are equally unhelpful* due to loss of reactivity in patients with anergy, especially those with severe systemic diseases and those with HIV infection. Early, transiently negative skin tests may be due to pericardial and pleural sequestration of PPD-reactive T-lymphocytes. A "therapeutic test" may be employed *as a last resort* by giving appropriate antimycobacterial agents to patients who are critically ill with persistent constitutional signs and no other demonstrable etiology. Uptake of radionuclides, like gallium 67 and indium 111, may indicate pericardial inflammation, but these measures are nonspecific since such uptake also occurs in purulent and viral pericarditis, leukemic infiltration and even mesothelioma.

More recently, high levels (over 40 IU/L) of *adenosine deaminase* (ADA) activity in pericardial fluid have been shown to be quasispecific for tuberculous pericarditis. (Very high ADA levels appear to portend eventual constriction). Indeed, differentiation of neoplastic effusions is virtually absolute with *low* levels of ADA accompanying high levels of carcinoembryonic antigen (CEA). Complement-fixing antimyolemmal and antimyosin type *antibodies* have been found in most patient with acute tuberculous pericarditis, but these decrease in late and constrictive stages. *Mycobacterial antigens* have been increasingly detected by enzyme-linked immunoabsorbent assay (ELISA) with very high specificity and relatively high sensitivity. Probably the optimal test, although costly and labor-intensive but giving a rapid answer, is the *polymerase chain reaction* (PCR), which amplifies mycobacterial DNA, thereby "fingerprinting" individual strains of *M. tuberculosis* in pericardial fluid with excellent specificity. This is particularly useful in patients infected with AIDS/HIV who have adenopathy and tend to have atypical mycobacteria, especially *Mycobacterium avium* complex. Clinical specimens are assayed for an insertion element yielding a DNA sequence unique for the *M. tuberculosis* complex of organisms. Moreover, because there is a 100% sensitivity for *active* tuberculosis, a negative result excludes active tuberculosis. Indeed, a negative result in patients with no tuberculous history implies no tuberculosis anywhere. Specificity is virtually 70% for active tuberculosis, but for any tuberculous infection, it approaches 90%, as it will be positive in some patients with prior tuberculosis, treated tuberculosis or myocardial tuberculosis. While false positives occur and blood in pericardial fluid may lead to false negatives through enzyme inhibition, the PCR is superior to bacteriologic methods. Yet, because of its high sensitivity and the need for *drug susceptibility testing*, cultures should be obtained.

Finally, a promising serologic assay is being developed utilizing ELISA based on monoclonal antibodies against specific epitopes on a protein antigen. If successful, this would obviate obtaining test specimens from the pericardium.

Management

Antimycobacterial treatment has greatly decreased mortality in tuberculous pericarditis, although frequently not preventing constriction. All isolates of *M. tuberculosis* should be tested for antimicrobial susceptibility. *Effective multiple drug therapy is mandatory* and severely ill patients can benefit from prednisone or other corticosteroids which will shorten the course, dramatically decrease symptoms and signs in the acute phase, and reduce the death rate. However, corticosteroids only modestly reduce the incidence of constriction, at least in the short run (whether even this is optimistic depends on very prolonged follow-up). Some atypical mycobacteria, like the *M. avium* complex, tend to be resistant to chemotherapy and require determined efforts to find appropriate combinations. Cardiac tamponade must be relieved, preferably by surgical drainage, under chemotherapeutic "cover" to prevent extrapericardial spread. Persistent hypotension warrants adrenal function testing because of possible adrenal tuberculosis. Any tendency to nonresolution of worsening over 6 to 8 weeks, significant pericardial thickening, or manifestations of constriction mandate *pericardiectomy* as soon as possible because results are much better in every respect when this is performed at earlier stages. If pericardiectomy is not needed in the acute stage, the long-term outcome is often satisfactory. However, *all patients who have had tuberculous pericarditis must be observed for years* to detect constriction or reactivation.

FUNGAL PERICARDITIS

General Considerations

In the United States, pericarditis due to fungus infections may be broadly divided into disease mainly due to two "geographic" fungi, *Histoplasma* and *Coccidioidomyces*, and two "nongeographic" fungi, *Candida* and *Aspergillus* (*Blastomyces* and *Cryptococcus* are comparatively rare, as is *Pneumocystis carinii*, DNA-classifiable as a fungus). To these may be added two "semifungi" (between bacteria and fungi), *Actinomyces* and *Nocardia* (Table 16.1). The geographic fungi are endemic in certain areas, whereas the nongeographic fungi are largely opportunistic invaders, depending on reduction in host defenses against infection. However, all fungal invaders occur preferentially in immunocompromised and severely burned patients, debilitated individuals, those taking broad-spectrum and multiple antibiotics, drug addicts, elderly individuals, infants (especially if premature) and patients taking corticosteroid agents that impair antifungal defenses, including phagocyte activity.

Histoplasmosis, coccidioidomycosis and aspergillosis may involve the pericardium during pneumonia, endocarditis or myocardial abscesses due to these agents. However, histoplasmosis is relatively benign compared to all of the others, which rarely have spontaneous remissions but have more slowly developing effusions with a tendency to chronicity (i.e., prolongation over months). Tamponade is less common in them than in histoplasmosis, while a tendency to constriction requiring pericardiectomy is far more common. Indeed, apparent cardiac decompensation during fungal infections may be due to tamponade or to constriction or fungal myocarditis (more common in children). *Precise diagnosis is crucial, particularly for the nongeographic fungi*, because amphotericin B, a principal antifungal agent, is very toxic. Pericardiectomy is usually crucial for the patient's survival.

GEOGRAPHIC FUNGI: HISTOPLASMOSIS AND COCCIDIOIDOMYCOSIS

Histoplasmosis

Histoplasmosis is the most common of the "naturally" acquired fungal infections. Subclinical histoplasmosis is frequent in endemic areas, the Ohio and Mississippi valleys and the western Appalachians. Pericarditis usually occurs late, well after the illness is established elsewhere with or without a diagnosis. In acute symptomatic illness, pericarditis is uncommon but not rare; clinically recognizable cases may be the most acute.

Pathogenesis

Microfoci of histoplasmosis with viable organisms can exist for a decade or more in contaminated areas. The conidiospores tend to be carried by the wind, especially in rural areas, with infection by inhalation from droppings by birds like starlings and bats. In urban areas, the infection is associated with excavations and demolitions. Infection is only rarely hematogenous from other foci; apparently, pericardial involvement is most often a noninfectious (irritative or immunopathic) complication of infection of adjacent mediastinal lymph nodes. *Histoplasma pneumoniae* myocarditis and endocarditis occur more often than pericarditis. However, pleural effusions are more common with pericarditis than with primary pulmonary histoplasmosis and may accompany immunopathic outpouring of pericardial fluid similar to the postpericardiotomy and post-myocardial infarction syndromes (Chapters 20 and 21).

Distinctive Clinical Features

Histoplasma pericarditis is relatively common in younger, usually immunocompetent patients, especially males between 20 and 40 years of age. In contrast, disseminated histoplasmosis, like other fungal infections, is more common in immunosuppressed patients.

Many cases are discovered during urban or rural outbreaks, which bring to mind this etiology. Pericardial involvement is often relatively benign, resembling idiopathic pericarditis and resolving within 2 weeks. However, while they are uncommon, almost half of *Histoplasma*-induced effusions develop hemodynamic compromise, frequently with clinical signs of cardiac tamponade. *In contrast to other forms of fungal pericarditis, effusion with or without tamponade can be rapid and massive.* The fluid is serous, xanthochromic or hemorrhagic with a predominance of leukocytes. Because of the frequency of pleuropulmonary involvement, there are mixed clinical manifestations: preceding respiratory illness is common, along with pleuritic pain, cough and dyspnea, especially in occasional cases that resemble viral or tuberculous pericarditis, and such patients may also have typical ECG changes (page 43). Only occasional patients develop constrictive pericarditis or pericardial calcification with or without constriction; rarely, constriction is the presenting syndrome.

If the acute pericarditis resolves, recurrences occur quite variably. Rarely, there is prolonged disseminated infection with fever, anemia, leukopenia and pneumonitis, including cavitation.

The diagnosis should be considered in endemic geographic zones. Skin tests are not valuable and may interfere with serology; rising complement fixation titers and the immunodiffusion test are helpful. However, although histoplasmosis probably accounts for some "viral" and "idiopathic" pericarditis in endemic areas and in travelers leaving them, *other causes of pericarditis must be considered in endemic areas*, even in seropositive patients. With any persistent illness, *biopsy of lymph nodes*, particularly mediastinal nodes, with cultures and methonium silver stains may be decisive. Ideally, histoplasma should be identified, since granulomas alone are nonspecific; indeed, tuberculosis may be associated in some patients. However, the organisms are difficult to find in pericardial fluid and even in biopsies. The principal differential diagnoses are pericarditis due to viruses, tuberculosis, brucellosis, Hodgkin's disease or sarcoid.

Management

In those patients whose condition resolves spontaneously or with anti-inflammatory agents without antifungal medication, pericardial involvement is almost certainly "immunopathic" or "irritative," without actual infection, including some who develop cardiac tamponade. Unless they appear to be recovering, are in no distress and have a "dry" pericardium on imaging, patients should be hospitalized due to the infrequent possibility of cardiac tamponade. Antifungal treatment with amphotericin B or ketoconazole is rarely indicated and then only for disseminated histoplasmosis or severe pericardial inflammation. For reduction of chest pain, fever, effusion and suppression of the pericardial rub, NSAIDs tend to be sufficient. Tamponade and constriction, of course, require cardiac decompression. Corticosteroids predispose to dissemination but may be added if other treatment does not succeed and the patient is severely ill. If there is disseminated histoplasmosis, *adrenal function should be assessed*, since, as in tuberculosis, the adrenals may be involved, and this will require appropriate steroid treatment.

Coccidioidomycosis

Coccidioides is endemic in the southwestern United States, particularly the San Joaquin Valley, and also in Argentina. Some cases are discovered at autopsy. The spores are inhaled from soil. Blacks, Filipinos and Chicanos appear most susceptible, perhaps because of occupational exposure.

Pathogenesis

Coccidioidomycosis of the pericardium is usually a complication of progressive disseminated infection. Rarely, it seems to be "primary," i.e., confined to the pericardium. Hilar nodes are involved, resembling tuberculosis. The infection causes a serofibrinous effusion with a potential for adhesions. Eosinophils are rarely increased in effusion fluid and in blood.

Clinical Features

The clinical spectrum is wide, from classic acute pericarditis to chronic adhesive pericarditis, and rarely progression to effusive–constrictive pericarditis. *Acute pericardial coccidioidomycosis usually accompanies pneumonia from the same organism*, with obvious mediastinal node involvement in some patients. Some develop pulmonary infiltrates, systemic adenopathy, osteomyelitis or meningitis. The main symptoms may be pneumonitic: cough, dyspnea, fever, and pleuritic pain. Patients are usually chronically ill, debilitated, malnourished and often immunocompromised. Diagnosis requires histologic documentation but is suggested by pericarditis occurring in the endemic zone, especially if there is disseminated coccidioidomycosis, but this must be differentiated from idiopathic and viral pericarditis and a spectrum of pulmonary lesions. Infection is reflected in positive serum precipitant tests, increasing complement fixation IgG antibody titers, IgM immunodiffusion titers, and the skin test, which in endemic areas is probably nonspecific. Cultures are made on Sabouraud's medium. Progress of the infection may be followed with gallium scans, which are diagnostically nonspecific, but once the diagnosis is established, they should reflect success or failure of management.

Management

Pericarditis may resolve without specific therapy. However, anticoccidioidal agents like fluconazole may be necessary, depending on severity and progress. Complications like tamponade and constriction must be treated by decompression.

"NONGEOGRAPHIC" FUNGAL INFECTIONS

These are due mainly to *Candida* and *Aspergillus*, which are usually opportunistic invaders that tend to be very necrotizing. They produce local vascular thromboses, including involvement of coronary bypass grafts, both venous and arterial. *Candida* myocarditis is not rare.

Predisposing factors for these fungi include (1) antibiotic treatment for bacterial infection, particularly with multiple and broad-spectrum agents, (2) systemic defects in antifungal host defenses, as in immunocompromised and postsurgical patients (for example, patients following cardiac surgery given corticosteroid treatment to prevent cerebral edema) and (3) patients with indwelling catheters, including central venous lines. Postoperative patients with sterile or purulent pericarditis may have secondary invasion by fungi; with severely impaired host defenses and fulminant fungal pericarditis, there is a high death rate. Treatment includes definitive antifungal agents, extensive surgical drainage and even pericardiectomy if feasible.

THE "SEMIFUNGI": ACTINOMYCES AND NOCARDIA

Once established in the pericardium, these related organisms produce similar clinical pictures. (Although *Actinomyces israelii* is a member of the normal oral flora, pericarditis due to it is rare.) Actinomycosis may occur with fistulas and sinus tracts from the skin and other organs as well as contiguous spread along tissue planes in the thorax and mediastinum. Pericarditis tends to be insidious until signs of a complication like tamponade or constriction appear. However, acute pericarditis may be followed by chronic effusion with pericardial thickening and adhesions. Indeed, acute tamponade may respond to medical and surgical management, only to be followed by rapid constriction. These agents can also cause concomitant endocarditis and myocarditis.

Diagnosis and Therapy

Diagnosis is suggested in appropriate patients by infection elsewhere, but specific diagnosis is by staining and culturing pericardial fluid. Actinomyces, the more common infection, yields gram-positive branching filaments that fluoresce with appropriate antibody techniques; biopsy of pericardium or nodes may show the typical "sulfur granules." Infection with either semifungus is fatal unless treated medically and surgically. *Actinomyces* responds to penicillin and other antibiotics. *Nocardia* responds also to sulfonamides, particularly sulfisoxazole. Optimal therapy is with combined antimicrobial therapy, surgical drainage and pericardiectomy as indicated.

PERICARDIAL DISEASE IN AIDS AND AIDS-RELATED COMPLEX (TABLE 16.2)

General Considerations

Immunocompromised patients with AIDS and AIDS-related complex respond as do other kinds of patients who are immunosuppressed, such as those receiving corticosteroid therapy and cytotoxic agents—mainly patients on cancer chemotherapy, those with serious inflammatory disorders and patients after organ transplantations. Fungal pericarditis (pages 274) is a good example of opportunistic organisms preying on such patients, who actually have an acquired immunosuppression, i.e., "AIDS" not due to HIV virus from intravenous drug abuse, sexual or accidental transmission.

Severe immunosuppression characteristic of AIDS predisposes to infection by multiple organisms, many of them opportunistic, and to disseminated malignancies like Kaposi's sarcoma and non-Hodgkin's malignant lymphoma. The

Table 16.2   Pericardial Lesions in Aids

Manifestations:	Clinically dry pericarditis
	Effusion/tamponade
	Constriction
	Myopericarditis
Pathogenesis:	Idiopathic (possibly HIV)
	Infectious
	Mycobacterial, *esp*. M. avium intracellulare and M. tuberulosis
	Viral: Herpes simplex, types 1 and 2
	Cytomegalovirus
	Other
	Fungal: Cryptococcus neoformans
	Histoplasma capsulatum
	Toxoplasma gondii
	Pneumocystis
	Aspergillus
	Nocardia
	Chlamydia
	Staphylococcus
	Other organisms
	Malignant
	Kaposi's sarcoma
	Lymphoma
	?Other

primary cause of death in AIDS is opportunistic infection, most often involving the respiratory system and frequently involving the myocardium and the pericardium. The recent increasing incidence of less common manifestations can be ascribed to spread of the disease by intravenous drug abuse and maternal transmission as well as the partial success of new treatments that permit patients to live longer and so to display the less common signs and symptoms.

The complications of AIDS, probably including infection by the HIV virus itself, affect the endocardium, myocardium and pericardium and occur significantly more often with AIDS than with AIDS-related complex; patients with cardiac involvement have lower T4 counts. While pericardial disease, particularly effusion, is relatively frequent, it is more often discovered at autopsy or by echocardiography or other imaging modality. In general, *late AIDS-related pericardial effusions have a grave prognosis, suggesting end-stage HIV disease.* Indeed, the most frequent cardiac lesion at autopsy is sterile pericardial effusion. Patients with definite pericarditis often also have myocarditis.

Pericardial involvement in AIDS occurs in six forms:

1. *Silent: Fibrinous* and *effusive pericarditis* with or without adhesions, or apparently *sterile pericardial effusion* as part of a generalized serous effusive process, including ascites and pleural effusion ("capillary leak syndrome"). In this group the specific etiology is often uncertain or unknown.
2. *Classic acute pericarditis*: Typical pain, rub, and often ECG changes. If effusive, the fluid may be clear, purulent or sanguineous. A determined search for infectious etiology is often rewarded. Mycobacteria, fungi and other opportunistic organisms are frequent, although nonspecific inflammatory changes are not rare in tissue specimens.
3. *Cardiac tamponade*: Although tamponade usually occurs with chronicity, it may be the presenting syndrome and is seen as such frequently in Africa.
4. *Constrictive pericarditis*: (Chapter 15).
5. *Pericardial neoplasia*: Mainly Kaposi's sarcoma, aggressive Hodgkin's lymphoma or non-Hodgkin's malignant lymphoma.
6. *Myopericarditis* (Chapter 9).

Nonmalignant Pericardial Disease in AIDS

Most often a specific cause of the pericardial lesion itself is not found in the absence of an aggressive syndrome, particularly if it is the initial manifestation. With definite inflammatory signs, there tends to be lymphocytic infiltration of the pericardium. Sterile effusions may be due to uremia or to congestive heart failure from associated myocarditis or cardiomyopathy. Most pericardial effusions in AIDS outpatients are small and symptomatic. However, pericardial effusions of any size are associated with shortened survival.

While asymptomatic effusions are apparently of uncertain or unknown etiology, *symptomatic pericardial involvement nearly always accompanies myocardial involvement*. Large effusions may be tuberculous or fungal. Indeed, AIDS predisposes to all species of mycobacterial infection, mainly *M. tuberculosis* and *M. avium*. Nontuberculous mycobacterial infection occurs late, usually after AIDS has been diagnosed. AIDS patients are at risk for both reactivation and active primary tuberculosis, with the incidence of the latter increasing. Yet AIDS seems to blunt the inflammatory reaction to the tubercle bacillus, producing atypical symptoms and, even for this aggressive organism, relatively less cardiac tamponade and constriction. *Coexisting infections*—for example, tuberculosis with cytomegalovirus infection—are not rare.

Neoplasia in AIDS

At least two forms of malignancy are clearly related to AIDS: Kaposi's sarcoma and non-Hodgkin's malignant lymphoma; Hodgkin's and other lymphomas also occur. *Kaposi's sarcoma* involves both the visceral and parietal pericardium with a particular predilection for epicardium and subepicardial fat; it produces effusion and occasionally pericardial constriction. This malignancy is usually disseminated but in AIDS may appear to be primary in the pericardium, with a strong tendency to cause tamponade. Similarly, *malignant lymphoma* is usually multicentric and only rarely primary in the heart, where it typically affects the myocardium and less often the pericardium. Occasionally an Epstein-Barr viral genome may be discovered.

In AIDS patients when there is simultaneous infection or malignancy in other organs and in the pericardium, pericardial effusions may not be demonstrably related by etiology.

Clinical Aspects

At any time, most patients with AIDS have no overt pericardial disease; it may be truly "silent" or dominated either by signs of disease in other systems or by myocardial involvement, which typically accompanies severe pericardial disease. Yet cardiac tamponade or tuberculous pericarditis can be the presenting syndrome. Indeed, young patients, particularly males—in whom pericardial effusions are much more common than in females with AIDS—who have cardiac tamponade, especially in city hospitals, should always be considered for possible HIV infection.

Chest pain with or without apparent cardiomegaly may lead to discovery of a pericardial effusion on imaging. Dyspnea, a common presenting symptom, is often ascribed to pneumonia and pleural effusions. However, *cardiopericardial involvement should be suspected, particularly if dyspnea seems to be out of proportion to any pleuropulmonary lesions*. Electrocardiograms are usually nonspecifically changed but may be typical of acute pericarditis (page 43), especially when the patient has typical painful acute pericarditis (page 97). Low voltage may be related to effusions in the pericardium or pleurae or to myocardial involvement. Kaposi's sarcoma and lymphoma are more likely than infectious lesions to produce hemorrhagic effusion. Mediastinal lymph nodes are frequently involved; special imaging like computed tomography or magnetic resonance may be needed to demonstrate them. *In AIDS, tamponade of any pathogenesis often is accompanied by cardiac as well as pericardial disease*; infective agents like *Toxoplasma* and cytomegalovirus tend to be accompanied by myocarditis. In many cases, disease in other systems, as indicated by uremia, may be responsible for pericardial involvement, although secondary infection of uremic effusions is well known.

   Tuberculosis should always be considered, both because of its potential severity, with occasional tuberculous lesions producing rapid or slow constriction, and also because there is specific chemotherapy. Indeed, under appropriate treatment, patients usually die of AIDS, not tuberculosis. Therefore, gene amplification techniques like the PCR and Southern blot hybridization should be used if classic techniques are negative.

PARASITIC PERICARDITIS

General Considerations

Pericardial parasitoses appear in endemic areas and in travelers from them, in whom milder attacks are often mistaken for idiopathic pericarditis syndrome (Chapter 23). However, the acute illness typically resembles suppurative bacterial pericarditis or occasionally viral pericarditis. Parasites that are frequent in the liver, like *Echinococcus*, and amebae, also may provoke sterile, presumably immunogenic ("sympathetic") pericardial effusions, which may even cause tamponade. Such parasites usually enter the pericardium from perforation through the diaphragm or from secondary lesions in the lung and pleura. In some parasitoses, fluid may be negative for the organisms, requiring biopsy for diagnosis. Frequently parasitosis elsewhere suggests the diagnosis ("guilt by association"). *Eosinophilia* in the blood or pericardial fluid always suggests a parasitic disease. As in other forms of pericarditis, arrhythmias and cardiac dysfunction indicate local involvement of the heart, like *parasitic abscess* or *diffuse myocarditis*, which are not rare. Individuals from endemic areas often have multiple parasitoses or a parasitosis with a chronic infection like tuberculosis, which may confound the diagnosis.

Toxoplasmosis

Toxoplasmosis (for example, due to *Toxoplasma gondii*) may be congenital or acquired. Acquired toxoplasmosis is transmitted by uncooked infected meat and feline carriers. Its prevalence is probably underestimated, and pericarditis is often found incidentally at autopsy in patients with more obvious *Toxoplasma* myocarditis. Pericardial, like myocardial, affection is mainly chronic—often a chronic pericardial effusion and rarely constriction. Rare also is acute pericarditis with or without tamponade and including fever, rash and adenopathy; it can resemble systemic lupus erythematosus. Indeed, lupus patients with positive ANA may produce a false-positive humoral antibody titer with IgG-*T. gondii* antibodies characteristic of the real disease. Pericardial involvement may occur during miliary spread, particularly in patients with leukemia and other disorders treated with chemotherapeutic agents or corticosteroids. Localized and "glandular" types are ordinarily benign and simulate infectious mononucleosis. Manifest toxoplasmic disease is characterized by occasional relapses after apparently successful treatment (usually with pyrimethamine and sulfamethoxazole).

Echinococcosis

Echinococcus (for example, *Echinococcus granulosus*) is an invasive and destructive sporozoan that occurs mainly in sheep-raising countries (a rare form may be transmitted by infected dogs). It produces *hydatid cysts* of the myocardium, pericardium and mediastinum, including great vessels. The pericardium is involved via rupture from an adjacent myocardial cyst or from a hepatic cyst that penetrates the diaphragm and often accompanies pulmonary and myocardial involvement. (The lungs may become seeded via further rupture into the right heart or the vena cava and the myocardium via the coronary circulation.) Chest pain and sharp anaphylactic reactions with eosinophilia are characteristic. Multiple intrapericardial rupture can produce striking symptoms or, surprisingly, only vague symptoms. Pericardial and mediastinal echinococcal cysts also compress the cardiac chambers or great vessels, producing corresponding abnormalities on cardiopericardial imaging, especially two-dimensional echocardiography, which shows well-defined unilocular (occasionally multilocular) cysts with trabeculations due to internal "daughter membranes." Rarely, apparently solid masses are seen due to necrotic matter and foreign-body inflammatory reactions that fill the cysts. Clinical syndromes match cyst locations, but anaphylactic reactions occur with any kind of involvement. Complications include secondary bacterial infections, tamponade and constriction. Surgical excision (enucleation) may be dangerous due to spillage of active parasites; removal of the pericystic fibrovascular layer may provoke severe hemorrhage. Evacuation of the cysts and instillation of silver nitrate is usually preferable.

Amebiasis

Amebiasis (for example, due to *Entamoeba histolytica*) occurs mainly in endemic areas and in travelers from them in whom the syndrome may appear years later. Although patients may also have intestinal amebiasis, liver abscesses, particularly in the left lobe, typically perforate the diaphragm and involve the pericardium, occasionally with lung and pleural involvement, simultaneously with or preceding pericarditis. Mortality is high, especially if the diagnosis is missed. While liver abscess is the most common nonenteric amebiasis, rarely a gastropericardial fistula with pneumopyopericardium produces a diagnostic challenge (pages 362–363). Serofibrinous ("presuppurative") pericarditis with straw-colored or sanguineous fluid can precede gross rupture into the pericardium and is often suspected to be tuberculous. Frank pericardial rupture can be insidious or dramatic with pain, shock, tamponade and cyanosis. The fluid is brownish, with *pus simulating anchovy paste*, the appearance of which is quasidiagnostic. Secondary bacterial infection can be a grave complication and must be considered in severely ill patients. Occasionally there is a classic acute pericarditis syndrome with ECG changes that are consistent with acute pericarditis, or there is subacute effusive-constrictive pericarditis with pericardial thickening, in which the inflammatory cell response is surprisingly mild. Survivors can develop full constriction. Patients often have diagnosed or undiagnosed chronic amebiasis with anemia, weight loss, low-grade fever and weakness; many have hepatomegaly and most have splenomegaly. Diagnosis is by fluorescent antibody tests or amebic enzyme immunoassay supported by a liver scan with technetium 99m. Medical therapy with antiamebic agents like metronidazole or dehydroemetine is highly successful in hepatic cases, but pericardial involvement requires drainage and, if necessary, resection.

Filariasis; Heartworm

Wuchereria bancrofti, for example, a nematode endemic in parts of Africa and India, produces hemorrhagic effusions in which microfilaria are easily found, as they are in blood smears obtained at night. Effusions may be clinically silent or massive with rapid or slow tamponade. Cough and constitutional symptoms are common. Persistent pericardial inflammation produces sanguinopurulent pericarditis with chronic lymphocytic inflammatory changes. Although survival may produce rapid constriction, even during chemotherapy, clues to the diagnosis include other manifestations of filariasis like elephantiasis, particularly of the limbs, scrotum and occasionally of the breasts.

Other Nematodes

Necator americanus is known to produce eosinophilic pericardial effusion, possibly an "allergic" effect. *Dracunculus* (guinea worm) has been found in constrictive pericardial scar.

Hypodermiasis

Hypoderma lineata or *Hypoderma bovis*, an organism, from a small area of western France, almost always affects children between 2 and 12 years of age exposed to bovine carriers. It provokes acute pericarditis or pleuropericarditis with a rub, appropriate ECG changes and effusion. Eosinophilia is a clue to parasitosis. However, organism-free immunopathic pericardial reactions occur, presumably due to "allergy" to passage of larvae. Patients may have painful swellings in various superficial body locations. A precipitin test is diagnostic. Nonsteroidal anti-flammatory drugs often suffice for treatment.

Schistosomiasis

Ova of *Schistosoma hematobium*, presumable hematogenously spread from the pelvic zone, have been found in granulomas from resected constrictive pericardial scar. Like disease due to *Dracunculus*, this may represent secondary invasion.

Chagas Disease

Pericardial involvement by *Trypanosoma cruzi*, mainly fibrosis with lymphocytic infiltration, is usually subclinical. It accompanies Chagas' cardiomyopathy.

SPIROCHETAL PERICARDITIS

Except for spirochetes transmitted during Lyme carditis and leptospirosis, spirochetal pericarditis (e.g., *Treponema pallidum* infection) is poorly characterized owing to the extreme rarity of its discovery in tissue, where its presence may be accidental.

Syphilitic Pericarditis

Treponema pallidum is identified only in the rare involvement of the pericardium by localized or miliary syphilitic gummas with a fibrotic reaction or accompanying a hemorrhagic effusion, which may or may not be luetic.

Chapter 16

Lyme Pericarditis

Lyme disease involves transmission, via tick bites, of the spirochete *Borrelia burgdorferi*, which can produce acute pericarditis, pericardial effusion and myopericarditis, particularly in young male patients who have been in tick-in-fested areas. Illness begins with a persistent migrating skin erythema either before or after nonspecific systemic symptoms. Fatal *myopericarditis may* ensue, its severity due mainly to myocardial and conducting tissue involvement. Silver stains of biopsied material may demonstrate the spirochetes. However, enzyme-linked immunoabsorbent assay can detect IgM and IgG antibodies to *B. burgdorferi*. Indium 111 antimyosin antibody scintigraphy may be helpful.

Leptospirosis

Although leptospirosis (for example, due to *L. icterohaemorrhagiae*, is mainly a tropical disease, it is reported at all ages from all over the world. Most cases are subclinical. The syndrome may simulate acute viral hepatitis (which is also a cause of pericarditis). Myocardial and pericardial involvement, often mild, seem more frequent in patients who are anicteric, although typical leptospirosis includes mild icterus as well as fever and myalgias. When these are severe, the syndrome is "Weil's disease." Infection arises from domestic or wild animals, particularly rats, through handling or swimming in contaminated water. Typical acute pericarditis, including a rub and ECG changes, may be due either to the organism itself or to an accompanying uremia when the kidneys are affected. The effects of myocarditis, with or without coronary and aortic arteritis, may dominate the picture. Conjunctival suffusion is a clue to the diagnosis, which can be made by a microscopic agglutination test for *Leptospira*.

RICKETTSIAL PERICARDITIS

Rickettsiae, particularly *Rickettsia rickettsii*, can produce pericarditis along with myocarditis and vasculitis via infected ticks in endemic areas, including South America, Africa, and the South Central and Atlantic States (Rocky Mountain spotted fever; RMSF). In Africa, tick-transmitted boutonneuse fever is due to *Rickettsia conorii*. Q fever, due to *Coxiella burnetii*, transmitted by sheep and cattle and their milk, has worldwide distribution. It appears to produce more obvious clinical pericarditis than does RMSF, and may present as a pericardial effusion.

The incidence of RMSF is increasing, especially in children. Exposure to ticks is one method of transmission of RMSF. The disease features abrupt onset of fever, with variable and diffuse changes due to vasculitis. Myocarditis and pericarditis can occur with or without vasculitis, the latter being a "toxic" or immunogenic process. The presence of appropriate cross-reactive antimyo-lemmal antibodies suggests that a number of cases with pericardial involvement are immunopathogenetic, with pericarditis following extension of myocarditis to the epicardium. Infections are discovered by appropriate serologic tests including Weil-Felix agglutinins and IgM and IgG antibodies.

CHLAMYDIACIAL PERICARDITIS (*CHLAMYDIA–PSITTACOSIS–LYMPHOGRANULOMA VENEREUM* GROUP)

These organisms produce classic acute pericarditis as well as large pericardial effusions. Rare until recently, Chlamydiaceae, especially *C. trachomatis, C. psittaci* and *C. pneumonitidis*, are increasingly found in overtly immunocompromised patients and patients with malignancies as well as otherwise healthy hosts. They produce pericarditis, myocarditis, pleuritis and pneumonitis. *Psittacosis* follows exposure to psittacine birds like parrots and nonpsittacine birds like pigeons, ducks and pheasants. Indeed, pericardial effusion is one of the commonest forms in affected birds themselves, making its comparative rarity in humans surprising. Acute pericarditis with or without myocarditis follows exposure to appropriate birds or dust from their cages, which usually first produces respiratory disease. For this group, specific diagnosis is by IgG antibody titers.

KEY POINTS

1. Every kind of infection and parasitosis that can reach the pericardium can inflame it. Acute viral and bacterial pericarditis are the commonest; if either is not conclusively demonstrated, a remarkably wide variety of etiologic agents must be considered.
2. Acute viral pericarditis probably accounts for the majority of "idiopathic" or "nonspecific"pericarditis. Absent any complications like tamponade and constriction, treatment is symptomatic and anti-inflammatory.
3. In adults, bacterial and fungal pericarditis may be hospital-acquired, particularly in surgical, severely ill and debilitated patients. Elderly patients may have few specific symptoms.
4. Classic tuberculous pericarditis due to *M. tuberculosis*, often difficult to diagnose, has become less frequent in developed countries. It is almost always serious from the outset, especially as a potent generator of debility, tamponade and acute, subacute and chronic constriction.
5. Tuberculin skin tests are of little help and may be misleading, while adenosine deaminase level in pericardial fluid is a relatively specific marker for tuberculous pericarditis. The polymerase chain reaction (PCR) backed by fluid and tissue culture is optimal. Culture is essential for determining antimicrobial susceptibility, so as to design multiple drug therapy.

6. Immunocompromised patients are susceptible to all common infectious agents, fungal and chlamydial infections and many opportunistic, rare and atypical microorganisms, particularly atypical mycobacteria. These have multiplied the variety of pericardial inflammations.
7. Patients with AIDS/HIV infection develop uncommon pericardial malignancies, particularly Kaposi's sarcoma and non-Hodgkin's malignant lymphoma. They also develop uninfected pericardial exudates and transudates, sometimes related to myocardial inflammation or failure.
8. Parasitic, rickettsial and spirochetal forms of pericarditis must be considered following appropriate geographic exposure and in patients with otherwise unexplained eosinophilia.

BIBLIOGRAPHY

Agner, R.C., Gallis, H.A. Pericarditis—Differential diagnostic considerations. Arch. Intern. Med. 1979; 139:407–412.

Anguita, M., Diaz, V., Bueno, G., et al. Brucella pericarditis: Two different forms of presentation for an unusual etiology. Rev. Espanola Cardiol. 1991; 44:481–484.

Brown, R. Clostridial pericarditis diagnosed antemortem. Am. Heart J. 1965; 70:801–805.

Carrel, T.P., Schaffner, A., Schmid, E.R., et al. Fatal fungal pericarditis after cardiac surgery and immunosuppression. J. Thorac. Cardiovasc. Surg. 1991; 101:161–164.

Cohen, J.I., Bartlett, J.A., Corey, G.R. Extraintestinal manifestations of Salmonella infections. Medicine 1987; 66:349–388.

Corey, G.R., Campbell, P.T., VanTrigt, P., et al. Etiology of large pericardial effusions. Am. J. Med. 1993; 95:209–213.

Drugs for tuberculosis. Med. Lett. 1995; 37:67–70.

Dupuis, C., Gronnier, P., Kachaner, J., et al. Bacterial pericarditis in infancy and childhood. Am. J. Cardiol. 1994; 74:807–809.

Edwards, J.E. Jr., Filler, S.G. Current strategies for treating invasive candidiasis: Emphasis on infections in nonneutropenic patients. Clin. Infect. Dis. 1992; 14(suppl. 1): S106–S113.

Evans, M.E., Gregory, D.W., Schaffner, W., McGee, Z.A. Tularemia: A 30-year experience with 88 cases. Medicine 1985; 85:251–269.

Flum, D.R., McGinn, J.T. Jr., Tyras, D.H. The role of the "pericardial window" in AIDS. Chest 1995; 107:1522–1525.

Fowler, N.O. Tuberculous pericarditis. JAMA 1991; 766:99–103.

Gallis, H.A., Drew, R.H., Pickard, W.W. Amphotericin B: 30 years of clinical experience. Rev. Infect. Dis. 1990; 12:308–329.

Greenberg, M.L., Niebulski, H.I.J., Uretsky, B.F., et al. Occult purulent pericarditis detected by indium-111 leukocyte imaging. Chest 1984; 85:701–703.

Guerot, E., Assayag, P., Morgant, C., et al. Pericardial manifestations of toxoplasmosis. Arch. Malad. Coeur Vaisseaux 1992; 85:109–111.

Holtz, H.A., Lavery, D.P., Kapila, R. Actinomycetales infection in the acquired immunodeficiency syndrome. Ann. Intern. Med. 1985; 102:203–205.

Kumakov, Yu. I., Kolodkin, B.A., Citvinenko, A.I. Dva sluchaya trikhinelleza (two cases of trichinellosis). Terap. Arkh. 1992; 64:99–100.

Lewis, W. AIDS: Cardiac findings from 115 autopsies. Prog. Cardiovasc. Dis. 1989; 32:207–215.

Lieber, I.H., Rensimer, E.R., Ericsson, C.D. Campylobacter pericarditis in hypothyroidism. Am. Heart J. 1981; 102:462–465.

Lorcerie, B., Boutron, M.C., Portier, H., et al. Manifestations pericardiques de la maladie de Lyme. Ann. Med. Interne 1987; 138:601–603.

Maisch, B. Myocarditis and pericarditis—Old questions and new answers. Herz 1992; 17:65–70.

Majid, A.A., Omar, A. Diagnosis and management of purulent pericarditis: Experience with pericardiectomy. J. Thorac. Cardiovasc. Surg. 1991; 102:413–417.

Mann-Segal DD, Shanahan A, Jones B, Ramasan D. Purulent pericarditis: rediscovery of an old remedy. J Thorac Cardiovas Surg 1996; 111:487–488.

Muir, P., Tilzey, A.J., English, T.A.H., et al. Chronic relapsing pericarditis and dilated cardiomyopathy: Serological evidence of persistent enterovirus infection. Lancet 1989; 1:804–807.

Naber, S.P. Molecular medicine: Molecular pathology—Diagnosis of infectious disease. N. Engl. J. Med. 1994; 331:1212–1215.

Odeh, M., Oliven, A. Chlamydial infections of the heart. Eur. J. Clin. Microbiol. Infect. Dis. 1992; 11:885–893.

Park, S., Bayer, A.S. Purulent pericarditis. Curr. Clin. Topics Infect. Dis. 1992; 12:56–82.

Querol, J.M., Farga, M.A., Granda, D., et al. The utility of polymerase chain reaction (PCR) in the diagnosis of pulmonary tuberculosis. Chest 1995; 107:1631–1635.

Sagrista-Sauleda, J., Permanyer-Miralda, G., Soler-Solder, J. Tuberculous pericarditis: Ten-year experience with a prospective protocol for diagnosis and treatment. J. Am. Coll. Cardiol. 1988; 11:724–728.

Satoh, T., Kojima, M., Ohshima, K. Demonstration of the Epstein-Barr genome by the polymerase chain reaction and in situ hybridization in a patient with viral pericarditis. Br. Heart J. 1993; 69:563–564.

Schrank, J.H. Jr., Dooley, D.P. Purulent pericarditis caused by Candida species: Case report and review. Clin. Infect. Dis. 1995; 21:182–187.

Spodick, D.H. Tuberculous pericarditis. Arch. Intern. Med. 1956; 98:737–749.

Spodick, D.H. Critical care of pericardial disease. In: Ripper, J.M., Irwin, R.S., Alpert, J.S., Fink, M.P. (eds.). Intensive Care Medicine, 2d ed. Boston: Little, Brown, 1991 pp. 282–295.

Spodick, D.H. Diseases of the pericardium. In: Parmley, W.W., Chatterjee, K. (eds.). Cardiology. Vol. 2. Philadelphia: Lippincott, 1992, chap. 43.

Tabrizi, S.J., Scott, J., Pusey, C.D., et al. Grand Rounds—Hammersmith Hospital—Nocardia pericarditis: A rare opportunistic infection. Br. Med. J. 1994; 309:1495–1497.

Taillefer, R., Lemieux, R.J., Picard, D., Dupras, G. Gallium-67 imaging in pericarditis secondary to tuberculosis and histoplasmosis. Clin. Nucl. Med. 1981; 6:413–415.

Ungerer, J.P.J., Oosthuizen, H.M., Retief, J.H., Bissbort, S.H. Signiificance of adenosine deaminase activity and its isoenzymes in tuberculous effusions. Chest 1994; 106:33–37.

Wang, C.Y., Snow, J.L., Daniel Su, W.P. Lymphoma associated with human immunodeficiency virus infection. Mayo Clin. Proc. 1995; 70:665–672.

Winkler, W.B., Karnik, R., Slany, J. Treatment of exudative fibrinous pericarditis with intrapericardial urokinase. Lancet 1994; 344:1541–1542.

17

Pericardial Disease in Metabolic Disorders

A variety of metabolic disorders (Table 17.1) that may involve the pericardium, often acutely, are precipitated by intercurrent stresses like excessive metabolic loads or infection. Moreover, especially in debilitated and immunocompromised patients, infective and malignant pericardial disease can masquerade as, or accompany, the metabolic variety. Numerically, the most important of this group is chronic renal failure.

RENAL FAILURE

Generalities

Chronic renal failure produces all morphologic forms of acute pericarditis, effusive and noneffusive, with and without tamponade and usually complicated by smaller or larger pericardial hemorrhages: *uremic pericarditis*. A more recent form of chronic recurrent uremic pericarditis, *dialysis pericarditis*, permits prolonged survival, and with it, constrictive and effusive-constrictive pericarditis. *Acute renal failure* also produces acute uremic pericarditis, usually of much less serious significance (page 295). Although nitrogen retention is necessary for uremic pericarditis, many patients escape pericarditis, so that the precise pathogenesis of all variants is uncertain; "toxic metabolites" are often invoked without direct proof. Contrary to early observations, crystal formation is absent in pericardial tissue and fluids.

Table 17.1   Pericardial Disease in Metabolic Disorders

Renal failure
   Uremic pericarditis with and without effusion/tamponade
      Acute renal failure
      Chronic renal failure
   Dialysis pericarditis with and without effusion/tamponade
      Acute
      Subacute/recurrent
      Constrictive/effusive-constrictive
   Nephrotic syndrome
   Severe renal transplant rejection
Hepatorenal failure
Myxedema/Hypothyroidism
Gout
Pericarditis associated with hypercholesterolemia
? Diabetic ketoacidosis
Adrenal failure
   ?Addisonian crisis
   Waterhouse-Friderichsen syndrome (probably meningococcal)
Pericardial amyloidosis (infiltration)

Pericardial involvement is not related to the etiology of renal failure (except for an immunopathic component in glomerulonephritis). While high blood urea nitrogen (BUN) levels are customary, usually over 60 mg/dL, there is no strict numerical relationship. Although echocardiography reveals excess pericardial fluid in many asymptomatic patients, the incidence of all forms of acute pericardial disease punctuating chronic renal failure has plummeted due to effective dialysis, hemoperfusion and renal transplantation. Small pericardial effusions and noninflammatory hydropericardium due to volume overload and congestive heart failure (Chapter 10) are common and, by themselves, usually not clinically significant.

In all forms of uremic pericarditis, *cardiac tamponade* is the main danger. It develops from increasing pericardial fluid, usually bloody, and often precipitated by critically increased bleeding. It may appear as an unexplained fall in blood pressure to a level that varies widely between lower than previously, but still high, and shock levels. Initially, some patients are asymptomatic; in others a change in mental status may be the first clue. Fever is variable in the absence of infection and more common in dialysis than uremic pericarditis. Chest pain varies from severe to mild to absent. Uremic pericardial rubs, louder than in most other forms of pericarditis, and often palpable, frequently persist for some time after the biochemical abnormalities are ameliorated.

In uremic pericarditis due to acute and chronic glomerulonephritis and in dialysis pericarditis (especially when precipitated by viral infections), complement-fixing *antimyocardial antibodies* appear, including *antimyolemmal autoantibodies*, that may have a pathogenetic role as well as being diagnostic markers.

Uremic Pericarditis in Chronic Renal Failure

Uremic pericarditis resembles the spectrum of viral pericarditis with all of its acute complications, including the characteristics noted in the preceding paragraphs. There are few chronic complications because without dialysis the average prognosis for life is 1 month. Serum BUN is nearly always over 60 mg/dL. Despite comparable degrees of renal failure, only some, usually younger, patients develop uremic pericarditis, which can be precipitated by sepsis, trauma (including surgery), hypercatabolic states, acute myocardial infarction or hyperparathyroidism. A constant exacerbating factor is the pericardial and systemic *hemorrhage diathesis* induced by uremia, owing to abundantly vascular granulation tissue accompanying uremic pericardial inflammation and hematologic impairments that promote bleeding. Indeed, *pericardial effusions in uremic patients usually predict tamponade in proportion to their size*, since the unstable uremic hemorrhagic diathesis can precipitate it suddenly.

Pericardial contents are sterile unless secondarily infected. (Formerly infections were frequently pneumococcal, but more recently they appear to be viral.) Uremic exudates tend to be abundant, with considerable fibrin and inflammatory cells. Despite destruction of the pericardial mesothelium and gross hemorrhage, pure—that is, uninfected—*uremic pericarditis is unique in that the inflammatory cells do not penetrate the myocardium. This accounts for the customary absence of typical Stage I electrocardiographic (ECG) changes* which depend on subepicardial myocarditis (page 43). Indeed, *when the ECG is typical of acute pericarditis, intercurrent infection must be suspected*; any local changes should suggest ischemia. Most often, ECGs are grossly unchanged during uremic pericarditis and reflect associated abnormalities like left ventricular hypertrophy and "strain," any coronary artery disease, and metabolic abnormalities like hyperkalemia and hypocalcemia (Figure 17.1). While any of these would tend to buffer superimposed acute J (ST) changes, these are absent unless there is an infectious pericarditis. Fluid retention and pleural effusions, particularly left or bilateral, may reduce ECG voltages with or without pericardial effusion.

Differential diagnosis may be difficult, especially in mentally confused patients and because nonuremic intercurrent pericarditis of any cause is always possible. For example, where hypertension has not been well controlled, dissecting hematoma of the aorta (page 356) must be considered. Indeed, uremic

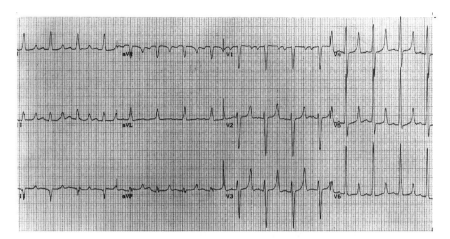

Figure 17.1 Uremic pericarditis. Electrocardiogram following appearance of a loud pericardial rub shows no evidence of pericarditis. Left ventricular hypertrophy by voltage as well as typical changes of hypocalcemia and hyperkalemia are seen.

tamponade may simulate any cardiocirculatory emergency, especially when with marked hypotension. Conversely, tamponade may be disguised by a relatively or absolutely high pressure level, although reduced from a previously higher level (high pressure tamponade; page 167). Confusion of tamponade with florid heart failure may arise from left ventricular hypertrophy, frequent in uremics, and any element of true myocardial failure, each of which can prevent pulsus paradoxus (page 198). Conversely, unexplained worsening renal function may actually be a clue to an element of cardiac tamponade. Sepsis of nonrenal origin may also coexist and precipitate tamponade; here, blood cultures may be positive for organisms and pericardial fluid negative. Hepatic congestion due to tamponade or heart failure may be confused with viral hepatitis. Finally, *in uremic patients, frequent autonomic impairment and decreased cardiac adenylate cyclase limits heart rate increases during pericarditis, even during tamponade*, so that *the heart rate may be deceptively slow* (60 to 80 beats per minute) despite any fever and hypotension.

   Treatment is clear: drainage of tamponading effusions, which should be gradual because of the possibility of "pericardial shock" in patients who may have underlying congestive failure or intercurrent myocarditis that predispose to postdrainage cardiac dilation (page 179). A neurogenic element may also contribute to postdrainage collapse because patients are vagotonic; therefore, pericardial drainage should be covered by atropine. Intrapericardial hydrocortisone, triamcinolone or an equivalent agent may accelerate improvement by suppressing inflammation. For uremia itself, of course, effective dialysis is mandatory, with careful monitoring of intravascular volume, since in the presence of excess pericardial fluid too rapid vascular volume reduction can precipitate florid tamponade.

Uremic Pericarditis in Acute Renal Failure

Patients with hypotension due to shock, sepsis, trauma or surgery may develop acute renal failure that can be self-limited under appropriate treatment. Yet with the BUN at 100 or higher, uremic pericarditis may appear. This responds to effective treatment of the etiologic condition, circulatory support and acute dialysis. Pericardial involvement is identified by discovering a rub and effusion or tamponade, although, as in chronic renal failure, obtunded or unconscious patients will not complain of chest pain. Unlike pericarditis or pericardial effusion following renal failure in chronic glomerulonephritis, this form of acute renal failure only rarely has an immunopathic component unless it is associated with acute glomerulonephritis.

Dialysis Pericarditis

Adequate renal dialysis effectively ends uremic pericarditis (sometimes still considered present in the first few months of dialysis). However, *classic uremic pericarditis* is reversed by dialysis, while *dialysis pericarditis*, usually appearing some time after dialysis is initiated, by definition resists dialysis. That is, pericarditis appears despite otherwise successful dialysis and even in stable patients with good biochemical control. Its pathogenesis is unknown, although dialysis pericarditis is much less common during peritoneal dialysis than during hemodialysis. Circulating immune complexes, which may be pathogenetic, are increased in dialysis patients, particularly those with various forms of serositis. They are less elevated with peritoneal dialysis. Indeed, immune complex-like material is found in the dialysate, and this "loss" may retard the pericarditis. A pathogenetic role for "middle molecules" has been proposed. Fortunately, dialysis pericarditis is becoming much less frequent owing to improved dialytic management.

Several factors are associated with precipitating dialysis pericarditis and effusion, above all *inadequate dialysis*. *Infection*, particularly viral, is frequent, with hepatitis and cytomegaloviruses common in dialysis units. Often such infections are systemic and the pericardial fluid is sterile. Thus, purely diagnostic pericardial drainage is rarely needed. Other factors, as in classic uremic pericarditis, include *hyperparathyroidism* and *hypercalcemia* (which may be responsible for stressful anorexia, nausea and vomiting) and *heparinization*, which increases the hemorrhagic tendency, although much less so with regional heparinization. Contributing factors include *catabolic loads*, including surgery and trauma.

Constitutional symptoms, especially fever, are more severe and more common than in uremic pericarditis, and dialysis pericarditis may be preceded by weight gain and hypotension. Some patients have unexplained clotting or bacterial infection of their blood access (e.g., shunts). Effusion, with or without hemorrhage, is the most important complication and tends to be recurrent; as in classic uremic pericarditis, *larger effusions predict subsequent cardiac tamponade*. The picture is further complicated by underlying myocardial involvement, which is more common than in uremic pericarditis and contributes to morbidity and mortality. Survival due to dialysis has allowed *uremic constriction* to appear. Uremic constrictive and effusive-constrictive pericarditis, subacute and chronic, are sequelae of pericardial hemorrhage and adhesions. Adhesions also produce fluid loculations, complicating echocardiography and other imaging.

Treatment is, basically, to intensify dialysis while avoiding hypotension. Any sign of tamponade calls for drainage of effusions with maintenance of an intrapericardial catheter for at least 2 or 3 days; repeated needle paracentesis may be especially dangerous. While there are no randomized controlled trials, an intrapericardial nonabsorbable steroid, like triamcinolone, appears to be effective. Of course, infections, including tuberculosis, should be ruled out. Because patients may be immunocompromised, systemic nonsteroidal agents for pain and fever should be used only if absolutely necessary. A trial of peritoneal dialysis for patients who have been on hemodialysis may be worthwhile. Finally, for intractable pericardial effusions, pericardial resection is the only effective approach.

Other Renal Conditions

While transplantation is usually successful for renal failure, severe *transplant rejection* has been accompanied by acute pericarditis. Patients with the *nephrotic syndrome* frequently have pericardial effusions associated with fluid retention (hydropericardium) or actual inflammation, with all the usual significance. Pericarditis in *hepatorenal failure* occurs at relatively low BUN levels and does not respond to dialysis; this is an almost uniformly fatal condition.

PERICARDIAL DISEASE IN HYPOTHYROIDISM/MYXEDEMA

Severe, usually primary hypothyroidism produce large, usually clear high-protein, high-cholesterol, high-specific-gravity pericardial effusions. These are constant in severe experimental and human myxedema and may precede other signs of the disease. Echocardiography reveals them in 5 to 30% of human hypo-thyroidism, the exact incidence and size depending on the severity, the duration and the stage of discovery. This is critical because many are apparently asymptomatic and may be discovered by chest x-ray taken for other purposes. The most conspicuous are some of the largest pericardial effusions and are nearly always chronic, due to very slow exudation. Indeed, some patients have over 2 L of fluid without obvious circulatory embarrassment. Clinical tamponade is rare because the slow tempo permits pericardial stretch. Two factors may precipitate tamponade: hemorrhage and, in some cases, cholesterol pericarditis (page 85) with an inflammatory reaction from precipitated cholesterol crystals. However, tamponade can occur without obvious precipitants, sometimes with high arterial pressure, presumably due to the increased catecholamines found in hypothyroidism.

In severe myxedema there may be pleural effusions, ascites and anasarca similar to chronic cardiac failure and constrictive pericarditis. In such cases, the blood volume is usually increased, whereas in uncomplicated myxedema it tends to be decreased. Large effusions also induce a restrictive pulmonary defect with dyspnea on exertion, which may be overlooked by the patient until reversed by drainage or treatment of hypothyroidism. The serous effusions are probably due to increased capillary permeability to protein, lymphatic obstruction and sodium and water retention, although myocardial compression by some level of chronic tamponade may contribute. Since serum thyroxine and thyroid-stimulating hormone levels in hypothyroidism are no different with or without effusion, it is not certain what role these play. In some cases, high sedimentation rates suggest an inflammatory component, which has been seen on electron microscopy, but the fluid typically has few leukocytes and erythrocytes. The ECG may not be visibly altered. However, bradycardia is the rule and severely myxedematous patients have distinctly low-to microvoltage of the QRS. The T waves are typically nonspecifically flattened or somewhat inverted (Figure 17.2); in some cases, low voltage, especially without effusion, suggests a myocardial component due to coronary disease or attendant cardiomyopathy. The latter account for true cardiomegaly with or without pericardial effusion.

Treatment is *thyroid hormone replacement*, which is nearly always followed by steady regression of the effusion. If this is given sufficiently early, any cholesterol precipitation is avoided. Mild degrees of tamponade should be monitored while the patient is responding to thyroid treatment. Except for florid tamponade, drainage is rarely needed. Rare patients with severe hypothyroid cholesterol pericarditis require further management (page 85). Timely diagnosis and treatment of hypothyroidism has reduced the incidence of significant pericardial disease in hypothyroidism and especially myxedema.

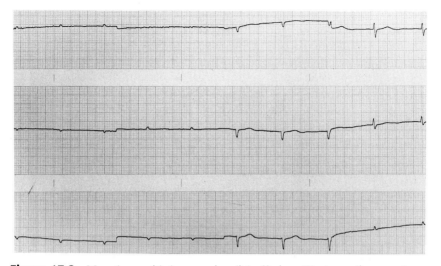

Figure 17.2 Myxedema with large pericardial effusion. Electrocardiogram shows bradycardia, low to microvoltage and nonspecific T-wave abnormalities. Q waves in leads II, III and a VF are consistent with inferior myocardial infarct of indeterminate age; however drastic voltage reduction may have eliminated preceding r waves.

OTHER METABOLIC DISORDERS

Definite pericarditis has been reported repeatedly during severe crises in patients with *diabetic ketoacidosis* and *adrenal failure* and in a number of patients with hyperuricemic *gout*. (Renal failure may occur with hyperuricemia and a high pericardial fluid urate level.) In each case, although bacterial infection—specifically in *Addisonian crisis* or tuberculosis—has been ruled out, there has not been convincing evidence that the pericarditis did not represent an intercurrent inflammation, often viral, that precipitated the diabetic or adrenal crisis. In one such patient, hepatitis was conspicuous and could have accounted for the pericarditis. In adrenal failure due to *Waterhouse-Friderichsen syndrome*, an accompanying pericarditis is almost undoubtedly meningococcal. In *diabetic ketoacidosis*, ECGs resembling stage I acute pericarditis (page 43) have been repeatedly observed both with and more often without clinical evidence of pericarditis (Figure 17.3).

To the extent that *amyloidosis* may be consider a "metabolic" defect, selective amyloid infiltration of the *pericardium* has produced a form of constriction. More often, there is a hydro-pericardium simply due to congestive heart failure in patients with amyloid *heart* disease.

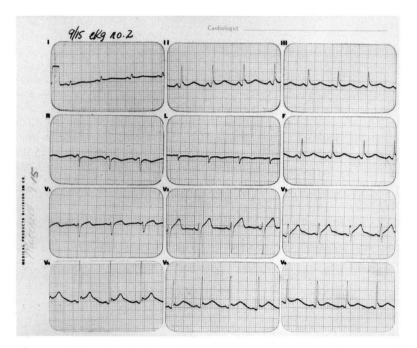

Figure 17.3   Diabetic ketoacidosis (DKA). Stage I ECG of acute pericarditis (repeatedly seen during DKA). J(ST) and PR segment deviations. T waves typical of hypokalemia.

Purely metabolic *cholesterol pericarditis* occurs in exceptional patients with high serum cholesterol but none of the usual inciting causes like hypothyroidism, tuberculosis, rheumatoid arthritis or other granulomatous lesions. Perhaps here pericarditis can be ascribed to the specific metabolic abnormality with intrapericardially precipitated cholesterol crystals inflaming the pericardium and with the consequences described in Chapter 7.

KEY POINTS

1. Renal failure of all pathogenetic types, usually with severe nitrogen retention, can provoke pericarditis of all varieties, the chronic and constrictive forms depending on life-prolonging dialysis and dialysis pericarditis. Cardiac tamponade is the main danger, especially because of intra-pericardial hemorrhage.
2. Intercurrent infection, usually viral, can cause pericarditis during any metabolic abnormality that is itself capable of involving the pericardium. In uremia, infections can cause a typical stage I ECG, which does not occur in purely uremic pericarditis.

3. Concomitant cardiovascular abnormalities like hypertension, myocardial failure and ventricular enlargement complicate the differential diagnosis of pericardial effusions and especially tamponade during uremic and dialysis pericarditis.

4. Protein-rich pericardial effusions in hypothyroidism and especially myxedema (rare today) develop slowly and only rarely critically compress the heart, although usually large and accompanied by ECG microvoltage. Some hypothyroid patients develop a form of cholesterol pericarditis. Thyroid hormone replacement characteristically rapidly reverses hypothyroidism-associated pericardial disorders.

5. Significant pericardial involvement in amyloidosis, in acute and chronic adrenal failure and the confusing typical stage I pericarditis ECG in diabetic ketoacidosis are all rare.

BIBLIOGRAPHY

Buselmeir, T.J., Davin, T.D., Simmons, R.L. Treatment of intractable uremic pericardial effusion: Avoidance of pericardiectomy with local steroid instillation. JAMA 1978: 240:1358–1360.

Frame, J.R., Lucas, S.K., Pederson, J.A., Elkins, R.C. Surgical treatment of pericarditis in the dialysis patient. Am. J. Surg. 1983; 140:300–305.

Frommer, J.P., Young, J.B., Ayus, J.C. Asymptomatic pericardial effusion in uremic patients: Effect of long-term dialysis. Nephron 1985; 39:296–301.

Maisch, B., Kochsiek, K. Humoral immune reactions in uremic pericarditis. Am. J. Nephrol. 1983; 3:264–268.

Morlans, M. Pericardial involvement in end stage renal disease. In Soler-Soler, J., Permanyer-Miralda, G., and Sagrista-Sauleda, J. Pericardial Disease: New Insights and Old Dilemmas. Dordrecht, The Netherlands: Kluwer, 1990, pp. 123–139.

Rutsky, E.A., Rostand, S.G. Treatment of uremic pericarditis and pericardial effusion. Am. J. Kidney Dis. 1987; 10:2–8.

Spodick, D.H. Pericarditis in disorders of metabolism. In: Spodick, D.H. Acute Pericarditis. New York: Grune & Stratton, 1959, chap. 23.

Spodick, D.H. Pathogenesis and clinical correlations of the electrocardiographic abnormalities of pericardial disease. In: Rios, G., (ed). Clinico-Electrocardiographic Correlations. Philadelphia: Davis, 1977, pp. 201–214.

Spodick, D.H. Pericarditis in the diabetic patient. In: Scott, R. (ed.). Clinical Cardiology and Diabetes. Vol. 3. Part I. Mount Kisco, N.Y.: Futura, 1981, pp. 151–171.

Spodick, D.H. Pericarditis in systemic diseases. Cardiology Clinics. 1990; 8:709–716.

18

Neoplastic Pericardial Disease

Neoplastic diseases affect the pericardium in three general categories: (1) *primary pericardial tumors*, benign or malignant, comparatively rare; (2) *nonneoplastic pericardial effusions* of uncertain origin accompanying malignancy elsewhere in the body; and (3) *secondary malignancies*, either metastatic and/or by extension from neighboring structures, relatively common.

SECONDARY PERICARDIAL MALIGNANCIES: METASTATIC AND INFILTRATIVE NEOPLASIA

Every kind of metastasizing and multicentric malignancy—solid, cystic, hematogenous—can affect the pericardium with or without concomitant involvement of the heart. (Secondary *cardiac* neoplasms are more often silent and for longer periods than pericardial malignancies.) Metastatic and infiltrative involvement of the pericardium may be the initial sign of malignant disease arising elsewhere and presenting as a pericardial effusion, or even more deceptively when a strong fibrinous reaction mimics "garden variety" acute pericarditis with a pain, a pericardial rub, typical electrocardiographic (ECG) changes and fever. (Leukemic, lymphomatous and myelomatous infiltrations are most likely to masquerade in this way, although solid tumors have also done so.) More often the ECG is nonspecific, but with "malignant pericarditis," the J-ST elevations sometimes last for days to weeks, implying persistent pericardial and myocardial irritation.

Pathogenesis

The cardiac lymphatic system seems to be the major pathway for tumor to reach the pericardium, often with mediastinal lymph node involvement. Indeed, in metastatic involvement of the heart by discrete tumor masses, the epicardial lymphatics are nearly always involved. Direct extension occasionally occurs from tumors of the lung, chest wall or esophagus. Solid tumors may be restricted to the pericardium, invade the myocardium or appear in each simultaneously. Lymphomas, Hodgkin's disease, leukemias, melanomas and especially multiple myeloma simultaneously infiltrate the myocardium and pericardium, although they can be isolated to the pericardium. Many of these are associated with local production of a variety of cytokines that can account for the associated pericardial inflammation. Rarely, such lesions are confined to the parietal pericardium and remain "silent" unless they erode a blood vessel. Melanomas very often invade the visceral pericardium with a very high incidence of cardiac involvement.

CLINICAL ASPECTS

Secondary pericardial neoplasia tends to be clinically insidious and difficult to diagnose unless cancer is recognized elsewhere in the patient. Neoplastic pericardial effusions are usually large (especially so in patients with hypoalbuminemia), with or without tamponade. With any neoplastic effusion, there is the constant menace of acceleration by intrapericardial hemorrhage due to critical tamponade precipitated by the disease or its management. Occasionally, a tumor duplicates a syndrome of constrictive pericarditis, especially effusive-constrictive disease, with the constriction due to neoplastic tissue, to adhesions and scarring or both. A tumor may also encase the heart, producing *elastic constriction* (page 254) with deceptive clinical sings (Figure 18.1). Equally deceptive are cardiac tumors involving the pericardium that can mimic the systemic and local signs of members of the vasculitis-connective tissue disease group (Chapter 19). Neoplastic effusions may become suppurative, suggesting infectious pericarditis, especially in patients who are immunocompromised due to treatment or to AIDS, including Kaposi's sarcoma; the organisms are either common or opportunistic pathogens, especially atypical mycobacteria and fungi.

Pericardial malignancy should be strongly suspected, particularly in patients with known malignancy elsewhere: (1) with any large, recurrent and especially hemorrhagic pericardial effusion or (2) syndromes, including refractory "heart failure," with markedly raised venous pressure, superior vena cava syndrome or (3) unexplained hepatomegaly. In addition to symptoms and signs of the preceding, dyspnea (including orthopnea, the most common symptom), unexplained chest pain and nonproductive cough should raise the question of peri-

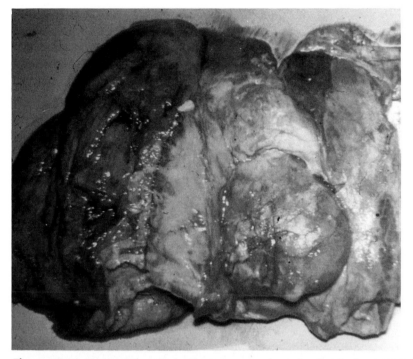

Figure 18.1   Pericardial neoplasia. Postmortem specimen showing the heart protruding from encircling neoplastic tissue (partly dissected), discovered at operation for elastic constriction.

cardial involvement. Patients with breast and lung malignancy, unless these lesions first appear in the pericardium, may have obvious pulmonary lesions, hypoxia and pleural effusions. Patients with lymphomas and related neoplasms may have enlarged lymph nodes in the mediastinum and elsewhere.

DIAGNOSIS AND DIFFERENTIAL DIAGNOSIS (TABLE 18.1)

In addition to the symptoms and history of allied disease, imaging modalities in their broadest application may point to the diagnosis utilizing one or more of standard chest films, echocardiography, magnetic resonance imaging (MRI), computed tomography (CT) and radionuclide scanning with indium 111, Gallium 67, or technetium. Irregularities or masses demonstrated by any of these may compress one or more cardiac chamber. Both CT and MRI are also ideal for determining tumor contents and texture. Typical imaging findings of a very large effusion (Figure 18.2) or of cardiac tamponade, particularly on echo-

Table 18.1   Neoplastic Pericardial Effusions: Diagnostic Procedures

History and physical examination
Radiologic and isotopic studies: nuclear scans
Echocardiography; computed tomography; magnetic resonance imaging
Routine examination of pericardial fluid
   Appearance
   Specific gravity
   Protein content
   Lactic dehydrogenase
Additional tests
   Amylase
   Carcinoembryonic antigen (CEA)
   Immunologic constituents
   Cytologic studies; chromosomal analysis
   Hormone receptor study
Biopsy; subxiphoid or video-assisted thoracoscopy
   Exploratory thoracotomy

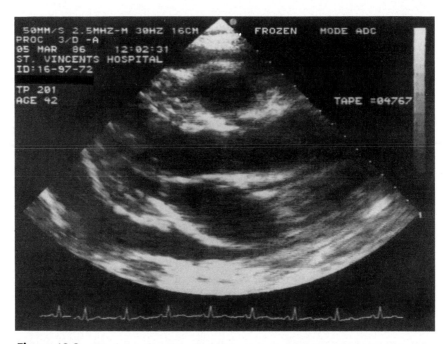

Figure 18.2   Massive pericardial effusion due to metastatic bronchogenic carcinoma. Typical of large and high-pressure effusions, the fluid has penetrated behind the left atrium (bottom of echo sector).

Doppler study, may necessitate sampling of fluid or tissue to demonstrate the malignancy. Some sarcomas produce floating tumor masses in pericardial fluid, visible by echocardiographs. Occasionally, pericardial fluid within pericardial recesses (page 8) simulates tumors and cysts. Finally, because they can cause pericardial effusions and obstruct one or both venae cavae, right atrial masses—tumors and thrombi—may simulate the behavior of pericardial neoplasms.

The *differential diagnosis* includes (1) cardiomyopathy due to treatment with antineoplastic agents, with or without a hydropericardium related to actual congestive heart failure, and (2) nonmalignant pericardial effusions of uncertain pathogenesis, which are relatively frequent with malignancy elsewhere in the body. The *ECG* is usually abnormal but nonspecific. There may be only ST-T wave changes and QRS changes related to the effusion itself, with the exception of remarkable mimicry of the acute pericarditis ECG by some malignancies. Rarely, a tumor encasing the heart (Figure 18.1), with or without compressive signs, may cause the Stage I electrocardiogram to remain indefinitely, i.e., widespread J-ST elevations. These may evolve with terminal T wave inversions but the J-ST elevations do not resolve (Figure 18.3). The presence of *electric alternation* on the ECG helps establish a significant, usually large, effusion, most often with tamponade. Electric alternation is itself a nonspecific indicator, since it may occur most often in malignant effusions.

Pericardial fluid obtained either by paracentesis or surgical drainage should be intensely studied for cells, including histochemical staining (Figure 18.4). Carcinoembryonic antigen (CEA) should be sought. (Table 18.1 summarizes the diagnostic approaches.) Unsatisfactory diagnostic results require *biopsy*; the

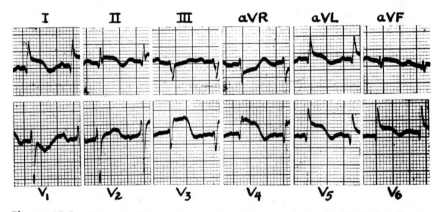

Figure 18.3 Electrocardiogram in a patient with extensive pericardial infiltration by lymphoma. There are ubiquitous J (ST) deviations, as seen in Stage I ECGs, but with simultaneous atypical T-wave inversions. These abnormalities resemble some seen with myopericarditis. This pattern was stable for at least 2 weeks.

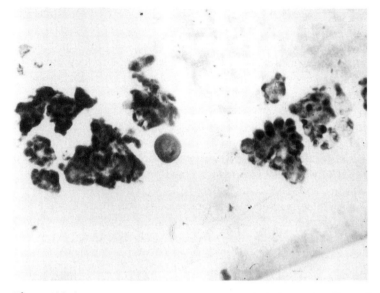

Figure 18.4   Squamous-cell carcinoma metastatic to the pericardium: clumps of malignant cells in pericardial fluid.

largest possible specimen should be obtained via the subxiphoid route or thoracoscopically. Indeed, when refractory effusions necessitate pericardial resection, the tissue obtained may give the answer. Pericardial fluid hematocrits may be misleading in distinguishing frank blood from bloody pericardial fluid (page 82) because cancer patients often have low hematocrits.

PRIMARY PERICARDIAL NEOPLASIA

Table 18.2 summarizes the primary neoplasms of the pericardium, most of which are uncommon enough to be termed "curiosities." The benign primary growths are found especially in infancy and childhood, whereas the primary malignancies are discovered mostly in the third and fourth decades. Lipomas and fibromas, discovered in mid and later life, may grow to giant proportions before discovery. Congenital or developmental pericardial cysts (Chapter 6) may require differential diagnosis, especially if they are atypically located and if imaging (even MRI) gives an illusion of solid tumor.

The most important primary malignancies are *mesotheliomas* and *sarcomas* (particularly angiosarcoma), which arise from the pericardial serosa and vasculature and, apparently, do not metastasize (although pleural mesothelioma can metastasize to the pericardium). They spread aggressively throughout the peri-

Table 18.2   Primary Pericardial Neoplasms

Mesothelioma, solitary or diffuse
  Benign/fibrous
  Malignant
Fibroma
Lipoma
Neuroma
Primary pericardial lymphoma (AIDS patients)
Sarcoma
  Angiosarcoma
  Fibrosarcoma
Lymphangioma
Lymphangioepithelioma
Hemangioma
Malignant hemangioepithelioma
Hamartoma
Pleochromocytoma

Pericardial tumors of infancy and childhood (also in adults)
Teratoma
  Benign
  Malignant
Dermoid
Bronchogenic cyst
Pericardial cysts (Chapter 6)
Pleochromocytoma
Neuroblastoma
Neurofibroma
Thymoma
  Benign
    Cystic
  Malignant

Pseudotumors
Pericardial venous varices
Heterotopic bone marrow (myeloproliferation)
Heterotopic thyroid tissue
Mesothelial hyperplasia

cardium and often invade the myocardium. *Mesotheliomas* (Figure 18.5)—recently apparently increasing in incidence—are strongly related to asbestos or fiberglass exposure, although there are numerous cases without either history.

In general, the signs and symptoms of the secondary metastatic and infiltrative malignancies (pages 302–303) also apply to the primary benign and malignant tumors of the pericardium.

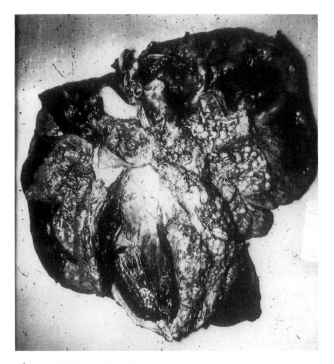

Figure 18.5 Pericardial mesothelioma—postmortem specimen with heart and lungs. Nodular tumor masses encase the heart and have invaded the adjacent visceral pleural surfaces.

CLINICAL PECULIARITIES

The benign tumors of infancy and childhood (which can also occur in adults) usually provoke large pericardial effusions, even in neonates in whom a cardiorespiratory distress syndrome may appear at or shortly after birth. *Teratomas* are nearly always found in infants presenting with large pericardial effusions, the fluid is usually a transudate, although occasionally sanguineous and rarely a pyopericardium. These tumors may have a blood supply via a pedicle from the aortic root or the pulmonary artery, producing technical problems for operative excision. They often compress the right atrium and ventricle and may have detectable calcifications, teeth and bones. *Intrapericardial bronchial cysts* may resemble teratomas on imaging (that is, with radioopaque contents), but pericardial effusion is not common.

Pheochromocytomas (paragangliomas) and related *neurofibromata* and *neuroblastomata* may appear first with sympathetic hormonal effect leading to detection by chemical or special imaging techniques, such as blood and urine tests for catecholamines and localization with iodine-131 metaiodo-benzyl-guanidine (^{131}I-mbg). Because they are hypervascular, intravenous contrast material can localize these tumors. *Thymomas* can cause pericardial effusions but may themselves be so large as to be confused with pericardial effusion and difficult to identify by imaging when they are isodense with surrounding structures. *Malignant thymomas* may present as multisystem disease and autoimmune syndromes as well as cardiac tamponade and superior vena cava obstruction; immunocompromised patients are more susceptible. Thymomas and other large tumors may rarely simulate cardiac tamponade or constriction and obstruct the superior vena cava. Some *large cystic tumors* can compress cardiac chambers, with the tumor itself responding to the respiratory phases and causing a pseudo–pulsus paradoxus.

The most important primary pericardial tumors remain mesothelioma and sarcoma, especially angiosarcoma. *Mesotheliomas* may give all the symptoms and signs mentioned for metastatic and infiltrative tumors, but they may be great imitators, mimicking idiopathic acute pericarditis with effusion (usually hemorrhagic) or growing without much fibrinous or effusive reaction to overspread the heart, causing atypical or even classic constriction (Figure 18.5). These pericardial effusions contain very high levels of hyaluronic acid. *Angiosarcomas* grow in bloody locules within the pericardial cavity, may or may not deform the cardiopericardial silhouette while enlarging it and, because they are composed of masses of larger and smaller blood-filled spaces, imitate hemopericardium of other origin.

TREATMENT (TABLES 18.3 AND 18.4)

Drainage of tamponading or refractory large effusions is mandatory. *Pericardiocentesis* has a high failure rate except for immediate temporary relief of tamponade. Percutaneous *balloon pericardiotomy* or a *subxiphoid surgical "window"* may be successful in some patients with predictably limited survival. The window is ideal for direct inspection and biopsy; balloon pericardiotomy avoids the discomfort and risk of surgery. A *pericardioperitoneal shunt* may provide prolonged palliation.

Extensive or complete *pericardial resection* is mandatory for persistent recurrence or for malignant pericardial constriction. In patients with a particularly poor prognosis or in whom operation would be hazardous, *sclerosing therapy* with tetracycline or other agents often palliates effusions. Frequently,

Table 18.3 Neoplastic Pericardial Effusions:
Therapeutic Approaches

Nonsurgical
  Pericardiocentesis
  Radiotherapy
  Intracavitary (local) therapy
    Newer chemotherapeutic agents
    Nitrogen mustard
    Quinacrine (atabrine)
    5-Fluorouracil
    Sclerosants; bleomycin, tetracycline, mitomycin
      C, "OK-432," other
    Radioisotopes
      Gold, yttrium 90, ^{32}Chromic phosphate, i.e.
        (Cr PO$_4$ labeled with radioactive ^{32}Cr)
    Talc poudrage
  Systemic chemotherapy
  Immunotherapy
    τIL-2
Surgical drainage/resection/biopsy
  Transthoracic
    Thoracoscopy (video-assisted)
    Subxiphoid
      Incision; biopsy
      Scope-assisted

*indwelling pericardial drainage tubes or catheters provoke a similar reaction
rendering sclerotherapy unnecessary.*) Intrapericardial nonabsorbable corticosteroid may be used in a similar nonspecific manner. Unfortunately, there is no
convincing evidence that intrapericardial treatment with therapeutic agents mod-
ifies the prognosis for life, which averages 4 months over all secondary malignancies except for occasional tumors that are especially sensitive to radiation
or systemic chemotherapy.

    Table 18.4 summarizes the advantages and disadvantages of the six prin-
cipal therapies of malignant pericardial effusion.

Table 18.4 MALIGNANT PERICARDIAL EFFUSIONS: TREATMENT

Pericardiocentesis	Pericardiocentesis + intrapericardial tetracycline or chemotherapeutic agents	Subxiphoid pericardiotomy	Pleuropericardial window	Pericardiectomy/ resection	External beam irradiation
Advantages					
Relieves tamponade	Relieves tamponade	Relieves tamponade	Can evaluate extent of disease	Can evaluate extent of disease	Noninvasive
Local anesthesia yields fluid for study	Local anesthesia	Local anesthesia	Excellent for diagnosis	Excellent for diagnosis	
	Lower recurrence than pericardiocentesis alone	Yields fluid for study	Can be done by balloon catheter		
	Controls most malignant effusions	Yields pericardial biopsy			
		Permits examination of pericardial space			
Disadvantages					
Very frequent recurrence	Occasional recurrences	Sometimes logistically difficult	General anesthesia unless by balloon	General anesthesia	Nondiagnostic
No biopsy	No biopsy			Thoracotomy morbidity significantly less if thoracoscopic	Tamponade unchanged

KEY POINTS

1. A wide variety of metastatic and infiltrative malignancies constitute the majority of pericardial tumors in adults; they tend to begin insidiously without specific symptoms and signs and so can provoke very large effusions unless accidentally discovered. *Malignant effusions are in danger of decompensating to critical tamponade from active bleeding.* Bronchogenic and mammary carcinomas and lymphomas are most common. Patients with AIDS may develop unusual tumors of the pericardium, including Kaposi's sarcoma.
2. Dyspnea is the commonest single symptom of pericardial tumors in adults. Recognized extrapericardial neoplasia should initiate diagnostic measures, particularly imaging, in such patients who develop unexplained dyspnea, chest pain or cough.
3. In patients without an etiologic diagnosis, extensive evaluation of pericardial fluid and tissue is mandatory. Though blood is a frequent component of pericardial effusions, it is diagnostically nonspecific.
4. Benign primary neoplasms and cysts are most common in childhood and infancy.
5. The most important malignancies, especially in adults, are mesotheliomas and sarcomas. Mesothelioma can simulate acute nonspecific pericarditis, constrictive pericarditis and tamponade of other etiology.

BIBLIOGRAPHY

Chan, H.S., Sonley, M.J., Moes, C.A., et al. Primary and secondary tumors of childhood involving the heart, pericardium and great vessels. Cancer 1985; 56:825-831.

Collins JJ Jr, Pins MR. Case 5 - 1996. Case records of the Massachusetts General Hospital. New England J Med 1996; 334: 452-458.

Engberding, R., Schulze-Waltrup, N., Grosse-Heitmeyer, W., and Stoll, V. Transthoracic and transesophageal 2-D echocardiography in the diagnosis of peri- and paracardiac tumors. Dtsch. Med. Wochenschr. 1987; 112:49-55.

Hawkins, J.W., Vacek, J.L. What constitutes definitive therapy of malignant pericardial effusion? "Medical" versus surgical treatment. Am. Heart. J. 1989; 118:428-432.

Maisch, B., Druge, L. Pericardioscopy—A new diagnostic tool in inflammatory disease of the pericardium. Eur. Heart J. 1991; 12(suppl):2-6.

Montalescot, G., Chapelon, C., Drobinski, G., et al. Diagnosis of primary cardiac sarcoma: Report of 4 cases and review of the literature. Int. J. Cardiol. 1988; 20:289-296.

Segawa, D., Yoshizu, H., Haga, Y., et al. Successful operation for solitary fibrous tumor of the pericardium. J. Thorac. Cardiovasc. Surg. 1995; 109:1246-1248.

Shepherd, F.A., Morgan, C., Evans, W.K., et al. Medical management of malignant pericardial effusion by tetracycline sclerosis. Am. J. Cardiol. 1987; 60:1161-1166.

Spodick, D.H. Diseases of the pericardium. In: Parmley, W.W., Chatterjee, K. (eds.). *Cardiology*. Vol. 2. Philadelphia, Lippincott, 1992, chap. 43.

Theologides, A. Neoplastic cardiac tamponade. Semin. Oncol. 1978; 5:181-188.

Thomason, R., Schlegel, W., Lucca, M., et al. Primary malignant mesothelioma of the pericardium. Texas Heart Inst. J. 1994; 21:170-174.

Vaitkus, P.T., Hermann, H.C., LeWinter, M.M. Treatment of malignant pericardial effusion. JAMA 1994; 272:59–64.

Wilding, G., Green, H.L., Longo, D.L., Urba, W.J. Tumors of the heart and pericardium. Cancer Treat. Rep. 1988; 15:165-170.

Yazdi, H.M., Hajdu, S.I., Melamed, M.R. Cystopathology of pericardial effusions. Acta Cytol. 1980; 24:401–412.

19

Pericardial Disease in the Vasculitis–Connective Tissue Disease Group

Pericarditis, pericardial effusion, pericardial adhesions and constriction occur in a wide variety of systemic diseases. These include most chronic inflammatory disorders of the *vasculitis–connective tissue disease group* (Table 19.1), a designation for a heterogenous group of disorders that have in common an inflammation tending to damage blood vessel walls. In those with a high prevalence of clinical pericardial disease, like systemic lupus erythematosus, or with pericardial disease that is frequently discovered only postmortem, like rheumatoid arthritis, the etiology may seem clear. However, any primary pericarditis (e.g., viral or postmyocardial infarction pericarditis) may coincide with one of these systemic diseases. In others, in which pericarditis is uncommon, the systemic vasculitic illness may be either etiologic or "permissive" of increased susceptibility to an unrelated primary pericarditis, like viral (pages 260–265) or "idiopathic" (pages 417–421) pericarditis. In this disease group, *only specific histologic lesions in the pericardium confirm the etiology,* although *characteristic pericardial fluid constituents may be adequate* and *characteristic clinical behavior often points strongly to the diagnosis.* Nevertheless, diagnosis can be difficult due to overlap among some patients with manifestations of more than one syndrome (Table 19.1).

Table 19.1   **Pericardial Disease in the Vasculitis–Connective Tissue Disease Group**

1. Rheumatoid arthritis (RA), including:
   Juvenile RA
   Still's disease, juvenile and adult
   Felty's syndrome
2. Rheumatic fever (ARF)
3. Systemic lupus erythematosus (SLE), including drug-induced SLE
4. Progressive systemic sclerosis (scleroderma) including
   CREST syndrome
5. Sjögren's syndrome
6. Polymyositis (dermatomyositis)
7. Mixed connective tissue disease (MCTD) and other "overlap" syndromes
8. Seronegative spondyloarthropathies
   a. Ankylosing spondylitis
   b. Psoriatic arthritis
   c. Reiter's syndrome
   d. Intestinal arthropathies
      (1) Crohn's disease
      (2) Ulcerative colitis
      (3) Whipple's disease
9. Vasculitides
   a. Giant-cell arteritis
      (1) Temporal (cranial) arteritis
      (2) Takayasu's arteritis
   b. Polyarteritis (*esp.* HBsAg-positive)
   c. Systemic necrotizing vasculitis
   d. Bürger's disease
   e. Kawasaki's disease (mucocutaneous lymph node syndrome)
   f. Hypersensitivity vasculitides
      (1) Allergic granulomatosis
      (2) Churg-Strauss syndrome
      (3) Hypereosinophilic syndromes
   g. Hypocomplementemic urticarial vasculitis syndrome (HUVS)
   h. Henoch-Schönlein purpura
10. Behçet's syndrome
11. Stevens-Johnson syndrome
12. Non-RA granulomata
    a. Wegener's
    b. Sarcoidosis
13. Panmesenchymal reaction of steroid hormone withdrawal
14. Periodic polyserositis (familial Mediterranean fever; FMF)

(*continued*)

Table 19.1 Continued

15.	Thrombohemolytic thrombocytopenic purpura (TTP)
16.	Serum sickness
17.	Polymyalgia rheumatica
18.	Eosinophilic fasciitis
19.	Osteogenesis imperfecta
20.	Other

Pathogenetic Considerations

"Vasculitis–connective tissue disease" is a classification of convenience, owing to features not equally shared by all group members. All develop variable abnormalities of collagen and inflammation and necrosis of blood vessels (*vasculitis*), affecting arteries of calibers often characteristic of each entity. The primary immunopathogenic event leading to vasculitis is probably *deposition of immune complexes*. Indeed, most group members have definite immunopathic, including autoimmune, features based on immunoglobulin or complement deposition and/or inflammatory cell infiltration in blood vessels and pericardium. Sometimes, increased or decreased pericardial fluid complement components with normal serum complement levels suggest local complement activation or consumption. In conditions with arthritis, synovial tissue and joint fluid abnormalities may resemble those of pericardium and pericardial fluid.

Some of this group's heterogeneity is due to *conditions related directly or indirectly* to exposure to infectious agents (e.g., streptococcal antigen in acute rheumatic fever; hepatitis B antigen in polyarteritis), to unrelated pericardial trauma (e.g., arthritic manifestations with pericarditis in postpericardiotomy syndrome and the postmyocardial infarction syndrome) or hypersensitivity—"allergic"—reactions (e.g., drug-induced lupus) that provoke immunologic responses. Finally, neoplasia can provoke vasculitis as well as pericarditis.

Depending on category, inflammation and necrosis may be mediated by immune complex deposition or cell-mediated immune reactivity or both. Some, like Wegener's granulomatosis and rheumatoid arthritis, are characterized by granuloma formation. Sarcoidosis, also granulomatous, is less well understood and not strictly a vasculitis but is included for convenience, particularly because its differential diagnosis is important. Many patients develop serologic evidence, including hypergammaglobulinemia, cryoglobulinemia, hypocomplementemia, circulating immune complexes and rheumatoid factor, each of which may also be found in pericardial fluid.

Most entities of the vasculitis–connective tissue disease group affect a clear preponderance of females, yet males form a disproportionately large part of those with pericardial involvement. This reflects the male preponderance in almost every form of pericarditis, a susceptibility that may ultimately prove to have a genetic basis.

Problems of Classification

Complicating any comprehensive classification in this disease group are the preceding pathogenetic considerations, overlap among syndromes (e.g., mixed connective tissue disease, polyarteritis with hepatitis B virus) and intriguing relations to conditions that are clinically classifiable elsewhere. Examples include pericarditis with or without arthritis, Crohn's disease and ulcerative colitis (classifiable under gastrointestinal disorders), leptospirosis classified with coronary arteritis and pericardial effusion, and Rocky Mountain spotted fever with infectious pericarditis. The classification in Table 19.1 thus remains one of convenience, since in most members of the vasculitis–connective tissue disease group *the diagnosis is initially suspected from their clinical behavior*. Various laboratory studies, e.g., antinuclear antibodies (ANAs), support and often confirm some diagnoses but, taken alone, are not entirely specific.

Finally, *some benign and malignant cardiac tumors, including myxoma, may be associated with systemic syndromes resembling those of members of the vasculitis–connective tissue disease group*. When accompanied by pericarditis or effusion, the mimicry is particularly deceptive.

PERICARDIAL DISEASE IN RHEUMATOID ARTHRITIS

General Considerations

Rheumatoid arthritis (RA) and all its variants, juvenile and adult, as well as adult-onset Still's disease, is probably the biggest single "generator" of pericardial disease. Incidence statistics are affected by referral bias, with only the severest forms coming under hospital scrutiny. Yet almost half of autopsy patients with rheumatoid arthritis have significant pericardial adhesions, and in the living population echocardiography shows approximately half to have excessive pericardial fluid. *Moreover, all morphologic forms of pericarditis are associated with rheumatoid arthritis.*

Clinical Considerations

Acute fibrinous pericarditis, usually subclinical, is demonstrable mainly in patients dying for any reason during severe arthritic flares. *Pericardial effusions*, also usually subclinical and small to moderate-sized, can become quite large, chronic and even tamponading. *Adhesive pericarditis*, usually generalized, but occasionally localized or with loculated fluid, can provoke all variants of *constrictive* and *effusive-constrictive* pericarditis.

Pericardial involvement is most common in middle-aged white males, in whom RA pericarditis tends to constrict more often than in females. All forms of pericardial disease become clinically more overt with severe rheumatoid arthritis, particularly in patients with strong serologic evidence, and only rarely in quiescent, well-controlled disease. Constriction occurs more often within 4 to 5 years of the onset of severe RA and is comparatively rare with chronicity.

Clinical Features

While recurrent acute and effusive pericarditis can develop, most patients undergo only a single acute event. The most common presentation is a pericardial rub, usually confined to systole, that may last from days to years and is accidentally discovered in a patient without chest symptoms. The other most common discovery is an asymptomatic effusion on echocardiography. Rarely, manifest acute pericarditis, clinically significant effusion or even constriction has been the first manifestation of rheumatoid arthritis. Recognition of rheumatoid pericarditis is confounded not only by its many variants but by intercurrent diseases, like viral pericarditis or drug-induced pericarditis (e.g., by phenylbutazone), by possibly increased susceptibility to other infections as well as viruses and the excellent substrate for bacterial infection afforded by chronic pericardial effusions (page 433). In general, clinical manifestations depend on the type of pericardial involvement. Also confounding is the rare presence of rheumatoid myopericarditis or myocardial granulomas. Uni- or bilateral pleural effusions, pleural rubs and lung lesions (including even Caplan's syndrome) are common with active disease. Any patient with rheumatoid arthritis and systemic congestion ("right heart failure") should raise the question of rheumatoid constriction or tamponade, although the more common causes of systemic congestion (e.g., true heart failure) are more likely in most RA patients.

Laboratory Data

While acute RA pericardial effusions may have more fibrin, acute and chronic effusions resemble arthritic synovial fluid and rheumatoid pleural effusions. They are mainly serous, occasionally serosanguinous, rarely frankly hemorrhagic and characterized by low glucose (under 45 mg/dL), a wide range of leukocytosis (mainly over 15,000 cells/mm^3) with many cells showing cytoplasmic inclusions that stain for IgM, and soluble immune complexes, including IgG; complement levels are very low; latex fixation titers are high.

Protein is increased (usually over 5 g/dL) and cholesterol, including cholesterol crystals, is frequently increased. Electrocardiographic changes are nonspecific; indeed, any significant changes suggest myocardial disease. Severe

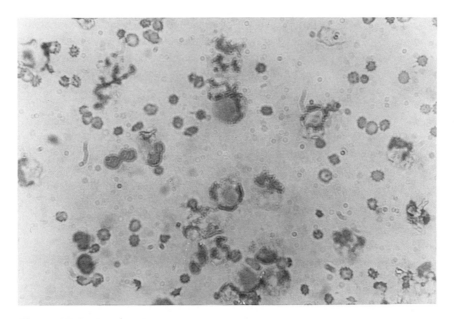

Figure 19.1 Systemic lupus erythematosus; Giemsa stain of pericardial fluid showing spontaneous formation of large, multinucleated "lupus cells."

cases must be differentiated from tuberculous and bacterial pericarditis, malignancy, and, rarely, other etiologies of cholesterol pericarditis (Chapters 7, 25).

Management

Treatment, in addition to management of RA itself, is necessary only for symptomatic pericardial disease (page 107). Unfortunately, constriction has occurred in RA patients despite established antiarthritic treatment with corticosteroids, high-dose aspirin and other anti-inflammatory agents.

PERICARDITIS IN ACUTE RHEUMATIC FEVER

General Considerations

Pericarditis in rheumatic fever (RF) has declined in proportion to its decrease in incidence in the developed world. Although mainly a disease of children and adolescents, (as well as some adults who mainly do not have cardiac involvement), the brief resurgence in the United States in the late 1980s of RF with severe carditis in young adults emphasizes its potential significance. Rheumatic fever is clearly associated with antecedent infection and has features of immuno-pathies and the vasculitis–connective tissue disease group; its pericardial lesions include extensive deposition in the pericardium and its vessels of IgG, IgM, and C3. At necropsy or surgery, most patients have at least discrete fibrotic "milk patches" on the epicardium; most of those with chronic valvular disease, with or without active carditis, also have pericardial adhesions, frequently obliterative, which for unknown reasons do not appear to cause constrictive pericarditis. Clinically, in the vast majority of cases, pericardial involvement is minimal or asymptomatic. Yet, *diagnosable pericardial involvement in acute rheumatic fever usually indicates severe and sometimes fatal pancarditis*, especially if accompanied by significant effusion, which may be partly or entirely related to RF myocarditis or congestive heart failure. Moreover, pericarditis without valve disease is rarely due to ARF and another cause must be sought (e.g. other connective tissue disease or infection.)

Diagnosis and Differential Diagnosis

Acute pericarditis is a sign of active rheumatic carditis. It usually occurs at the onset of the initial episode with symptoms and signs in the first week following the appearance of fever and arthritis; chest pain varies from mild to severe; there may be a secondary temperature rise and disproportionate tachycardia; dyspnea is probably related to myocarditis and pulmonary congestion or edema. The pericardial rub may be intense and last several days. Some degree of effusion is the rule, with amber fluid containing considerable fibrin. Tamponade is rare but must be differentiated from congestive failure.

Differential diagnosis from other vasculitis–connective tissue disease group members is essential, particularly juvenile rheumatoid arthritis in adults who have lymphadenopathy, systemic lupus, and also endocarditis (all forms), Lyme disease, and sickle cell crisis. Occasionally, pericarditis is the first sign of acute rheumatic fever; therefore *in any child with pericarditis, ARF must be ruled in or out*, especially if there is a rash and arthralgias, which also occur in viral pericarditis and childhood exanthemata. Without definite carditis, the diagnosis of RF pericarditis is circumstantial; (1) fever and arthritis, usually preceding pericarditis, (2) relative youth in most cases, and (3) serologic positivity for beta-hemolytic streptococci.

Management

Nonsteroidal agents may suffice; in young children aspirin should be avoided if possible. Corticosteroid therapy may be used if these fail and may be marginally better, but there is no conclusive proof of its superiority. Tamponading effusions must be drained (page 173).

PERICARDITIS IN SYSTEMIC LUPUS ERYTHEMATOSUS (SLE)

General Considerations

Pericarditis is the most common cardiac manifestation of this multisystem autoimmune disease. The pericarditis of SLE is characterized by epicardial microvasculitis and necrosis, and a number of antibodies to nuclear components and phospholipids that form pathogenic antigen-antibody complexes. *Systemic lupus erythematosus causes the entire spectrum, and all stages—acute, subacute, chronic and recurrent—of anatomic and pathophysiologic pericardial abnormalities.* This spectrum includes acute, clinically dry pericarditis and exudative pericardial effusion—serous, serosanguinous or hemorrhagic—pericardial adhesions, and constrictive pericarditis. Immune complexes are deposited in the pericardium, including IgG, IgM, C3 and rarely hematoxylin bodies. Most patients with SLE develop some form of pericarditis, either clinical or subclinical; precise statistics are influenced by institutional referral bias or population bias, e.g., postmortem observation. Pericardial effusion, often large, is common, although cardiac tamponade and constrictive pericarditis are comparatively uncommon. (Anticoagulant therapy is potentially dangerous in such patients.)

Males are relatively overrepresented, especially among patients who develop constriction, in this typically "female disease." Yet *all females with acute pericarditis should be tested for SLE.* This is imperative because any form—acute pericarditis, pericardial effusion, cardiac tamponade and even constriction—may be the very first clinical manifestation of SLE. However, pericarditis typically accompanies severe lupus and is often diagnosed during an acute flare, which may be painful or painless but virtually always with serologic evidence of active disease.

Lupus nephropathy is often present, so that *uremic pericarditis with effusion may be mistaken for or accompany SLE pericarditis* (page 292). Increased susceptibility to a wide range of common and opportunistic bacteria and fungi can be due to the effects of anti-inflammatory, immunosuppressive or cytotoxic treatments and can lead to contamination of previously sterile effusions. Even with infective purulent effusions, blood cultures tend to be negative and some grossly purulent fluids are explained by a very high white cell content. Patients receiving methysergide treatment may develop constrictive pericarditis or, more often, an imitative fibrosing mediastinitis.

Drug-induced SLE (page 413) is not rare and produces all the pericarditic forms of idiopathic lupus from acute to constrictive. However, acute forms clear after discontinuing the offending drug, usually procainamide, isoniazid, hydralazine, methyldopa, or penicillin. In *silica-associated connective tissue disease* expressed as SLE, pericarditis is as frequent as in non-silica-associated SLE.

Congenitally acquired SLE pericarditis is rare, occurring in infants of mothers with the disease.

Diagnosis

In SLE patients, an enlarged cardiopericardial silhouette may represent pericardial effusion, myocardial lupus, or both. Echocardiography is very efficient for diagnosing effusion and may also show valvular Libman-Sacks vegetations. *Pericardial fluid* shows high-protein, low-glucose and variable white blood cell counts, from low to very high, mainly polymorphonuclears with spontaneous formation of "lupus cells" (Figure 19.1); these are not specific for lupus. Higher leukocyte counts appear to correlate with anticardiolipin antibody. As in pleural and synovial fluids, whole (hemolytic) complement is characteristically low to absent. Appropriate *antinuclear antibody* responses can aid diagnosis, (although not pathognomonic) but titers decrease with advancing age. The *electrocardiogram* (ECG) may show typical Stage I changes of pericarditis or may be nonspecific, including presentation in Stage III (page 41); the latter always raises the question of lupus myocardiopathy. In all cases blood should be cultured and tests for tuberculosis performed, particularly in patients on anti-inflammatory and immunosuppressant therapy. Although, like arthritis, pericarditis tends to subside between episodes, patients should be followed for the development of constrictive pericarditis. Constriction is only rarely an initial manifestation.

Management

In general, therapy is the same as for the systemic disease. Critical tamponade, of course, requires drainage and constrictive pericarditis requires pericardiectomy. However, occasional patients with less than critical tamponade respond to high-dose corticosteroid therapy and even a trial of nonsteroidal anti-inflammatory therapy.

PERICARDITIS IN PROGRESSIVE SYSTEMIC SCLEROSIS (PSS): SCLERODERMA

General Considerations

Scleroderma provokes uncontrolled fibroblastic activity leading to abnormal collagen deposition in the microvasculature, skin, synovia, gastrointestinal tract, lungs, heart, kidneys and pericardium, occurring diffusely or in limited systemic scleroderma—the CREST syndrome—*C*alcinosis, *R*aynaud's phenomenon, *E*sophageal dysfunction, *S*clerodactyly and *T*elangiectasia. Although myocardial involvement with congestive failure is common, *pericardial scleroderma is the most common cardiac form*, with the pericardium involved in most patients at autopsy. Pericardial effusion is revealed in almost one-half the patients by echocardiogram, but relatively few patients have clinical manifestations of pericardial scleroderma. These, however, run the gamut of pericardial disease from acute fibrinous pericarditis (always raising the question of intercurrent infection), to pericardial effusions, which may be chronic or tamponading, to constrictive pericarditis. Any of these may recur over long periods. Constriction results from relentless fibrosis (and can recur after pericardiectomy, though fortunately rarely). Usually scleroderma has already declared itself, particularly in the skin, and esophagograms may have already shown reduced peristalsis and narrowing before cardiac or pericardial involvement becomes manifest. Rarely, acute and chronic pericardial effusions and even tamponade have preceded the diagnosis of scleroderma, including the CREST syndrome. Finally, eosinophilic fasciitis with pericarditis may resemble scleroderma.

Pericardial effusion attributable to scleroderma is an exudate that contrasts with acute exudates in other forms of vasculitis because of the *absence of autoantibodies, immune complexes or complement deposition,* along with very few white blood cells and a variable protein level. Pericardial transudates and pleural effusions are more likely to result form congestive heart failure or uremia. While pericardial fibrosis (rarely calcification) facilitates cardiac tamponade with smaller fluid accumulation, pericardial scarring in scleroderma is typically slow and associated with a gradual obliteration of small vessels that contributes to tissue hypoxia.

Pericardial involvement occurs with or without myocardial scleroderma, but ECGs, almost always abnormal, are nonspecifically changed and probably reflect involvement of myocardium and conducting tissue. Consequently, in scleroderma a typical Stage I ECG of acute pericarditis (page 41) and, indeed, some cases with clinical acute fibrinous pericarditis, should always raise the question of intercurrent infection.

Because of the systemic nature of the disease, confounding factors frequently must be considered. Thus, the patient's hemodynamics may be affected by pulmonary lesions producing pulmonary hypertension, right ventricular hypertrophy and systemic congestion; these often dominate the clinical picture. Myocardial scleroderma occasionally produces a restrictive cardiomyopathy, which can masquerade as pericardial constriction; moreover, just as in radiation pericarditis, both constrictive pericarditis and restrictive cardiomyopathy may coexist (page 250). Pericardial effusion may also be a transudate, due to congestive heart failure; pleural effusions are probably on this basis. Renal scleroderma can introduce an element of uremic pericarditis.

Management

Symptomatic pericardial disease is associated with poor prognosis. In the absence of specific antisclerodermic therapy, symptoms should be treated and tamponade or constriction relieved by drainage or pericardiectomy respectively.

SJÖGREN'S SYNDROME

This "sicca syndrome" (dry eyes and dry mouth due to destructive lymphocytic infiltration of exocrine glands) occurs in isolation or in association with connective tissue disorders like SLE, rheumatoid arthritis or scleroderma. Pericarditis is of the types associated with the dominant connective tissue disorder, which is usually severe.

POLYMYOSITIS/DERMATOMYOSITIS

These apparently related chronic inflammatory autoimmune diseases of skeletal muscle and skin also affect the heart and pericardium with or without established skeletal muscle involvement. Both cardiac and pericardial involvement is usually asymptomatic. Pericarditis, more common in children than adults, is usually discovered incidentally as a pericardial effusion on echocardiography, or at autopsy as an effusion, or, occasionally, fibrinous pericarditis. Here, as in Sjögren's syndrome, pericarditis appears to be more frequent in patients with *"overlap syndromes,"* i.e., with complicating manifestations of other connective tissue disorders. Effusions, however, are occasionally large although rarely tamponading. Particularly rare is manifest acute pericarditis at the time dermatomyositis is discovered, raising the usual question of an intercurrent more common form of pericarditis, particularly viral. Because it is equally rare, constrictive pericarditis must raise the same etiologic consideration. Moreover, SLE and scleroderma can occur with a predominantly myositic syndrome; this, as well as the frequency of pericarditis in mixed connective tissue disease syndromes, could lead to misclassification.

PERICARDITIS IN MIXED CONNECTIVE TISSUE DISEASE (MCTD)

Mixed connective tissue disease (MCTD) is a set of "overlap syndromes" with variably combined features of systemic lupus, scleroderma, and dermatomyositis/polymyositis. The patients present combinations of polyarthritis, Raynaud's phenomenon, lymphadenopathy, esophageal dysmotility, skin and muscle involvement and frequent pulmonary disease with pulmonary artery hypertension, which may be marked; mitral valve prolapse is frequent, often with mitral regurgitation. Occasional components include asymmetric ventricular septal hypertrophy and left ventricular dilation, as well as intimal hyperplasia and perivascular leukocytosis of the intramural coronary arteries and focal myocarditis. *Pericarditis is the most frequent cardiac finding*, and it is particularly common at autopsy with pericardial effusions (often symptomatic) of all sizes. Pleuritis is also common and *acute pericarditis or pleuritis can be a presenting feature*. One difference from other connective tissues diseases is relative lack of renal involvement. There are high titers of speckled fluorescent ANA and especially circulating antibodies against nuclear ribonucleoprotien (nRNP). Echocardiograms frequently show effusion, usually small, and there may be apparent pericardial thickening, consistent with postmortem findings of patchy epicardial fibrosis that suggests repeated pericarditic episodes. With the widespread cardiac and pericardial involvement, it is not surprising that the ECG is nearly always abnormal. Compared to the other connective tissue diseases, the *ECG is particularly sensitive to pericarditis in MCTD*, relatively frequently showing characteristic ST segment deviations. This is not surprising because of the relative frequency of acute fibrinous pericarditis in MCTD. The pericardial fluid is serous or serosanguinous but only rarely becomes tamponading. While dyspnea may be due to tamponade, it is more commonly the result of pulmonary involvement or myocardial failure. The prognosis, however, is generally surprisingly good in mixed connective tissue disease, since pericardial involvement responds readily to short courses of low- to moderate-dose corticosteroid therapy.

PERICARDITIS IN THE SERONEGATIVE SPONDYLOARTHROPATHIES

The members of this quite complex group are outlined in Table 19.1. They have the following in common: (1) *arthritis* with a predilection for involvement of the sacroiliac, apophyseal and lumbosacral joints of the spine and the entheses (ligamentous and capsular insertions); (2) *absence of serology* positive for rheumatoid arthritis (e.g., rheumatoid factor); (3) *male* predominance; (4) *extra-atricular manifestations* including iritis, uveitis, enteric inflammations, pericarditis, myocarditis and lesions of the aortic root and valve that often produce aortic regurgitation; (5) association with haplotype histocompatibility *antigen B27* (HLA-B 27). Indeed, the amino acid sequence of HLA-B27 is imitated by proteins from enteric bacteria. Recognized syndromes include, particularly, *ankylosing spondylitis, Reiter's disease and the intestinal arthropathies* (Table 19.1), all of which are associated with dysentery and sometimes urethritis. The dysentery at times is related to specific organisms (which may not be causative), including *Yersinia, Shigella, Salmonella* and *Campylobacter. Psoriatic arthritis* should be included with this group because constrictive pericarditis has been reported in it. Iritis and cardiac involvement are found primarily in those with definite B27 positivity.

Ankylosing spondylitis is particularly seen in relatively young males with a painful stiff back due mainly to sacroiliitis. In them, while pericarditis is usually not prominent, pericardial rubs are discovered and constrictive pericarditis ensues in those with severe acute toxic polyarthritic episodes and particularly in early disease. Fibrous pericardial adhesions may be seen at necropsy. Some of the patients have had features of Reiter's disease. With chronicity, there is an increasing incidence of aortic regurgitation and atrioventricular blocks.

Reiter's disease, either venereally acquired or due to dysentery-inducing organisms, is marked by a sterile or occasionally chlamydial urethritis, conjunctivitis, arthritis and (particularly in Europe) diarrhea. Cardiac involvement is relatively frequent, particularly acute pericarditis with a pericardial rub, and myocarditis with murmurs, gallops and conduction abnormalities, all of which may be transient. Pericardial effusion with improved complement levels may accompany any of these as well as "Reiter's aortitis."

The *intestinal arthropathies* present inflammatory bowel disease including *Crohn's disease* and *ulcerative colitis,* in which acute pericarditis is unusual but may occur with or without cardiac tamponade. The presence of erythema nodosum, arthritis and uveitis, which are more common, can confuse identification of the syndrome, especially if they all precede the appearance of the intestinal manifestations. Yet, *Whipple's disease*, a multisystem disorder, has a high proportion of pericardial lesions at necropsy. Serofibrinous pericarditis, sometimes with pleurisy, may accompany seronegative migratory polyarthritis and gastrointestinal symptoms or may appear only after establishment of the intestinal syndrome. Pericardial constriction has also preceded or followed abdominal complaints but is sufficiently rare to raise the question of an intercurrent primary pericarditis. Pericardial histology (PAS-positive material) may be required to implicate Whipple's pericarditis.

PERICARDITIS IN THE SYSTEMIC VASCULITIDES

Giant-cell arteritis (GCA) affects medium and larger arteries in any organ system, including the heart and pericardium. Although the occurrence of pericarditis with or without effusion is of uncertain pathogenesis, possibly due to an immunopathy, this is also true of the more frequent pleuritis, both lesions sometimes presenting with pleuritic chest pain. Infections frequently precede GCA, so that any early pericardial syndromes could be mistaken for viral or other infectious pericarditis. Moreover, dissecting aortic aneurysms associated with GCA can rupture into the pericardium with often lethal hemotamponade (page 356).

Temporal (cranial) arteritis, particularly common in the elderly, is accompanied by pericarditis and pericardial lesions at necropsy and only occasionally presents clinically acute pericarditis, always raising the question of intercurrent infection. *Takayasu's arteritis* ("pulseless disease," aortic arch syndrome) is a chronic idiopathic inflammation of large vessels, often with corresponding arterial bruits, occurring particularly in relatively young females. Clinically, there may be acute pleuritis and pericarditis, sometimes recurrent. More common is postmortem discovery of pericardial scarring. Any tamponade is more likely due to rupture of a coronary sinus aneurysm. In these forms of arteritis, therapy with anti-inflammatory, particularly corticosteroid, agents will reduce the inflammation and lower the elevated sedimentation rate but without effect on ischemia due to arterial lesions.

Polyarteritis

Polyarteritis (periarteritis nodosa) only occasionally shows acute pericarditis or effusion in the absence of uremia. This appears to be more common in patients who are positive for HBsAg, with an associated chronic active hepatitis in some patients. Hemopericardium is occasional. Patients with coronaritis producing myocardial infarcts develop epistenocardiac pericarditis (page 336).

Hypersensitivity Vasculitides

This group includes allergic granulomatosis, the Churg-Strauss syndrome and various hypereosinophilic syndromes, all of which have some relation to polyarteritis and produce acute pericarditis, pericardial effusion with, or usually, without, tamponade and constrictive pericarditis, congestive heart failure and acute myocardial infarction. With persistent hypereosinophilia, *restrictive cardiomyopathy* may result due to endocardial involvement.

The *Churg-Strauss syndrome* is a multisystem vasculitis with necrotizing arteritis and eosinophilic infiltrates including extravascular granulomata, particularly in the epicardium. Epicardial and pericardial involvement is relatively frequent, producing all forms of pericarditis and myopericarditis, complicated by ischemia due to the vasculitic lesion. Pericardial effusion is due either to inflammation, myocardial failure or both. Characteristically, patients have a history of asthma and allergic rhinitis, often with nasal polyposis, each of which may be transient and episodic. There are both *peripheral eosinophilia and pericardial fluid eosinophilia.* Tissue eosinophilia includes pulmonary infiltrates, as well as pericardial infiltrates (identified by biopsy); some patients have circulating immune complexes. Tissue injury in this syndrome may be directly caused by the eosinophils, particularly the occasional degranulated eosinophils that can bind IgG (although these cells and higher levels of blood eosinophils are more characteristic of the hypereosinophilic syndromes). Diagnosis and differentiation from polyarteritis may be suggested by the history but are made by finding necrotizing granulomas with intense eosinophilic infiltration along with the blood eosinophilia.

Hypereosinophilic syndromes broadly include any condition with increased numbers of eosinophils anywhere. They have considerable overlap with polyarteritis and the Churg-Straus syndrome and include Loeffler's syndrome, which may also induce fibroplastic endocarditis and a restrictive cardiomyopathy. Pericardial involvement here must be differentiated and is complicated by the potential occurrence of simultaneous myocardiopathy and endocardiopathy. Indeed, patients with persistent eosinophilia have developed constrictive pericarditis without any other defined syndrome, presumable due to the histotoxicity of eosinophils. Comparable findings may be due to parasitoses, particularly in endemic areas (pages 282). Pericardial involvement in eosinophilic fasciitis has accompanied colitis and carpal tunnel syndrome.

Other Vasculitides

Other conditions that may be conveniently grouped among the systemic vasculitides include *Kawasaki's disease*, occurring worldwide but especially in Japanese children and only occasionally provoking pericarditis, which may be obscured by accompanying myocarditis or endocarditis. Ruptured coronary aneurysms have caused hemopericardium in these children. Occasional acute pericarditis is seen in *relapsing polychrondritis* and *necrotizing aortitis* of uncertain origin. Sporadic cases of pericarditis in *systemic necrotizing vasculitis, Bürger's disease, mucocutaneous lymph node syndrome* and *adult Henoch-Schönlein purpura* are difficult to characterize and may be due to intercurrent disease.

Hypocomplementemic Urticarial Vasculitis Syndrome (HUVS)

Acute pericarditis with and without effusion, asymptomatic pericardial effusion and pericardial effusion with tamponade are recognized parts of this syndrome. They appear to result from lymphocytic infiltration of the pericardium and pericardial vasculitis, although in some cases pericardial tissue changes have been minimal. This disease presents as a dermatologic syndrome primarily in women between 30 and 50 years of age, characterized by chronic urticaria which on skin biopsy proves to be a necrotizing venulitis. The systemic disease may resemble lupus, but without the antibodies to native DNA, although the serum is characterized by profound hypocomplementemia. This syndrome tends to be recurrent, with recurrent pericardial manifestations and exudative pleural effusions. There may be circulating IgG antibodies to the collagenlike region of Clq (probably not pathognomonic). Although some form of dyspnea may be due to acute pericarditis or cardiac tamponade, many of these patients also have emphysema and reversible airway obstruction of uncertain pathogenesis.

PERICARDITIS IN BEHÇET'S SYNDROME

This disorder is characterized by painful oral and genital ulcers (in contrast to the painless ulcers of Reiter's disease) and by recurrent hypopyon iritis, sometimes with skin and central nervous system involvement. Arteritis—including aortitis and coronary arteritis, gastrointestinal tract involvement from esophagus to colon and steroid-responsive arthritis in some patients—reveals its relation to the systemic vasculitides. Although some patients develop myocarditis, *the most common cardiac lesion is acute pericarditis, fibrinous or effusive*, including pleuropericarditis, each of which may be recurrent. Although some cases are related to myocardial infarctions and aneurysms, the pericarditis of Behçet's syndrome is usually self-limited or responsive to the anti-inflammatory agents used for the disease itself. However, Behçet's sometimes provokes thrombosis of major veins and may mimic constriction; this has also been attended by chylopericardium (page 84) and chylothorax. Occasionally, pericarditis precedes other manifestations. There is a male predominance throughout the syndrome, which may be even greater among those developing pericardial lesions.

PERICARDITIS IN WEGENER'S GRANULOMATOSIS

Wegener's granulomatosis is characterized by necrotizing local and systemic granulomatous vasculitis of the upper and lower respiratory tracts and glomerulonephritis; there is overlap with polyarteritis and both the giant-cell and hypersensitivity arteritides. Diagnosis is suspected on clinical grounds but often requires biopsies, particularly of the lung or kidney. Serologic tests include antineutrophil cytoplasmic antibody and plasma thrombomodulin, which reflects the extent of vascular injury. Cardiac involvement occurs in up to 20 percent of cases, including granulomatous myocarditis, endocarditis (including valvulitis) and aortitis; *pericarditis occurs in at least half of these* and, with its complications, ranges from acute fibrinous pericarditis to serous or hemorrhagic effusion and occasionally tamponade or constriction. Because myocardial infarction and uremia in this syndrome may also provoke pericarditis, these must be considered in the differential diagnosis. The frequency of arrhythmias and blocks testifies to the relative frequency of myocardial involvement by the disease itself. At postmortem, in addition to generalized pericardial disease, there may be focal pericarditis along with patchy myocardial fibrosis and occasional epicardial granulomas, including giant cells.

PERICARDITIS IN SARCOIDOSIS

Cardiac involvement in sarcoidosis is much more common at postmortem examination than clinically, since the granulomata may be microscopic and not strategically located. Widespread active granulomatous myocarditis and pericarditis, fortunately rare, produce serious and often fatal disease. Pericardial effusions with serous or serosanguinous fluid are relatively common by echocardiography and have occurred even during corticosteroid therapy. Tamponade is rare but may be particularly serious if there is also extensive myocardial involvement. The vast majority of pericardial effusions are probably transudates due to myocardial disease, including heart failure. Constrictive pericarditis has been reported.

PERICARDITIS IN SERUM SICKNESS

Serum sickness—with fever, urticaria, lymphadenopathy, myalgia, arthritis, neuritis, vasculitis and glomerulonephritis—can provoke acute pericarditis of a benign type or may be due to some of these diffuse lesions. The mechanisms are probably related to pericardial deposition of soluble antigen-antibody complexes when there is an excess of antigen. Severe disease may require corticosteroid therapy.

PERIODIC POLYSEROSITIS
(FAMILIAL MEDITERRANEAN FEVER: FMF)

Familial Mediterranean fever is a clinical syndrome of recurrent attacks of fever associated with pleuritis, peritonitits, arthritis and erysipelaslike erythema occurring in individuals of Mediterranean ethnic origin. Pericarditis is comparatively rare in FMF unless it is associated with development of renal amyloidosis leading to azotemia and uremic pericarditis. Electrocardiographic signs may be the only evidence. However, pericarditis has been the initial manifestation of FMF.

VASCULITIS-RELATED SYNDROMES

Sporadic pericarditis, raising the question of an intercurrent more common form, has been reported in *Stevens-Johnson syndrome, polymyalgia rheumatica, thrombohemolytic thrombocytopenic purpura (TTP)* and *panmesenchymal reac-*

tions to steroid hormone withdrawal. The latter may be a rebound phenomenon producing clinical eruption of subclinical pericarditis. Pericarditis has been reported in adult *celiac disease*, even as a presenting feature, as a result of disturbed humoral and cell-mediated immunity, including autoimmune reactions. Deposition of circulating immune complexes originating from the small intestine make this resemble the pericarditis described in serum sickness (page 330) and inflammatory bowel disease (page 326). Response to a gluten-free diet makes an etiologic association more convincing. *Osteogenesis imperfecta* has been associated with numerous valve disorders and aortic dissection with hemopericardium.

Finally, some pericarditis-inducing *rickettsioses*, like Q fever and Mediterranean spotted fever (MSF), produce infection-associated vasculitis in affected organs.

KEY POINTS

1. Pericarditis of all morphologic types and physiologic consequences occurs throughout the vasculitis–connective tissue disease group, with highest incidence in rheumatoid arthritis and systemic lupus. Histologic study is confirmatory. However, in most cases, characteristic clinical behavior often indicates and pericardial fluid abnormalities strongly support specific diagnoses sufficiently for treatment.
2. The primary immunopathic event leading to vasculitis and injury is probably immune complex deposition in the pericardium which, with cell-mediated immune reactivity, accounts for inflammation and necrosis. These processes sometimes require exposure to infectious agents—specific, as in rheumatic pericarditis, or nonspecific—in variable proportions of this disease group.
3. *Diagnosis of pericardial involvement in this group is confounded by myocardial failure with pericardial transudates and renal failure with uremic pericarditis or transudate from fluid retention.*
4. Pericarditis is frequent in all varieties of rheumatoid arthritis, adult and juvenile, but is usually subclinical and discovered postmortem or by a pericardial rub or a pericardial effusion on echocardiography in patients who have had no chest symptoms. Occasional RA patients develop (and may present as) cardiac tamponade or constriction.
5. Pericarditis in acute rheumatic fever usually indicates severe pancarditis, especially in children. In any child with acute pericarditis, ARF must be ruled in or out.
6. Pericarditis appears to be the most common cardiac manifestation of systemic lupus, scleroderma, mixed connective tissue disease and Behçet's syndrome. *All female patients with any form of acute pericarditis should be tested for SLE.*
7. Pericarditis in the seronegative spondyloarthropathies, including the "intestinal arthropathies," has a wide spectrum of clinical manifestations.
8. Pericarditis occurs throughout the range of systemic vasculitides, not only those involving the microvasculature. Vasculitides affecting the aorta or coronary vessels may cause hemopericardium.

BIBLIOGRAPHY

Alpert, M.A., Goldberg, S.H., Singsen, B.H., et al. Cardiovascular complications of mixed connective tissue disease in adults. Circulation 1983; 69:1182.

Beier, J.M., Nielsen, H.L., Nielsen, D. Pleuritis-pericarditis—An unusual initial manifestation of mixed connective tissue disease. Eur. Heart J. 1992; 13:859–861.

Birnbaum, Y., Shpirer, Z. Cardiac involvement in inflammatory bowel disease. Harefuah 1989; 1:235.

Browning, C.A., Bishop, R.L., Heilpern, R.J., et al. Accelerated constrictive pericarditis in procainamide-induced systemic lupus erythematosus. Am. J. Cardiol. 1984; 53:376–377.

Cathcart, E., Spodick, D.H. Rheumatoid heart disease: A study of the incidence and nature of cardiac lesions in rheumatoid arthritis. N. Engl. J. Med. 1962; 266:959–964.

Davison, A.G., Thompson, P.J., Davis, J., et al. Prominent pericardial and myocardial lesions in the Churg-Strauss syndrome (allergic granulomatosis and angiitis). Thorax 1983; 38:793–795.

Diderholm, E., Eklund, A., Orinius, E., Widstrom, O. Exudative pericarditis in sarcoidosis. Sarcoidosis 1989; 6:60.

Ehrenfeld, M., Asman, A., Shpilberg, O., Samra, Y. Cardiac tamponade as the presenting manifestation of systemic lupus erythematosus. Am. J. Med. 1989; 86:626.

Erol, C., Sonel, A., Candan, I., et al. Pericardial involvement in familial Mediterranean fever. Postgrad. Med. J. 1988; 64:453.

Escalante, A., Kaufman, R.L., Quismorio, F. P., Jr., et al. Cardiac compression in rheumatoid arthritis. Semin. Arthritis Rheum. 1990; 20:148.

Fitzpatrick, A.P., Lanham, J.G., Doyle, D.V. Cardiac tumours simulating collagen vascular disease. Br. Heart. J. 1986; 51:592–595.

Gladman, D.D., Gordon, D.A. Urowitz, M.B., Levy, H.L. Pericardial fluid analysis in scleroderma (systemic sclerosis). Am. J. Med. 1976; 60:1064.

Hiraishi, S., Yashiro, K., Oguchi, K., et al. Clinical course of cardiovascular involvement in the mucocutaneous lymph node syndrome: Relation between clinical signs of carditis and development of coronary arterial aneurysm. Am. J. Cardiol 1981; 47:323–330.

Jamieson, T.W. Adult Still's disease complicated by cardiac tamponade. JAMA 1983; 249:2065.

Janosik, D.L., Osborn, T.G., Moore, T.L., et al. Heart disease in systemic sclerosis. Semin. Arthritis Rheum. 1989; 19:191.

LeRoy, E.C. The heart in systemic sclerosis. N. Engl. J. Med. 1984; 310:188.

Martin, J.C., Harvey, J., Dixey, J. Chest pain in patients with rheumatoid arthritis. Ann. Rheum. Dis. 1996; 55:152–153.

Maryhew, N.L., Bache, R.J., Messner, R.P. Wegener's granulomatosis with acute pericardial tamponade. Arthritis Rheum. 1988; 31:300.

McWhorter, J.E., LeRoy, E.C. Pericardial disease in scleroderma (systemic sclerosis). Am. J. Med. 1974; 57:566.

Russo, M.G., Waxman, J., Abdoh, A.A., Serebro, L.H. Correlation between infection and the onset of the giant cell (temporal) arteritis syndrome. Arthritis Rheum. 1995; 38:374–380.

Sattar, M.A., Guindi, R.T., Vajcik, J. Case report—Pericardial tamponade and limited cutaneous systemic sclerosis (CREST syndrome). Br. J. Rheumatol. 1990; 29:306–307.

Shah, A., Askari, A.D. pericardial changes and left ventricular function in ankylosing spondylitis. Am. Heart J. 1987; 113:1529.

Spodick, D.H. Still's syndrome: Atypical juvenile rheumatoid arthritis. Arch. Pediatr. 1953; 70:1–19.

Spodick, D.H. Pitfalls in the recognition of pericarditis. In: Hurst, J.W. (ed.). Clinical Essays on the Heart. New York: McGraw-Hill, 1985: pp.95–111.

Spodick, D.H. Pericarditis in systemic disease. Cardiol. Clin. 1990; 8:709–716.

Spodick, D.H., Southern, J.F. A 55-year old man with recurrent pericarditis and pleural effusions after aortic valve replacement: Case records of the Massachusetts General Hospital, Case 23-1992. N. Engl. J. Med. 1992; 326:1550–1557.

Tamir, R., Pick, A.J., Theodor, E. Constrictive pericarditis complicating dermatomyositis. Ann. Rheum. Dis. 1988; 47:961.

Wolf, R.E., King, J.W., Brown, T.A. Antimyosin antibodies and constrictive pericarditis in lupus erythematosus. J. Rheumatol. 1988; 15:1284.

Yale, S.H., Adlakha, A., Stanton, M.S. Dermatomyositis with pericardial tamponade and polymyositis with pericardial effusion. Am. Heart. J. 1993; 126:997–999.

20

Pericardial Involvement in Diseases of the Heart and Other Contiguous Structures

The structures abutting the pericardium are usually good, or at last quiet, neighbors. However, disease in any of them can invade the pericardium, and each may be involved simultaneously by the same disorders or by their treatment; rarely, disease of the pericardium itself involves one or more of its neighbors (Table 20.1).

MYOCARDIAL INFARCTION–ASSOCIATED PERICARDITIS (TABLE 20.2)

Problems of Recognition and Timing

As with so many kinds of pericarditis, clinical detection of pericardial involvement lags behind the degree of postmortem discovery. In general, "early" and "delayed" kinds of infarct-associated pericarditis have been identified. There is no absolute temporal separation—in some cases, because of the apparent continuation of one form into the other; in other cases, the very early appearance of pericarditis with all the characteristics of the delayed form; in a few cases, recurrence of a pericardial rub after it had disappeared. Despite uncertainty as to the precise onset of infarction processes, their clinical and pathologic behavior makes the two forms clinically and pathogenetically distinct, although not al-

Table 20.1 Pericardial Involvement in Diseases of Contiguous Structures

I.   Myocardial infarction:
     A. Acute myocardial infarction
        1. Infarct (epistenocardiac) pericarditis
        2. Pseudoaneurysm
        3. Right ventricular infarction
           a. Physiologic effect of intact pericardium
           b. Loculated effusion, right ventricular tamponade
     B. Postmyocardial infarction syndrome (PMIS)
II. Dissecting aneurysm (hematoma) of the aorta; intramural aortic hemorrhage (IAH)
     A. Mimicking acute pericarditis
     B. Hemopericardium/tamponade
     C. Late pericardial constriction
III. Pleuropulmonary disorders
     A. Pneumonia/empyema
     B. Pulmonary embolism
        1. Direct (adjacent) pericardial involvement
        2. PMIS-like pericardial syndrome (exudative pericarditis)
        3. Pericardial transudate
        4. Acute cor pulmonale
           a. Conus rub
           b. Physiologic effect of pericardial constraint on right ventricle
     C. Pleuritis/pleurodynia
VI. Mediastinal disease
     A. Mediastinal lymph nodes
        1. Inflammatory
        2. Malignant
     B. Mediastinal abscess
     C. Mediastinal fibrosis
        1. Postinflammatory
        2. Of uncertain/toxic origin
V.   Esophageal disorders: pericardial irritation/penetration/fistula/pneumopericardium
     A. Benign ulcer disease
     B. Achalasia/Barrett's esophagus
     C. Malignancy
        1. Pericardial encroachment
        2. Radiation effects
     D. Esophagitis
        1. Reflux esophagitis
        2. Infectious: tuberculous, other

(*continued*)

Table 20.1 Continued

E. Ingestants: chemical trauma
   1. Lye, other caustics
   2. Sclerotherapy of esophageal varices
   3. Medications: aspirin; enteric coated KCl
F. Physical trauma
   1. Chest trauma: blunt/sharp
   2. Foreign bodies
   3. Instrumentation: endoscopy (including TEE), bougienage
   4. Esophageal surgery
      a. Resection and anastomosis
      b. Colonic substitution with ulcer/necrosis
   5. Sword swallowing
G. Esophageal diverticula

VI. Diaphragmatic disorders
   A. Intra- or juxtapericardial hernias of abdominal organs
      1. Congenital defects of diaphragm and/or pericardium (includes hiatal hernia)
      2. Traumatic disruption
         a. Sharp trauma
         b. Blunt trauma
         c. Iatrogenic
            (1) Surgery of chest and/or abdomen
            (2) Subxiphoid pericardial surgery
               (a) Drainage
               (b) Epicardial pacemaker implant
   B. Inflammatory perforation
      1. Ulcers: stomach; small and larger intestine
      2. Subphrenic abscess
VII. Liver disease (*esp.* abscess)
VIII. Primarily pericardial disorders (rare)
   A. Purulent pericarditis with external penetration
   B. Malignancy with external penetration
   C. Pericardial calcification eroding esophagus
   D. "Foreign-body pericarditis"

---

ways accurately diagnosed. "Delayed" pericarditis is the post–myocardial infarction (Dressler's) syndrome (PMIS; pages 349–356). Since the true "early" form is confined to the infarction zone, it is known as "infarct pericarditis," or *epistenocardiac* pericarditis—a more descriptive Greek-derived term meaning "pericarditis on top of the infarct." "Epistenocardiac" is literally exact, because transmural myocardial infarcts are roughly pyramidal, with a base on the endocardium and an apex erupting through the epicardium, there to be capped

Table 20.2   Infarct-Associated Pericardial Disease

1.	Infarct (epistenocardiac) pericarditis
2.	Postmyocardial infarction (Dressler's) syndrome (PMIS); recurrences
3.	Pericardial effusion with either 2 or 1; rarely, tamponade unless hemopericardium
4.	Hydropericardium (congestive failure) with or without 1 or 2
5.	Hemopericardium with or without antithrombotic therapy
	-With 1
	-With 2
	-With 3
	-With myocardial rupture
6.	Pericardial adhesions: following epistenocardiac pericarditis; following PMIS
	-Nonconstrictive
	-Constrictive
	-Effusive-constrictive
7.	Ventricular pseudoaneurysm

by a relatively small zone of direct pericardial injury. This occurs in almost half of transmural infarcts but is clinically discovered in many fewer due to varying diligence in the auscultatory pursuit of pericardial rubs—virtually the only objective sign in the vast majority.

The principal confounding factor in distinguishing epistenocardiac pericarditis from the PMIS is uncertainty as to the actual age of any acute infarct. Patients with ventricular rupture—where the moment of death is known—frequently have infarcts which, by their histopathology, preceded the onset of symptoms by as much as 7 to 14 days. Indeed, the symptoms of progressive rupture (usually a slow, sinuous myocardial penetration) may be the first sign of an otherwise "silent" infarction. Thus, while recognition of pericarditis on the day of admission for infarction usually means that we are dealing with infarct pericarditis, in some cases the behavior of the lesion reveals the PMIS.

INFARCT PERICARDITIS (EPISTENOCARDIAC PERICARDITIS)

Clinical Characteristics

Infarct (epistenocardiac) pericarditis occurs with anatomically *transmural or nearly transmural infarction* and is *localized* to the zone of infarct eruption on the epicardium. Thus any electrocardiographic (ECG) reflection should be localized or overshadowed by infarct changes. For this reason, generalized Stage I ECG changes of pericarditis during infarction always raise the question of the PMIS (Figure 20.1A and B). These are mostly Q-wave infarcts. Of course,

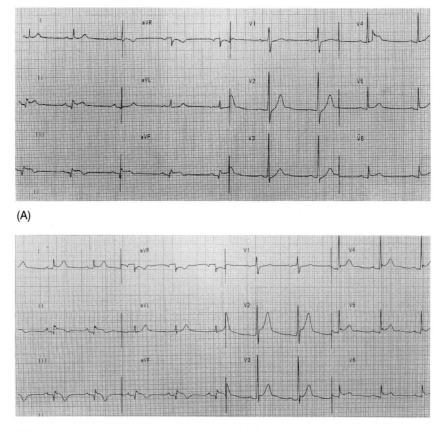

(A)

(B)

Figure 20.1 A. Acute inferolateral myocardial infarction. Day 1: J (ST) elevations in leads II, III, aVF, V5 and V6; depressions in aVL, V2 and V3. Abnormal Q waves in II, III and aVF. B. (Same patient as in Figure 20.1A). Day 2: the patient has a pericardial rub and ECG now shows J (ST) elevations in I, II, III, aVF, V2 to V6 characteristic and virtually diagnostic typical variant of the Stage I ECG; ST isoelectric in aVL associated with nearly isoelectric QRS (see Chapter 5). This extent of ST deviation is unusual, suggesting either a large infarct or "early" postmyocardial infarction syndrome (PMIS).

confinement of the ECG to only 12 leads means that some Q-wave infarcts will be considered non-Q-wave infarcts; other transmural infarcts do not generate Q waves. Acute pericarditis accompanying "non-Q-wave" infarcts therefore may be either an early PMIS or a true epistenocardiac pericarditis. (It is uncertain why pericarditis with Q-wave infarcts, like most forms of pericarditis, preponderantly occurs in males, whereas with non-Q-wave infarcts, pericardial involvement among males and females is approximately equal.)

The pericardial exudate over a transmural infarction is fibrinous, with few or no white cells, and is sterile except in rare cases of infected infarction, usually from septic coronary emboli during bacterial endocarditis (page 267). The late consequence with healed infarcts is a collagenized overlying pericardial scar. Because infarcts causing epistenocardiac pericarditis are transmural and relatively large, ventricular thrombi, especially apical and right ventricular thrombi, are relatively common and probably the reason that *systemic embolism is more common* in *patients who have had infarct pericarditis* and, with right ventricular infarcts, *pulmonary embolism.* Moreover, there are more ventricular aneurysms in patients with infarct pericarditis and more mural thrombi in these aneurysms. Such complications reflect the strong tendency for infarct pericarditis to be discovered with larger infarcts and therefore associated with *higher Killip class and more atrial and ventricular arrhythmias than in patients without pericarditis.* The atrial arrhythmias are related to heart failure or atrial infarction. Ventricular arrhythmias are also related to the infarct rather than the pericarditis. They reflect greater infarct size in patients with infarct pericarditis as compared to those without pericarditis; larger infarcts with pericarditis appear to cause *fever:* temperature exceeds 99°F more frequently and lasts longer than without pericarditis. During the first week of myocardial infarction, infarct pericarditis is also probably the most common cause of *new chest pain* that is distinguished from ischemic pain by certain characteristics, mainly its respirophasic and positional ("pleuritic") fluctuation (page 101 and Table 8.2).

The importance of larger infarct size with easily discoverable (i.e., rub-producing) pericarditis is reflected in the late mortality statistics. Surprisingly, despite higher Killip classes in infarct patients with pericardial rubs, the *in-hospital prognosis* is no different with or without pericarditis, although patients with epistenocardiac pericarditis dying in hospital mainly do so from power failure. However, the *late prognosis*—6 months to a year and after—is distinctly worse in those who have had infarct pericarditis. Moreover, patients with non-Q-wave infarctions and "early" pericarditis are at increased risk of death over those with non-Q-wave infarctions without pericarditis. Thus, it is no surprise that *patients with infarct pericarditis reflect larger infarct size by greater* (1) myocardial enzyme release, (2) number of ECG leads with elevated ST segments, (3) degree of J-ST elevation, (4) number of leads with infarct Q waves and other QRS abnormality, (5) echocardiographic estimate of infarct size, (6) aggregate wall motion abnormalities and (7) radiographic score for extravascular lung water. There is equally no surprise that with epistenocardiac pericarditis, anterior and multisite infarctions are much more frequent than with the usually smaller inferior infarcts. Moreover, with inferior infarcts, there are approximately twice as many with pericarditis when there is anterior recorded

ST depression (Figure 20.1A)—a sign of a more serious process—compared to patients with inferior infarcts without pericarditis.

Patients with infarct pericarditis have lower ejection farctions, which continue to fall up to the sixth to tenth day, whereas in survivors without pericarditis, initially depressed ejection fractions tend to rise by the sixth to tenth day. With pericarditis, there are also more frequent signs of congestive heart failure and increased pulmonary capillary wedge pressures. Thus, detection of pericarditis is associated with a relatively poor ultimate prognosis. However, epistenocardiac pericarditis is not independently predictive when adjusted for left ventricular function; indeed, with Q-wave infarcts, global ejection fraction remains the best independent risk predictor. On the other hand, although early thrombolytic therapy has decreased the incidence of epistenocardiac pericarditis, should pericarditis appear despite thrombolysis it is a marker of greater damage and increased in-hospital mortality.

Pericardial Effusion

In acute myocardial infarctions, pericardial effusions can be irritative (pericarditic) or due to hydropericardium. Hydropericardium is more common and unrelated to pericardial irritation, which usually produces very little exudate. Strictly irritative effusions are mostly small, with or without a rub; there is probably increased microvascular permeability, associated in some patients with increased extravascular lung water. Increased myocardial interstitial fluid and obstruction of cardiac lymph and venous drainage probably produce the occasional larger irritative effusions that resemble or coincide with hydropericardium. Effusions tend to develop early, mainly from the first to third day. The majority occur without any evidence of pericardial irritation and are only small to moderate-sized by echocardiography.

Hydropericardium should be suspected with most effusions above minimal echo-detectable size and indicate some degree of heart failure with fluid retention. Hydropericardia are more frequent with larger Q-wave anterior and right ventricular infarcts; they are associated with higher pulmonary capillary wedge pressures, left ventricular dyssynergy, increased right atrial pressures and increased pulmonary alveolar-arterial oxygen difference. They are only slowly absorbed over days to weeks. Although tamponade is rare in the absence of bleeding, hydropericardium—detectable pericardial effusion *without signs of pericardial inflammation* (rub;ECG changes; pleuritic pain)—presages increased short-term infarct mortality because of its association with the foregoing factors.

Finally, *anteriorly loculated effusions* may cause isolated right heart tamponade by selectively compressing the right ventricle, atrioventricular (A-V) groove or right atrium. Patients develop new hypotension and pulsus paradoxus is absent (pages 169 and 158). Rarely, right and left constrictive hemodynamics and syndrome are provoked.

Hemopericardium

Hemorrhagic pericardial effusion or frankly bloody hemopericardium occurs "spontaneously" or, more often, with thrombolytic and antithrombotic therapy and, of course, myocardial rupture. Any patient with rapid "cardiac" enlargement and a loud or persistent pericardial rub or an unexplained drop in hemoglobin or hematocrit—with or without signs of tamponade—should be observed for pericardial hemorrhage due to excessive anticoagulation or subacute ventricular rupture. Indeed, it is probably pericardial bleeding that ultimately produces the few cases of constrictive pericarditis due to myocardial infarction. Yet it is amazing how uncommon any significant or detectable pericardial bleeding is with infarct pericarditis despite antithrombotic therapy of all kinds. With subacute ventricular *rupture*, the patient can survive and echocardiography may show echodense material—organizing blood or clots—simulating the texture of intracardiac thrombi but interposed between the heart and the parietal pericardium, sometimes with a distinct layered effect; such clotting and organization can occur within pseudoaneurysms (page 346) and may also produce an early elastic form of pericardial constriction (page 254). *Acute ventricular rupture* produces rapid tamponade and death, usually with a vagally mediated bradycardia culminating in electromechanical dissociation, comparable to the consequences of intrapericardial rupture of aortic dissecting hematoma (page 356). Only immediate pericardiotomy and repair offer any hope of survival.

Pericardial Friction

A pericardial rub is the most specific sign of infarct pericarditis. It is usually faint and monophasic with peak incidence from day 1 to day 3 after onset; the great majority occur within 4 days. Rubs are not rare at admission, particularly after resuscitation, and may represent either epistenocardiac pericarditis or, much less often, when the true onset of infarction had been earlier and silent, the PMIS (page 349). Rubs may be heard with any infarct location, since the exudate can spread through the pericardium (for other reasons, nearly all rubs are best heard at the left mid-to-lower sternal border; Chapter 4). Postural and breathing maneuvers may be necessary to elicit rubs, which should be diligently sought because most are faint and fleeting. Indeed, a persistent (days to weeks), loud, or widespread rub may indicate the PMIS or at least unusually intense infarct pericarditis, requiring intensified observation if the patient is on antithrombotic therapy. Tri- or biphasic rubs are often quite obviously pericardial, but with infarction pericarditis *the majority are monophasic, usually systolic,* and can resemble or coexist with murmurs of mitral and tricuspid regurgitation or ventricular septal rupture, all serious complications of infarction. Disappearance followed by recurrence of a rub may indicate the PMIS either as a new lesion or in continuity with the original epistenocardiac pericarditis. As with pericardial effusions, pericardial rubs with an inferior infarction are more frequent with right ventricular involvement (usually proximal right coronary artery lesions) and more easily detected due to proximity of the right ventricle to the anterior chest wall.

Electrocardiographic Correlations

Epistenocardiac pericarditis occurs with transmural, usually Q-wave infarcts and therefore is usually not separately detectable by ECG because it is localized. For the same reason, *atrial fibrillation is more common following P-R segment deviations*, a sensitive sign of atrial myopericarditis of unknown specificity that is not rare during epistenocardiac pericarditis. Failure of evolution of acute ST-T changes of infarction or reversals of ST-T evolution in the infarct zone has been associated with infarct pericarditis and impending rupture. Rare patients with apparent infarct pericarditis and a typical Stage I ECG (page 41), probably, have an early PMIS or, possibly, an intercurrent acute pericarditis, perhaps viral. (Note: recent upper respiratory infection is more frequent in patients with myocardial infarction than in matched control patients.) *Patients with infarct pericarditis ultimately have more arrhythmias, more second- and third-degree atrioventricular block, more bundle branch and other fascicular blocks—* all correlated with larger infarcts rather than the pericarditis per se. Frank myocardial rupture appears as a typical catastrophic hemopericardium: sinus bradycardia, sometimes alternating with junctional rhythms, going on to electromechanical dissociation and agonal rhythms. Strangely, QRS amplitude may not be low.

Effects of Thrombolysis

Thrombolysis, the most effective antithrombotic therapy when administered sufficiently early during an infarct, usually reperfuses the culprit artery and produces a smaller infarct, better left ventricular function, better survival and less pericardial involvement. Indeed, *the incidence of epistenocardiac pericarditis is decreased by at least one-half with very early thrombolysis,* along with a reduced incidence of clinical signs of congestive heart failure among patients with pericarditis. *Thrombolysis also decreases the incidence of PR segment depression* (page 41) *while accelerating ECG resolution* either toward normal or to completion of characteristic infarct findings. Moreover, in patients with inferior infarction, those with precordial ST segment depressions no longer have a greater incidence of pericarditis than those without them. The rarity of significant pericardial bleeding is remarkable because of the customary throm-bolytic state usually accompanying aggressive antiplatelet treatment. However, *thrombolysis appears to have increased the number of ruptured infarcts* and made this form of hemopericardium occur earlier. Rarely, recanalization of an artery supplying a very necrotic infarct zone produces a bloody pericardial effusion and even tamponade.

Diagnosis

Demonstration of a pericardial rub firmly diagnoses infarct-associated peri-carditis. It appears that even without a rub, *typical pleuritic pain is strong evidence, while pain in one or both trapezius ridges (page 10), is almost as pathognomonic.* Classic ECG changes of pericarditis (page 41) are uncommon with epistenocardiac pericarditis and should suggest "early" PMIS, while the recent demonstration of failure to evolve or "resurrection" of previously ter-minally inverted T waves strongly suggest pericarditis. Rarely, "hyperacute" ST changes of infarct resemble those of Stage I pericarditis, though usually with telltale signs of infarction (Figure 20-2). Absence of effusion on imaging or a clear pericardial tap excludes subacute (i.e., not immediately fatal) ventricular rupture, but an effusion, even if bloody, does not prove it. High-density intra-pericardial echoes parallel to the cardiac surfaces with or without right atrial or right ventricular compression suggest subacute rupture. In contrast, intra-pericardial echoes due to adhesions are angled or perpendicular to the cardiac surface and may be mobile.

Differential Diagnosis (Table 20.3)

Certain conditions must be distinguished from infarct pericarditis, although they may coexist: pulmonary embolism, recurrent ischemia or infarction, acute stress ulcer, mitral and tricuspid regurgitation, ventricular septal rupture and primary pericarditis without infarction. *"Early" PMIS* is principally distinguished by more diffuse ST and PR segment changes and especially more severe symp-toms, louder and more persistent rubs and greater tendency to pericardial hem-orrhage. *Primary, noninfarction pericarditis* may resemble infarct if the ECG is atypical (Chapter 5); however, in the absence of myopericarditis (Chapter 9), any ST elevations are *not accompanied by reciprocal changes* as they usually are in infarction. (Note: Computer interpretations often miss this and mistake pericarditis for acute anterolateral or inferolateral infarction.) *Rare exceptions* exist among atypical ECGs in which rS complexes (especially in leads aVL and aVF) show pseudoreciprocal ST depressions (Figures 5.11, 5.12).

Pulmonary embolus, which can also accompany a right ventricular infarct with pericarditis and mural thrombi, may require a lung scan or an angiogram.

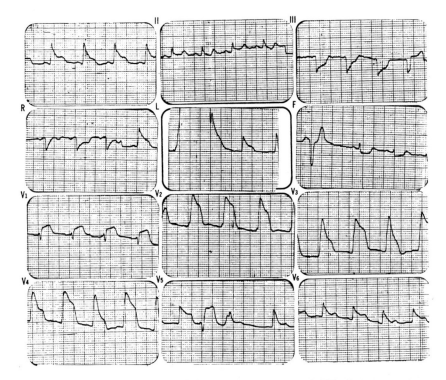

Figure 20.2 Acute myocardial infarction. "Hyperacute" J (ST) changes mimicking stage I ECG of pericarditis. Degree of J-point deviation is not seen with uncomplicated acute pericarditis. ST depression in aVF and lead II appear to be reciprocal. Monophasic QRS-T in I, III, L and V2-V6 is characteristic of acute myocardial infarction. There are no PR segment deviations.

Recurrent ischemia should respond to nitrates, whereas pericardial pain and J (ST) changes will not do so; there will also be new ST-T- and/or Q-wave changes and reciprocal changes in many recurrences. *Acute mitral and tricuspid regurgitation and ventricular septal defect* should be distinguishable by their particular murmurs and any thrills; however, their murmurs sometimes resemble rubs. Here the Doppler tracing is of great assistance. A pericardial rub mimicking *mitral regurgitation* is usually not accompanied by acute pulmonary congestion.

Fortunately, *tamponade is rare*. Yet, particularly in patients on antithrombotic therapy, tamponade must be distinguished from circulatory collapse due to other causes like shock and myocardial failure. Injured, low-compliance myocardium may also prevent pulsus paradoxus (Chapter 13), which is also

Table 20.3   Ischemia/Infarction Vs. Early/Late Pericarditis[a]

	Pericarditis: Epistenocardiac or PMIS[b]	Ischemia: Angina or Infarction
Pain		
Usual quality	Sharp; waxes and wanes	"Pressure"; steady
Usual duration	Persistent: hours to days	Limited: minutes to hours
In trapezius ridge(s)	Yes: quasispecific	No
Respiratory variation	Pleuritic	No
Body position	Worse in recumbency	No effect
Nitroglycerin	No effect	Frequent relief

Significant peri-
   cardial effusion
	Common in PMIS and peri-
	   cardial bleeding
		Rare without heart failure

Fever	Low to moderate	Low

Cardiac signs	Pericardial rub (often faint,
	   transient with episteno-
	   cardiac pericarditis)
		S4, S3 (heart failure)
		Mitral, tricuspid regurgita-
		   tion
		Kussmaul's sign (RV infarc-
		   tion)

Rales	Patchy when present (PMIS)	Diffuse when present
ECG	Rarely typical of pericarditis (Stage I) except "early" PMIS	Locates ischemia

[a]No findings obligatory. Symptoms and signs more intense with PMIS than epistenocardiac pericarditis. Ischemia/infarction signs often coexist with either kind of pericarditis.
[b]PMIS = post-myocardial infarction syndrome.

absent with local chamber compression by loculated fluid. Diagnosing tamponade thus may require evidence from imaging (particularly echo-Doppler cardiography) or cardiac catheterization. Even if intrapericardial blood has been drained with relief of tamponade, *pericardial clots* seen on echo or other imaging presage recurrence and demand special vigilance.

Pain in one or both trapezius ridges is definitely of pericardial origin, whereas new pleuritic pain strongly favors pericarditis, especially following effective antithrombotic therapy, which usually rules out pulmonary embolism. However, *with a large infarct, unexplained deterioration should always include cardiac tamponade in the differential diagnosis* since, although rare, hemopericardium can occur quite late. (This was formerly more of a problem due to intracoronary thrombolysis.) If the diagnosis of myocardial infarction is mistaken, thrombolysis may produce tamponade not only from inflamed pericardium but also from a missed aortic dissection, which can also mimic both infarct and acute pericarditis (page 357). Rarely, mediastinal hemorrhage will resemble cardiac tamponade, especially in postoperative patients; imaging should identify it.

Ischemia of any type must be differentiated from both epistenocardiac pericarditis and the PMIS (including the "early" form). The differential diagnosis is detailed in Table 20.3).

Treatment

Infarct pericarditis is usually mild and responds to aspirin, up to 650 mg every 4 hr for 5 to 10 days. Other nonsteroidal agents theoretically risk thinning an infarct, but this is not conclusively demonstrated in humans and ibuprofen (which increases coronary flow) is the agent of choice. Corticosteroid therapy may be used for refractory symptoms but should be avoided, if possible, due both to delayed infarct healing and the possibility of steroid side effects and dependence. Rarely, severe, persistently refractory pain has been treated by stellate ganglion block. All patients with pericardial pain should be reassured.

Although more frequent with thrombolysis, hemopericardium remains uncommon in epistenocardiac pericarditis, which therefore need not contraindicate heparin and other antithrombotic treatment (especially without a widespread or intense pericardial rub). Indeed, the risk of hemopericardium is probably outweighed by the benefits of preventing infarct extension and ventricular thrombi. Yet the problem is confounded by the possibility of "early" PMIS, with its less localized, diffuse pericarditis and much greater tendency to bleed (page 350). Since pericardial bleeding can occur even with clotting indices in the therapeutic range, these must be monitored and the patient watched for tamponade, especially if continued anticoagulation is strongly indicated, as in patients being catheterized or having angioplasty. Bleeding with significantly abnormal prothrombin time may call for vitamin K; protamine sulfate may be required to reverse excess heparinization. All are individualized decisions and all patients are closely monitored.

Pseudoaneurysm (False Ventricular Aneurysm); Pericardially Contained Myocardial Rupture

Pseudoaneurysms are uncommon, occurring with larger infarcts, usually within 5 weeks of infarction. They also occur after ventricular surgery, especially valve replacement. Pseudoaneurysms also follow endocarditis, penetrating wounds or cardiac surgery (including surgical resection of true aneurysms). They represent a *contained myocardial rupture*, most often posterolaterally, that is limited by the visceral pericardium with or without an adherent parietal pericardium or by the parietal pericardium (Figures 20.3, 20.4). (Occasional ruptures are relatively well contained when there is abundant epicardial fat.)

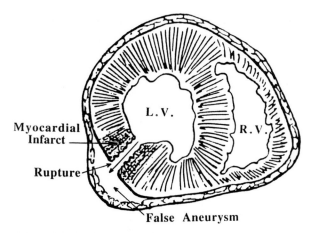

Figure 20.3 Left ventricular postinfarctional pseudoaneurysm. Through the narrow neck, blood from myocardial rupture is contained by visceral pericardium and a thin layer of epicardial fat. Adherent parietal pericardium can add to the wall. Pseudoaneurysms may rupture at any time; they constitute a surgical emergency.

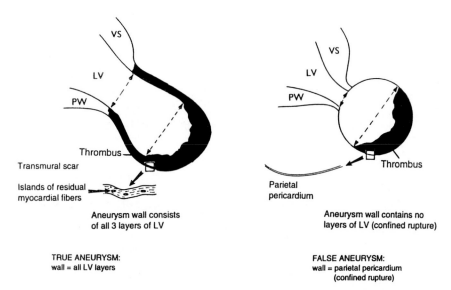

Figure 20.4 Comparison of true and false ventricular aneurysms. True aneurysm usually has a relatively wide neck and often contains thrombus with a wall of myocardial scar tissue, residual muscle and often endocardium. False aneurysm is limited only by pericardium (here, parietal pericardium but often visceral pericardium and epicardial fat); it can contain thrombus but is prone to rupture.

Pseudoaneurysms are distinguished by a narrow neck communicating with the ventricular cavity, with blood flowing bidirectionally: into the pseudoaneurysm in systole and out in diastole at fairly high velocity. Indeed, the neck may be so narrow as to be visible only on color Doppler recording (Figure 21.13B). Respiratory variation in peak velocity is frequent (Figure 21.13C). Rare pseudo-aneurysms communicating with both ventricles permit left-to-right shunting. The wall of the pseudoaneurysm is pericardium, epicardial fat and any scar tissue (Figures 20.3 and 20.4), producing globular, saccular or oddly angled shapes and usually containing thrombus (Figures 20.4 and 21.13A-C). (In contrast, the wall of a true aneurysm is aneurysmal muscle and fibrous tissue usually with a wide communication with the ventricular cavity; Figure 20.4 and Table 20.4). Only rarely is survival possible for a few years because of a strong tendency to spontaneous rupture. *This forces a surgical decision upon discovery.* (The rare chronic pseudoaneurysms may be protected by organized thrombi.) Indeed, mural thrombi as well as congestive heart failure, angina, ischemic pain, arrhythmias, emboli and bacterial endocarditis are more frequent than with true aneurysms.

Imaging usually makes the diagnosis, demonstrating an abrupt discontinuity from the adjacent myocardium rarely seen in true aneurysm. Diagnosis is easiest by echocardiography with spectral and color-flow Doppler (Figures 21.13B,C); transesophageal and transgastric scanning are superior to transthoracic. With TTE, careful subcostal scans are most useful. Sometimes an echo contrast study is useful. Radionuclide imaging (e.g., gadolinium), catheter ventriculography or cine-magnetic resonance imaging (MRI) will be decisive when echo-Doppler studies fail. Chest radiographs may show a local double density along the peri-

Table 20.4   Pseudoaneurysm vs. Aneurysm: Differential Features

	Pseudoaneurysm	True aneurysm
Wall	Pericardium (epicardium + clot/hematoma)	Myocardium + pericardium
	Avascular	Coronary vessels may be present
Usual location	Posterior and/or inferior LV; may involve RV	Anterior, anterolateral or apical LV, rarely RV
Orifice proportion to maximum dimension	<50%	≥ 50% usually
Orifice by echo-Doppler	Usually small; may not be detected without Doppler flow through it	Usually easily seen; may appear narrow in inferior or posterior aneurysms

cardial silhouette or retrocardiac density on lateral films. *Differential diagnosis* includes true aneurysm, pericardial cysts, and loculated pericardial effusions. There may be murmurs, either a systolic murmur through the aneurysm itself, or due to a damaged adjacent papillary muscle (especially the posterolateral) causing mitral regurgitation, or both. Sometimes the ECG shows persistent ST elevations resembling those of true aneurysms and probably due to ischemia or ischemic wall motion abnormality.

The Pericardium and Right Ventricular Myocardial Infarction

Pericarditis is relatively frequent when inferior myocardial infarction is accompanied by right ventricular infarction. However, both the normal and inflamed pericardium, via ventricular and atrioventricular interaction (page 20), constrain the injured right heart which tends to dilate. Right ventricular dilation raises intrapericardial pressure, decreasing left ventricular transmural pressure (page 21), and consequently reduces left ventricular filling, preload and stroke volume. (Pulmonary embolism may act similarly, acute right heart dilation imposing acute pericardial constraint.) This form of relative pericardial constriction has constrictive hemodynamics (pages 220–225), reduced blood pressure, jugular venous distention and occasionally a third heart sound or Kussmaul's sign. Even pulsus paradoxus may appear, possibly related to increased pericardial fluid or septal hyperresponsiveness to the respiratory cycle (page 226). *These signs may individually depend on the pathophysiologic "mix"—whether relative constriction due to pericardial tightening or increased intrapericardial pressure dominates.* Elevated right atrial pressure tends to equal or exceed pulmonary wedge pressure. Although left ventricular output is reduced, the lungs are usually clear. Thus, the clinical picture usually resembles constriction, or with a pericardial rub and pulsus paradoxus it can suggest tamponade (differential diagnosis detailed in Table 20.3). Sometimes, tricuspid regurgitation due to the right ventricular infarct simulates or obscures a pericardial rub. Naturally, both may be present.

POST–MYOCARDIAL INFARCTION SYNDROME (PMIS; DRESSLER'S SYNDROME)

First reported in France in 1953, this form of pericarditis was well described, beginning in 1956, by Dressler. Since then, the picture has become clearer, although its pathogenesis is not entirely elucidated. This infarct-associated pericarditis is distinct from epistenocardiac pericarditis directly caused by transmural infarction; PMIS does not require anatomically transmural infarction. Most cases are distinguished by fever, high sedimentation rate, considerable "pericardial" pain (page 110), pleuritis and sometimes pneumonitis. Its usual onset is between 1 week and several months after the clinical onset of infarction. Some patients have a remote history of pericarditis. Like epistenocardiac pericarditis, the PMIS occurs more often after larger infarctions, particularly anterior infarcts, inferior infarcts accompanied by right ventricular infarction, and infarctions with more complicated in-hospital courses. Moreover, the syndrome can appear as an extension of epistenocardiac pericarditis, with persistence or rapid recurrence of rub and fever, or as an exacerbation of the customarily low-grade "infarct fever" with considerable malaise, in contrast to typical infarct pericarditis which is comparatively mild and transient. Indeed, some early cases begin during initial hospitalization for acute infarction as severe pericarditis not resembling classic infarct pericarditis.

The usual gap from onset of infarct symptoms to the PMIS suggests a necessary latent period, in contrast to those patients in whom typical PMIS almost coincides with the infarct's apparent onset. However, *the symptoms and signs of recent infarct need not represent the actual onset of infarction.* This is demonstrated by patients with cardiac rupture in whom the moment of death is accurately established, but the histology of the infarct can place it as much as 10 days and even longer before the patient first recognized the appropriate symptoms—its clinical onset. In the same context are the 25 to 33% of patients with silent infarctions detected much later by ECG in the Framingham Heart Study. In such patients, a bout of pericarditis due to PMIS could have appeared as "idiopathic pericarditis" because the infarct was missed and PMIS often resembles viral pericarditis. Although originally reported in approximately 5% of patients with acute myocardial infarct, the exact incidence of PMIS remains uncertain but may be less. Yet this depends critically on the quality of follow-up after a myocardial infarct, so that absence of PMIS in hospital and often for several weeks afterwards prevents ascertainment of its real incidence. Actual incidence may also relate to the changing clinical "environment" since its original description. Although the syndrome occurs with and without antithrombotic treatment, it may be more frequent in patients with pericardial bleeding, which can occur during infarction with or without an anticoagulant or thrombolytic regimen. Indeed, Dressler reported prothrombin times above 30 sec in an era when longer prothrombin times were the rule, perhaps accounting for many cases. He also used dicumarol rather than coumadin, the chemical differences perhaps having some effect.

Pathogenesis

The PMIS has frequently been *considered an autoimmune process* based on the usual latent period and factors in common with other pericardial injury syndromes (notably the postpericardiotomy syndrome; page 403). These include (1) latent period, (2) development of antiheart antibodies, (3) preceding pericardial injury (most recognized PMIS cases have had epistenocardiac pericarditis with or without pericardial bleeding), although (4) PMIS occurs in a substantial number of patients with anatomically nontransmural infarctions, and therefore without the direct pericardial injury causing epistenocardiac pericarditis, (5) frequent recurrence, (6) typical prompt response to anti-inflammatory agents, (7) frequent associated pleuritis with or without pneumonitis, (8) changes in cellular immunity suggested by altered lymphocyte subsets compared to control patients, and (9) finally, there is evidence favoring immune complex formation incorporating antibody combined with myocardial antigen, complement pathway activation and evidence of cellular as well as humoral immunopathic responses.

Despite the attractive evidence and similarity to the postpericardiotomy syndrome (PPS), *numerous observations make the pathogenesis uncertain*. Patients develop PMIS at widely varying times after the index infarct and despite prior treatment of any epistenocardiac pericarditis with anti-inflammatory agents. Antibodies—antiheart (AHA), antiactin (AAA) and antimyosin (AMA)—are provoked both by cardiac surgery and infarction; surgery is more immunostimulating than infarction, evoking much greater quantities of them. However, *these are not antipericardial antibodies*—which have not been identified—so that the question arises, why should the pericardium (or the pleura or the lung) be the subject of an immunopathic response by antibodies stimulated by damage to very different cells? While the surgical *postpericardiotomy* syndrome appears to require a "permissive" viral infection, presumably developed preoperatively or intraoperatively (page 404), viral studies have been uniformly negative in the PMIS. Of course, since recognizable PMIS occurs in relatively few post-infarct patients, there may be questions, as yet unsettled, of unique susceptibility. Finally, some infarcts or cases of infarct-simulating myocarditis are precipitated by respiratory or systemic infections with a continuing inflammatory myocardial immunopathy that could involve the pericardium (Chapter 9).

Clinical Features

In occasional patients, an original infarct pericarditis may seem to worsen, appearing to be particularly severe, but eventually declaring itself as PMIS dating from the "clinical onset" of infarction. These patients have considerable malaise, marked pleuritic chest pain and severe chest discomfort, usually with a pericardial rub, frequent pericardial and pleural effusions, and either the appearance of fever de novo or exacerbation of "infarct fever" to as much s 104°F. The ECG occasionally shows ST- and T-wave changes suggesting pericarditis superimposed on evolving infarct, but it is usually dominated by evolutionary infarct changes. Telltale PR segment deviations are a strong clue (Figure 20.5). In contrast, some other patients with apparent "epistenocardiac

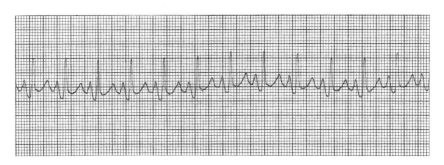

Figure 20.5 Postmyocardial infarction syndrome (PMIS) on postadmission day 11. Patient with severe malaise, new fever (104°F) and pericardial rub. The only ECG change was striking PR segment deviations.

pericarditis" (i.e., apparent early infarct pericarditis), who have a typical Stage I ECG (Figures 20.6A and B), can be considered to have the PMIS. In them, the actual onset of the infarct probably occurred before it surfaced clinically ("clinical onset"). Indeed, there is no reason why ordinary infarct pericarditis should have classic, diffuse stage I ECG changes, since the pericardial lesion is "epistenocardiac," that is, inflammation confined to the zone of eruption of anatomically transmural infarct onto the visceral pericardium.

More commonly, the PMIS occurs from a week to several months after the apparent onset of infarction, and many patients have already had characteristically mild epistenocardiac pericarditis. The PMIS now appears as a typical "new" acute pericarditis syndrome resembling viral pericarditis. Thus, it is nearly always much worse than the average case of infarct pericarditis. That is, *the PMIS is qualitatively similar but quantitatively worse than epistenocardiac pericarditis.* While it thus is usually a case of recurrent morbidity rather than mortality, *it is potentially life-threatening due to more frequent effusion, tamponade, hemorrhage, and association with larger infarcts and thrombosed ventricular aneurysms.*

Pericardial effusion occurs in at least half the patients. Indeed, a pericardial effusion with or even without a typical acute pericarditis syndrome occurring after an acute infarct should suggest the PMIS, particularly if there are pulmonary infiltrates and a pleural effusion (usually left-sided) and especially in the absence of heart failure. Both the pericardial and pleural effusions may be serous or hemorrhagic with or without antithrombotic treatment. Chest x-ray and echocardiography or other imaging will disclose such effusions. Laboratory examination show leukocytosis, typically mainly polymorphonuclear (occasionally with increased eosinophils) and mild anemia. The sedimentation rate is virtually always significantly high. These also typify exacerbations and

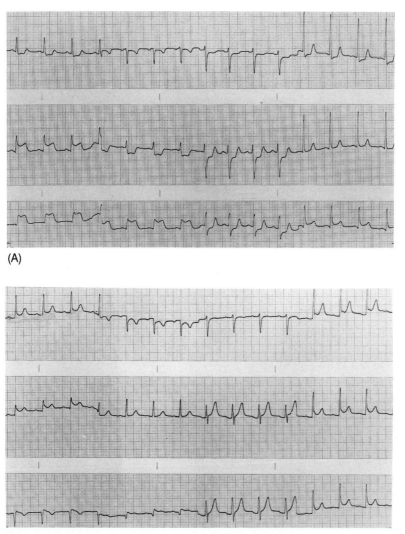

(A)

(B)

Figure 20.6 A. Acute inferoapical infarction: day 1. ST elevations in II, III, aVF and V6. Widespread ST depression in I, aVL and V1-V4 indicates severity. B. Same patient as in Figure 20.6A, day 2. Consistent with "early" postmyocardial infarction PMIS; typical Stage I ECG of acute pericarditis. Abnormal Q waves now in aVF (and III). J (ST) elevation in almost all leads, *including those formerly showing J (ST) depression*. J (ST) is isoelectric in aVL but it had been markedly depressed, producing a pseudo-S wave in Figure 20.6A that is now gone, with the newly isoelectric J-point over 3 mm higher than previously.

recurrences, which can be single or multiple, over weeks or even years after the index infarction.

Syndromes like PMIS have followed coronary angioplasty and both cardiac and pericardial injuries like catheter perforation, epicardial pacemaker implantation and even transvenous endocardial pacemakers with or without detectable myocardial perforation. Rarely, a similar syndrome follows *pulmonary embolism* with dominant pleuropulmonary manifestations, but also pericardial effusion, pericardial rubs or both (page 359).

Complications

Complications of the PMIS are uncommon but include both *tamponade* by serous or serosanguineous effusions and relatively early or late *constrictive or effusive-constrictive pericarditis,* accompanied by a moderate anemia of chronic disease. Constriction is not surprising because organization of pericardial exudate and clotting of blood in the pericardium has been detected in the PMIS. Indeed, in the acute phase, these can produce *loculated effusions* (page 208), making pericardiocentesis difficult.

Rarely, effusions in PMIS may look purulent because of a high concentration of neutrophils; taken with the customary fever, this mimics purulent pericarditis, but pericardial fluid is sterile. Rare cases of PMIS are accompanied by *Sweet's syndrome*, an acute febrile neutrophilic dermatosis that is ordinarily associated with solid neoplasia and chronic inflammatory bowel disease, both of which can themselves involve the pericardium; Sweet's syndrome responds to corticosteroid treatment, as does the PMIS. The PMIS has been observed in patients with ventricular aneurysms, particularly at autopsy, but this could be coincidental, since it is the larger and particularly anterior and apical infarcts that become aneurysmal. It is likely that it will also be observed with pseudoaneurysms.

Prognosis

Prognosis of patients with the PMIS is fundamentally that of the index infarction or any ventricular aneurysm and accompanying coronary heart disease unless it is complicated by tamponade or constriction.

Differential Diagnosis

The PMIS occurring during the index hospitalization is more easily recognized than at any time later when, despite the history of myocardial infarction, any etiologic variety of pericarditis could occur. Differentiation is particularly difficult when early pneumonitis or pleuritis dominates the picture and a pericardial rub or effusion is not yet discovered. Recognition *as PMIS* is, of course, even more difficult when the original infarct was not recognized. (Note: Up to one third of infarcts are clinically "silent.") Indeed, *any other kind of pericarditis*, particularly a viral or idiopathic pericarditis syndrome (page 260), is suggested when the index infarct has been missed. Moreover, the PMIS often resembles the pericarditis in many vasculitides (Chapter 19), with which it shares some immunopathic features. Pericardial hemorrhage complicating thrombolysis or systemic anticoagulation is another differential consideration.

Diagnostic problems also arise when only a pleural rub is present or if there is pleurisy and a parapneumonic effusion; pleural fluid in the PMIS is more likely to have a normal pH. Also to be considered are atelectasis, infectious endocarditis and sepsis, especially with marked or persistent fever.

Moreover, regardless of its time of onset—during the index myocardial infarction or long afterward—*the PMIS must be distinguished from extended or recurrent ischemia or infarction*. When the PMIS provokes either tamponade or eventual constriction, differential diagnosis includes congestive heart failure during recurrent ischemia and particularly recurrent infarction. With a late PMIS, any new cardiac enzyme rise should be absent or mild, new Q waves will be absent, and pain—recognizable or not as pericardial/ pleuritic—should not respond to nitrates. With uncomplicated recurrent infarction, a pleural rub is also much less likely, and pericardial and pleural effusions are much less common. Indeed, there may be true infarct pericarditis; the rub of any such epistenocardiac pericarditis is nearly always much softer and evanescent and less persistent than that of PMIS; the pericarditis itself is much less painful, and fever is not likely to be prominent. Indeed, these patients appear "less sick" than those with PMIS if the infarct itself is not severe.

Another important diagnostic consideration is *pulmonary embolism*, especially because this requires anticoagulation, whereas anticoagulation is best discontinued in patients with the PMIS, who can have hemorrhagic pericardial effusions. Here ventilation-perfusion lung scans may not be diagnostic because they can appear abnormal in both conditions; a pulmonary angiogram may be needed, especially in patients with right ventricular infarction or thrombophlebitis. Fortunately, the remarkable PMIS mimic in occasional cases of pulmonary embolism is uncommon. as is the concurrence of a pericardial rub (page 359).

Management

If the PMIS occurs after hospitalization, the patient should be rehospitalized to be observed for cardiac tamponade, differential diagnosis, and possible adjustment or discontinuation of anticoagulant treatment—an individualized decision. Bed rest and nonsteroidal anti-inflammatory drugs (NSAIDs) like aspirin or ibuprofen will usually be helpful. However, severely symptomatic patients will require opiates, and persistent recurrences may require a corticosteroid. Because of the possibility of chronicity and because of steroid complications, steroids should be employed only as a last resort and at the lowest possible doses with the earliest tapering to discontinuance. Colchicine as well as NSAIDs ease weaning from corticosteroid treatment. Cardiac tamponade or constriction should be managed by the appropriate mechanical interventions: drainage or pericardiectomy.

DISSECTING ANEURYSM (HEMATOMA) AND INTRAMURAL HEMORRHAGE OF THE AORTA

Dissecting aortic aneurysm, DeBakey types I and II, and aortic intramural hemorrhage (IMH) often rupture into the pericardium; perforating aortic ulcer occurs distally and appears not to involve the pericardium. Dissecting aneurysm and IMH are almost indistinguishable clinically and the discussion here mostly applies to both. Rupture is the most frequent cause of death due to aortic dissection, usually through tamponade by enough blood to also overwhelm the antithrombotic mechanisms of the pericardium (page 24). With survival, intra-pericardial clotting then prevents nonsurgical drainage (which in any case is dangerous). In terminal cases, there is always more than 100 mL of blood, usually between 400 and 1500 mL, depending on the rate at which the hemo-pericardium develops. This can be subacute and even chronic. Subacute and chronic bleeding are tolerated due to smaller leaks and mitigation of the aortic dissecting and shearing forces by medical treatment. Chronicity is the only way the larger hemopericardia can reach as much as 1500 mL. "Chronicity" is relative, sometimes taking weeks to months before discovery—and, rarely, reactivation—of an aborted dissection after many years. In catastrophically acute cases, pure blood fills the pericardium and patients are tamponaded by 100 to 150 mL. In contrast, a protracted course allows considerable dilution by peri-cardial effusion due to pericardial irritation and the osmotic effects of intra-pericardial hemolysis.

Clinical Aspects; Electrocardiography

Other effects of aortic dissection include pericardial irritation by blood that first dissects under the epicardium, provoking a rub and occasionally constricting coronary arteries sufficiently to cause myocardial ischemia and even to mas-querade as ordinary infarction. Occasionally, the ECG resembles the charac-teristic Stage I of pericarditis (Figure 21.7). Rarely, dissection into the coro-nary ostia may precipitate infarction. Occlusion of renal arteries combined with hypotension can produce acute uremic pericarditis (page 295), also complicat-ing the diagnosis. Indeed, *dissecting aneurysm may first present from hours to*

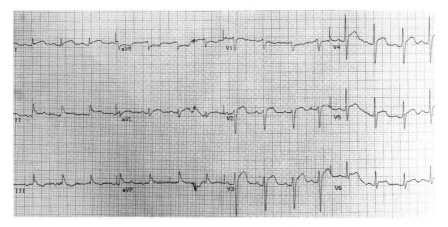

Figure 20.7   Dissecting aortic aneurysm with intrapericardial rupture. Electrocardiogram is a variant of the typical Stage I of acute pericarditis (Chapter 5). This occurred
before critical tamponade and represents subepicardial penetration of blood or epicardial irritation by blood constituents like potassium from hemolyzed red blood cells.

*many days before aortic rupture as apparent acute pericarditis and without pain
that is more typical of dissection.* These cases, some complete with pericardial
rub and ECG changes, suggest a diagnosis of idiopathic pericarditis—a much
more common disease. (Note: In *recognized* aortic dissections, pleuritic chest
pain and pericardial rubs—with or without ECG changes—are ominous signs;
these and hypotension should initiate immediate search for and relief of
tamponade.) In such dissections of relatively slow clinical onset, misleading
ECG changes may be due to release of potassium from hemolysis of
intrapericardial red blood cells; ST segment elevations are proportional to the
elevation of intrapericardial potassium above its concentration in circulating
blood. In any case, *in aortic dissection and intramural hematoma affecting the
pericardium, the ECG is seldom normal* and may show preexisting left ventricular hypertrophy, changes suggesting acute ischemia or infarction, acute pericarditis or any of these in combination.

Diagnostic Considerations

*In older patients with a history of hypertension, apparent acute pericarditis
should always be considered part of another syndrome. In younger patients,
where idiopathic pericarditis is generally more common, signs of Marfan's or
other inherited connective tissue disease or aortic coarctation*—each capable of
producing both painful and "silent" aortic dissections—*should be diligently
sought* by physical examination, including somatic features like body habitus

and auscultation for rubs or murmurs. (Note: A new murmur of aortic regurgitation is characteristic of proximal aortic dissection; both aortic regurgitation and dissecting aneurysms are more common in patients with bicuspid aortic valves, congenital aortic stenosis and coarctation with rib notching on the chest film.) Particular suspicion is also justified in hypertensive pregnant patients. Finally, patients with giant-cell (temporal) arteritis, which itself causes pericarditis, also have a propensity to aortic aneurysm and dissection (page 326).

Echocardiography, preferably omniplane transesophageal, to detect pericardial effusion, any aortic regurgitation, a false lumen and an aortic intimal flap is optimal for diagnosis. Apart from painful or painless acute pericarditis, the presence of apparent pericardial effusions or aortic regurgitation in such patients should always raise the question of aortic dissection. Moreover, because of the success of thrombolytic therapy early in acute myocardial infarction, candidates for thrombolysis should be carefully evaluated if there is the remotest chance of an aortic intramural hemorrhage or dissecting hematoma for which thrombolysis has been catastrophic. *Precise diagnosis as in all acute conditions should be as rapid as practicable*, because of the narrow "windows" for both aortic rupture and myocardial salvage. Extreme care must be taken since the most efficient technique *transesophageal echocardiography* (TEE), has appeared, at least once, to precipitate intrapericardial aortic rupture, ascribable to transmitted pressure during the scope manipulation and the common increases in blood pressure and heart rate and retching during TEE. These patients should be adequately anesthetized and sedated to reduce the gag reflex and minimize mucosal reactions. However, *TEE is the procedure of choice* because it is as sensitive as CT and MRI, the Doppler is sensitive to aortic regurgitation, and the equipment is portable. While TEE depends more on operator expertise and may be "blind" to parts of the aortic arch, transthoracic echocardiography (TTE) is much less sensitive, but may be more rapidly available.

If there is any question, especially after negative or indecisive echocardiography, which can be practiced almost anywhere, *computed tomography (CT), especially helical CT, or spin-echo magnetic resonance imaging* (MRI—time-consuming and logistically almost impossible) will usually define aortic mural hemorrhages or any intimal flap (absent in IMH). They are safer and more sensitive than *aortography*, which occasionally may become necessary but can miss both dissections and an intramural aortic hematoma. Depending on the site of dissection, a dissecting hematoma may produce a strictly anterior "effusion" in the pericardium, which could resemble epicardial fat on echocardiography (page 136). (In MRI and CT, true epicardial fat makes distinction of all pericardial effusions easier.) Indeed, all imaging techniques show pericardial effusions due to aortic dissection that are more often anterior than in any other location. In CT, intrapericardial attenuation values depend on the amount and age of the hemopericardium as well as the proportion of blood (often 100%) in the apparent effusion. For example, fresh acute hemopericardium has a Hounsfield number similar to the attenuation of blood in the heart. In any case, aortography is rarely needed, and in many cases it is not worthwhile to catheterize and visualize the coronary arteries, to avoid both provoking more dissection and loss of time.

The safest and most efficient management of patients in whom acute dissection is likely is to *carry on all diagnostic procedures in the operating room.* Too often, pericardial drainage gives only temporary or no relief of tamponade; subsequent increase in blood pressure disrupts sealing clots, accelerating intrapericardial leakage with eventual frank hemopericardium, shock, electromechanical dissociation and death. The definitive treatment is surgical relief of tamponade and repair of the aortic dissection. *Atropine* can be given to avoid vagally mediated bradycardia, hypotension and eventual *electromechanical dissociation* common in severe hemopericardium (page 82).

Only rarely does aortic dissection involving the pericardium heal spontaneously. Yet constrictive pericarditis has resulted from this process as early as 7 months later.

PLEUROPULMONARY DISORDERS

Diseases of the lungs and pleura, primarily inflammatory and neoplastic, may directly invade the pericardium or simultaneously involve the pericardium, the heart or both. These are mainly pneumonia and empyema (page 266) and pleuropulmonary carcinoma (page 302), which may be metastatic or primary in the lungs or pleura. Pleuritis, and particularly pleurodynia affecting the diaphragmatic pleura, can involve the pericardium by contiguity, although pleurodynia ("devil's grippe") is most attributable to Coxsackievirus infection (page 263). Less well known is pericardial involvement in pulmonary thromboembolism.

Pericardial Involvement in Pulmonary Thromboembolism

Direct Involvement

Pericardial involvement following pulmonary infarction is uncommon but is well known as (1) an apparently direct effect by contiguity, (2) a complication of antithrombotic therapy for pulmonary embolism, (3) a simultaneous event in posttraumtic pulmonary embolism and pulmonary embolism following cardiac or other surgery and (4) rarely, as an apparently immunopathic event with a pericardial component closely mimicking the PMIS (page 360).

Infarction of pulmonary segments adjacent to the pericardium can produce pleuropericardial rubs, sometimes strictly exopericardial rubs (page 27), and even classic pericardial rubs, which, rarely, may be the first sign of a pulmonary embolus. These occur with or without pleuritic pain, which by itself is nonspecific. When such pericardial signs follow blunt chest trauma, cardiac surgery or penetrating cardiac trauma (Chapter 21), the obviously mixed picture may be difficult to unravel. This is equally true of hemorrhagic pericardial effusions following any kind of antithrombotic treatment for acute myocardial infarction or pulmonary embolism. Such effusions are sufficiently rare that one might suspect a simultaneous clinically silent pericarditis. In any case, all of these conditions have sometimes produced *cardiac tamponade, to be distinguished from circulatory collapse due to the pulmonary embolism.* In other cases, massive pulmonary embolism has been attended by hydropericardium, presumably due to right heart failure. Such cases may have a *conus rub* (page 28) due to acute cor pulmonale without pericarditis. Finally, since pulmonary embolism can by asymptomatic, signs of acute pericarditis or pericardial effusion should alert physicians to search for it in patients who have risk factors for embolism and to anticipate pericardial bleeding, since antithrombotic therapy appropriate for pulmonary thromboembolism may be dangerous with pericardial inflammation.

Indirect Involvement

Acute pulmonary embolism raises intrapericardial pressure, probably because of right heart dilatation. This makes left ventricular (LV) transmural pressure better than LV end-diastolic pressure as an index of preload.

Post–Pulmonary Infarction Syndrome

Rarely, in the days to weeks after pulmonary embolism, acute pericarditis with or without effusion may appear with a syndrome closely resembling the PMIS (pages 349–356). Like those with the PMIS, these patients have pericardial rubs, fever, leukocytosis, elevated sedimentation rates, frequent pericardial and pleural effusions, and rarely even cardiac tamponade. Like the PMIS and other immunopathies, this syndrome responds sensitively to anti-inflammatory treatment and particularly rapidly to a corticosteroid. In the usual absence of a severe syndrome, NSAIDs should be tried first. This syndrome is poorly understood because few cases have been recognized (presumably many others have been missed or misdiagnosed as unrelated pericarditis) and because it tends to be milder than most cases of PMIS.

MEDIASTINAL DISEASE

Opportunities for direct or simultaneous pericardial involvement by mediastinal disorders, particularly inflammation and neoplasia, are obvious. These include involvement by mediastinal lymph nodes, as in tuberculous lymphadenitis with a "classic" point of pericardial penetration near the root of the great vessels. All conditions producing mediastinitis, mediastinal abscess and mediastinal fibrosis often involve the pericardium to some degree, including clinically insignificant involvement (with an exopericardial rub), acute inflammation and simulation of constrictive pericarditis by entrapment of the great veins and aorta near their communication with the heart.

When mediastinopathies do not involve esophageal structures hematogenously or by lymphatic spread, severe diseases of the pleura or esophagus erupting into the mediastinum can provoke mediastinitis, including mediastinal abscesses and eventual mediastinal fibrosis (which rarely may be on a toxic or immunopathic basis). In any case, such mediastinal syndromes, especially when acute, precede pericardial involvement. In less acute cases, pericardial involvement may be the first syndrome to surface, and any of the major responses of the pericardium to irritation or invasion can be detected. Chest x-ray films may show an unusually wide and irregular mediastinal shadow; CT and MRI should disclose the anatomic details.

PERICARDIAL INVOLVEMENT IN ESOPHAGEAL DISEASE (TABLE 20-5)

The normal esophagus is usually a quiet posterior neighbor opposite the third to the eleventh thoracic vertebrae. It overlies the pericardium covering parts of the left atrium and ventricle. Esophageal disorders can involve the pericardium and all it contains, often catastrophically, frequently with little or no warning due to insidious onset and progression, and almost always confusingly because of what appears to be isolated pericardial or cardiac disease or combined esophageal and cardiopericardial signs and symptoms. Rarely, the pericardium has struck back, as in a patient with densely calcific constrictive pericarditis in whom a pericardial calcific plaque eroded the esophagus.

Predisposing Factors

Although esophageal involvement is occasionally a surprise after the pericardial lesion has appeared, the vast majority of patients who are "candidates" for pericardial involvement include those who have had esophageal surgery and other trauma, gastroesophageal reflux, Barrett's esophagus, hiatal hernia (including the gastric fundus) and patients with esophageal strictures.

Pathogenesis: Direct and Indirect Pericardial Involvement

The pericardium is *directly* involved by fistulas from processes penetrating the esophageal wall, like inflamed esophageal diverticula, and less often by lymphangial spread. These include *inflammation—esophagitis and ulcers* of pep-

Table 20.5 Pericardial Involvement in Esophageal Diseases

A. *Predisposing factors*
   Esophageal trauma
      Surgery (including surgical colonic interposition)
      Instrumentation
      Other
   Gastroesophageal reflux
   Barrett's esophagus
   Hiatal hernia (including gastric fundus)
   Esophageal strictures
B. *Direct pericardial involvement: mainly esophagopericardial fistula*
   due to anterior esophageal penetration
   Esophagitis
   Esophageal diverticulitis
   Corrosive ingestants
   Neoplasia (*esp.* malignancies)
   Esophageal ulcers
      Peptic
      Bacterial
      Viral
      Fungal
   Foreign bodies
   "Spontaneous" esophageal rupture
   Postradiation therapy
C. *Indirect esophagopericardial involvement*
   Mediastinitis
   Mediastinal abscess
D. *Consequences*
   Pericarditis: acute; subacute; (rarely) chronic/recurrent
   Pneumopericardium/pneumohydropericardium/pneumopyopericardium
   Pericardial effusion; (rarely) tamponade
   Pericardial adhesions/loculation
   Cardiac involvement, *esp.*:
      Left atrial or left ventricular penetration
         Thrombosis
         Systemic embolism, including:
         Food
         Air/gas
         Debris

---

tic, bacterial, viral and fungal (especially candidal) origin—*neoplasms, perfo-rating foreign bodies, corrosive ingestants and "spontaneous" esophageal rup-ture.* Esophagopericardial fistulas also develop from inflamed *surgical and anastomotic suture lines* in the esophagus and in patients with *colonic interpo-*

sition for stricture and other esophageal lesions, resulting in a thoracic colon-pericardial fistula. The pericardium may be *indirectly* involved when *mediastinitis or abscess* results from esophageal perforations well away from the abutting pericardium (i.e., anywhere except anteriorly). Overall, such pericardial involvement is uncommon but not rare due to chronic peptic ulceration and after surgery of the esophagus. Penetrating tuberculous ulcers appear to have disappeared, but with increasing numbers of immunocompromised patients, their absence may not be permanent.

Clinical Aspects

Stokes (1854) listed ulcerated perforation of the pericardium among causes of secondary pericarditis, "most of which must be familiar to the clinical observer," suggesting an unusual frequency of these lesions in the 19th century. Symptoms and signs depend on the structures involved, including the pericardium itself. With penetration of the atria, nearly always the left, or of the left ventricle, mixed pictures develop. From the pericardial standpoint, *patients may present as having acute pericarditis, pericardial effusion, pneumopericardium, pneumohydropericardium or pneumopyopericardium with or without tamponade.* Any of these may be the presenting syndrome, including *purulent pericarditis*, which occasionally precedes discovery of the fistula, even by years. Such cases usually have small amounts of pericardial fluid, often loculated by pericardial adhesions from chronic inflammation. Indeed, such sealing of the intrapericardial portion permits the fistula to continue silently and later to penetrate the left atrium or ventricle with much more dramatic clinical pictures.

Esophagopericardial fistulas also occur due to a variety of chemical and physical traumata of the esophagus (Table 20.5) as well as to malignancies, either esophageal, pulmonary or, rarely, metastatic. Fistulation has also followed radiation therapy of such tumors.

Although the history is sometimes not helpful, most often there has been chronic peptic esophagitis, esophagogastric surgery or a malignancy. Patients present with pain, which can be retrosternal or in the left chest and can involve the shoulders and the interscapular zone. Most have fever, and many a pericardial rub with shock, dyspnea and cyanosis, any one of which can be the initial symptom. A clinical clue is discovery of a *pneumohydropericardium* or *pneumopyopericardium* with a splashing "mill-wheel sound" (page 38). While polymicrobial pericarditis is common, blood cultures may or may not be positive. Pleural effusions, particularly on the left, and occasional pulmonary infiltrates are common. Esophageal signs can be deceptively absent or the patient may have recent or long-standing odynophagia or dysphagia. *Cardiac involvement can simulate acute myocardial infarction and*, particularly with left ventricular penetration, present a picture equivalent to infarction with cardiogenic shock. Moreover, any intracardiac spread can produce *systemic embolization* by food, air and septic and necrotic debris. There may be localized bleeding,

unless sealed off by the pericardium. With penetration of the left atrium, cardiac bleeding is usually well contained by the extraordinary pericardial clasp
of that structure (page 11), which tends to prevent pericardial spread, so that
only an *esophagus–left atrial fistula* results.

Diagnosis

The ECG is frequently consistent with pericarditis, which, however, gives no
information as to the origin of the process. The ECG may reflect any other
cardiac injury, and any *pericardial rub* at least directs attention to the pericardium. *Key to diagnosis is all forms of imaging.* The *chest x-ray* can show an
increased cardiopericardial shadow or pneumopericardium, the "air" due to
swallowed air, or gas produced by infection and digestive tract contaminants.
Intrapericardial air or gas can contribute an element of pneumotamponade (page
88); however, unless there is bleeding, the tendency to relatively small effusions makes tamponade uncommon. *Contrast studies* are often essential to define fistulas from the esophagus and other hollow viscera as well as thickened
pericardium and any intrapericardially herniated organs. (Oral, water-soluble
contrast media can appear in the pericardium with or without actually defining
smaller fistulas.) Barium may be used but may be too dense for patients with
dysphagia. A *technetium* scan can confirm a fistula in doubtful cases. *Esophagoscopy* may show esophagitis or ulcer or may be "negative" with small lesions;
gas insufflation during the procedure can increase a pneumopericardium. *Esophageal biopsy* may be positive for infection or inflammation. *Pericardial drainage* with a low pH and bacterial flora (microscopic and by culture) as well as
debris point to an upper gastrointestinal fistula. Immunocompromised patients
may demonstrate fungi, particularly *Candida*. Oral methylene blue will appear
in the pericardial drainage. In any case, pericardial involvement should be
anticipated in a patient with anterior esophageal ulcers, esophagitis, malignancy,
herniated gastric fundus or a history of any kind of esophagogastric surgery who
develops pneumo- or pneumohydropericardium. Definitive treatment is surgical, although rarely an esophagopericardial fistula has closed after pericardial
evacuation. Rare, also, is subsequent constrictive pericarditis.

DIAPHRAGM AND LIVER DISEASE

Diaphragmatic defects may be congenital, traumatic or iatrogenic. Congenital
absence of a portion of the diaphragm may involve the pericardium either by
concomitant absence of a part of the pericardium or, more often, by herniation
of abdominal contents into the pericardial cavity. These are usually recognized
in childhood. It is equally evident that absence or disruption of any part of the
diaphragmatic "buffer" will permit direct transmission of inflammatory and
other gastrointestinal and intraperitoneal disease to the pericardium.

Inferior extension of surgical median sternotomies and the advent of sub-xiphoid incision for pericardial drainage (page 174) and to insert pacemakers and other devices rarely results in diaphragmatic defects owing to inadvertent inclusion of the diaphragm in the incision, permitting abdominal contents to herniate into the pericardial cavity. This also occurs due to blunt and sharp trauma (with diaphragmatic rupture and gaps that permit omentum, stomach, duodenum, colon, liver and even jejunum to herniate). *Any of these can compress the heart due to crowding by these organs with or without pericardial effusions.* Strangulation of intrapericardial bowel makes it gangrenous, producing a grossly and microscopically contaminated cardiac tamponade that can be acute or subacute. Pericardial adhesions to the herniated organs along with intestinal obstruction also complicate diagnosis and treatment. *Diagnostic clues* include a history of infradiaphragmatic surgery (including pericardial drainage procedures) and trauma, unilaterally—rarely bilaterally—elevated diaphragm, signs of bowel obstruction, abdominal organs discovered in the chest and pericardial effusion with or without tamponade.

Subphrenic abscesses involve the mediastinum either by direct extension or hematogenous spread, producing the physical findings of mediastinitis and pericarditis with pericardial rubs and, more often, pericardial effusion with or without a rub. The pericardium is penetrated either directly through the diaphragm or from the adjacent mediastinitis, which is often purulent. Myocarditis occasionally accompanies, complicating the diagnosis. Oddly, unless there are major complications, cardiovascular signs alone do not suggest a poor prognosis. However, significant pericardial effusion, and particularly tamponade, is ominous.

Liver disease is included for completeness because severe liver inflammations, particularly with abscess formation (page 282) can penetrate the diaphragm or involve the heart and pericardium hematogenously. Naturally, in cases of infectious hepatitis (page 263), liver and pericardial inflammation can be simultaneous, though they may be recognized sequentially.

KEY POINTS

1. Myocardial infarction–associated acute pericarditis occurs in two forms: *epistenocardiac pericarditis*, due directly to transmural infarction, and the *post–myocardial infarction syndrome* (PMIS), which behaves like an immunopathy and appears days to weeks after the onset of infarction. Occasionally, a more or less silent infarction precedes acute symptoms and the PMIS coincides with or follows rapidly after hospital admission, making it difficult to distinguish from epistenocardiac pericarditis.
2. *Epistenocardiac pericarditis* is usually mild, transient and easily treated. The PMIS tends to be more intense and much more symptomatic, prone to recur indefinitely and probably accounts for typical Stage I ECG changes, since the much more common epistenocardiac form is localized to the infarct surface. The fact that the PMIS

frequently appears after recovery, particularly if it follows a silent infarct, contributes to the tendency to mistake it for other forms of pericarditis (including epistenocardiac pericarditis).

3. Patients with epistenocardiac pericarditis have a worse posthospital prognosis than those without infarct pericarditis, consistent with its association with larger infarcts and higher Killip classes. Moderate-sized to large pericardial effusions usually signify heart failure. Thrombolytic therapy has reduced its incidence, while increasing and making earlier the incidence of ventricular rupture.

4. *Pseudoaneurysms* are ventricular ruptures contained by overlying pericardium, usually with a much narrower "neck" than true aneurysms and a strong propensity to rupture. Diagnosable by imaging, especially echo-Doppler study, they require surgical resection.

5. In right ventricular infarction, the pericardium tends to constrain the heart, increasing ventricular and atrioventricular interaction and imposing mainly constrictive (restrictive) hemodynamics with corresponding clinical findings.

6. The principal danger of dissecting hematoma (aneurysm) or intramural hemorrhage of the aorta (IMH) is acute hemopericardium with rapid tamponade and terminal electromechanical dissociation. *Diagnostic workup for such suspected aortic lesions is best done in the operating room*, especially because pericardiocentesis is hazardous and acute exacerbation is frequent. Subacute and chronic bleeding from such lesions is difficult to diagnose.

8. Pericardial involvement in mediastinal and pleuropulmonary disorders, especially pulmonary embolism, may be subtle or obvious. A rare postpulmonary infarction syndrome closely mimics the PMIS with pericardial findings.

9. Severe esophageal, stomach and intestinal disease, especially with ulceration, may penetrate the pericardium with dramatic inflammatory consequences, including variants of pneumohydropericardium.

10. Disorders of the diaphragm directly penetrate the pericardium or permit herniation of abdominal organs into it or next to it.

BIBLIOGRAPHY

Brack, M., Asinger, R.W., Sharkey, S. W., et al. Two-dimensional echocardiographic characteristics of pericardial hematoma secondary to left ventricular free wall rupture complicating acute myocardial infarction. Am. J. Cardiol. 1991; 68:961–964.

Calvin, J.E. Optimal right ventricular filling pressures and the role of pericardial constraint in right ventricular infarction in dogs. Circulation 1991; 84:852–861.

Chirillo, F., Cavalini, C., Longhini, C., et al. Comparative diagnostic value of transeosphageal echocardiography and retrograde aortography in the evaluation of thoracic aortic dissection. Am. J. Cardiol. 1994; 74:590–595.

Ersek, R.A., Chesler, E., Korns, M.E., Edwards, J.E. Spontaneous rupture of a false left ventricular aneurysm following myocardial infarction. Am. Heart J. 1969; 77:677–670.

Evans, J.M., O'Fallon, W.M., Hunder, G.G. Increased incidence of aortic aneurysm and dissection in giant cell (temporal) arteritis—A population-based study. Ann. Intern. Med. 1995; 122:502–507.

Friocourt, P., Benit, C.H., Batisse, J.P., et al. Pericardite et embolie pulmonaire. Arch. Mal. Couer Vaissaux 1984; 77:689–697.

Gammie JS, Katz WE, Swanson ER, Peitzman AB. Acute aortic dissection after blunt chest trauma. J Trauma 1996; 40: 126–127.

Gheorghiade M, Ruzumna P, Borzak S, Havstad S, Ali A, Goldstein S. Decline in the rate of hospital mortality from acute myocardial infarction: Impact of changing management strategies. Am Heart J 1996; 131: 250–256.

Giles, P.J., D'Cruz, I.A., Killam, H.A.W. Tamponade due to hemopericardium after streptokinase therapy for pulmonary embolism. South. Med. J. 1988; 81:912–914.

Isselbacher, E.M., Cigarroa, J.E., Eagle, K.A. Cardiac tamponade complicating proximal aortic dissection: Is pericardiocentesis harmful? Circulation 1995; 90:2375–2378.

Khan, A.H. Review—The postcardiac injury syndromes. Clin. Cardiol. 1992; 15:67–72.

Khogali SS, Bonser RS, Beattie JM. Concealed post-infarction left ventricular rupture—a diagnostic dilemma. Postgrad Med J 1996; 72: 121–122.

Krainin, F.M., Flessas, A.P., Spodick, D.H. Infarction associated pericarditis: Rarity of diagnostic electrocardiogram. N. Engl. J. Med. 1984; 311:1211–1214.

Oliva, P.B., Hammill, S.C., Talano, J.V. Effect of definition on incidence of postinfarction pericarditis. Circulation 1994; 90:1537–1541.

Robson, R.H. Hydropneumopericardium and oesophagitis: A nonfatal case. Thorax 1979; 34:262–264.

Silvey, S.V., Stoughton, T.L., Pearl, W., et al. Rupture of the outer partition of aortic dissection during transesophageal echocardiography. Am. J. Cardiol. 1991; 68:286–287.

Spodick, D.H. Pitfalls in the recognition of pericarditis. In: Hurst, J.W. (ed). Clinical Essays on the Heart. New York: McGraw-Hill, 1985, pp. 95–111.

Spodick, D.H. Pericardial complications of acute myocardial infarction. In: Francis, G.S., Alper, J.S. (eds.). Modern Coronary Care. Boston: Little Brown, 1990, pp. 331–339.

Spodick, D.H. Postmyocardial infarction syndrome (Dressler's syndrome). A.C.C. Curr. J. Rev. 1995; 4:35–37.

Widimsky, P., Gregor, P. Pericardial involvement during the course of myocardial infarction—A long-term clinical and echocardiographic study. Chest 1995; 108:89–93.

21

Traumatic Pericardial Disease: Accidental, Criminal, Surgical and Biological Trauma

The bony thorax affords only partial protection for the heart and pericardium. Thoracic resiliency permits their compression between the sternum and vertebrae, and their loose suspension may predispose to certain kinds of injury.

PERICARDIAL REACTIONS TO PHYSICAL TRAUMA

The remarkably broad range of pericardial injury (Table 21.1) evokes a set of one or more responses due to disruption of pericardial tissue and, frequently, adjacent and remote tissues. These may be *immediate* (cellular and vascular inflammation); *delayed*, including immunopathic (the *post–cardiac*—i.e., pericardial and myocardial—*injury syndrome; PCIS*); and due to *healing* (adhesions, constriction, effusive-constrictive pericarditis). The inflammatory response may be sterile or infective with or without significant pericardial effusion, which itself can develop slowly or rapidly and often with cardiac tamponade. *Traumatic tamponade*, the most common cause of early death with cardiac wounds, is usually due to bleeding, producing early or late cardiac compression or at least some degree of hemopericardium. Occult traumatic tamponade may be clinically "silent" only to suddenly decompensate with life-threatening consequences. Rapid bleeding overwhelms the antithrombotic mechanisms of the

Table 21.1   **Traumatic Pericardial Disease: Accidental, Surgical and Biological**

A. *Pericardial Responses to Injury*: with and without cardiac abnormality
    I. *Temporal*
        a. Immediate
            1. Cellular
            2. Vascular
        b. Delayed
            1. Immunopathic
            2. Reparative (scarring)
    II. *Tissue reaction*
        a. Inflammation: sterile/infected pericarditis
        b. Effusion
        c. Hemorrhage/hematoma
        d. Scarring (adhesions)
            1. Local
            2. General
            3. Constrictive/effusive-constrictive
    III. *Cardiac tamponade* (Note II b and c): Immediate; occult; delayed
    IV. *Pericardial rupture*
B. *Pericardial wounds*
    I. *Direct trauma*
        a. Penetrating
            1. Pointed instruments, weapons
            2. Bullets and other projectiles; "foreign-body pericarditis"
            3. Catheters: cardiac, PTCA, pericardial; central venous;
                radiofrequency ablation; endocardial pacing
        b. Epicardial pacing
        c. Automatic implanted cardioverter defibrillator (AICD)
        b. Surgical
            1. Surgery of the heart and pericardium
                (a) Direct effects
                    (1) Surgical pericarditis with and without effusion/tamponade
                    (2) Intrapericardial bleeding
        b. Delayed
            1. Surgical pericarditis
            2. Postpericardiotomy syndrome (cf. B III)
                (c) Adhesions
                (d) Postsurgical pericardial defects
                (e) Cardiac transplant/transplant rejection
                (f) Chylopericardium (cf. Chapter 7)
                (g) False aneurysm (cf. pages 346)

(*continued*)

Table 21.1 Continued

---

       2. Lung surgery (intrapericardial pneumonectomy)

       3. Open chest cardiac massage

       4. Removal of epicardial pacing wires

   c. Pericardial fistulation

       1. *Perforated viscera*: fistula to pericardium with *pneumopericardium* (see Chapters 7 and 11)

         (a) Esophagus

           (1) Ulcer, malignancy, esophagitis

           (2) Colon interposed after esophageal resection

         (b) Stomach

         (c) Duodenum

         (d) Bronchi

         (e) Transverse colon

       2. *Chemical*: communication with pericardial injury

         (a) Biliary tract

         (b) Pancreas

         (c) Esophagus

           (1) Ulcer

           (2) Sclerotherapy of varices

           (3) Dilation of esophageal structure

   d. Electrical

       1. Cardioversion/accidental shock

       2. Lightning

   e. Radiation

       1. Immediate (irradiation of contiguous masses): acute pericarditis—dry/effusive

       2. Delayed

         (a) Late acute

         (b) Late effusion

         (c) Adhesions/fibrosis/constriction

       3. Pancarditis: syndrome usually dominated by pericardial involvement

  II. *Indirect trauma*; blunt/nonpenetrating trauma causing cardiac/pericardial contusion, laceration, rupture

   a. Impact, crush, blast, deceleration

   b. Closed chest cardiac massage

  III. *Post-cardiac injury syndromes (PCIS)*:

   a. Post–myocardial infarction syndrome (PMIS; Dressler's)

   b. Post–pericardiotomy syndrome (PPS); due to surgery/wound

       1. With and without effusion/tamponade

       2. Constrictive/effusive-constrictive disease

C. *Foreign body pericarditis*

D. *Complications*

  I. Extrapericardial bleeding (slow/rapid) causing hypovolemia, permitting low pressure tamponade

---

Table 21.1 Continued

  II. Trauma to neighboring organs, surgical and accidental: intrapericardial
       wounds, hernias, fistulas
       a. Lung, pleura, bronchi: pneumopericardium, pyopneumopericardium,
           hemopneumocardium, pneumothorax, hemothorax
       b. Abdomen; liver and other organs
       c. Diaphragm
       d. Esophagus
       e. Mediastinum
       f. Chest wall/flail chest
       g. (Brain)
 III. Heart abnormalities: associated/unassociated/iatrogenic
       a. Myocardial disease/damage
       b. Conduction system damage; arrhythmias
       c. Coronary
           1. Transection/occlusion
           2. A-V fistula
       d. Cardiac (especially RV) thrombi
       e. Postsurgical paradoxic septal motion

  IV. Vascular injuries: great vessels, coronaries
   V. Infection: early, late
  VI. Pericardial sequelae
       a. Adhesive/constrictive/effusive-constrictive
       b. Recurrent pericarditis with or without effusion
       c. Pseudoaneurysm
       d. Pericardiolithiasis

---

pericardial mesothelium, which are also inhibited by any pericardial trauma itself, permitting intrapericardial clotting. Survival, aided or not by timely treatment, often produces pericardial adhesions, which can be local or general and not rarely succeeded by corresponding constrictive or effusive-constrictive pericardial disease (Chapter 15). The effects of blunt chest trauma, often more complex than penetrating trauma, can occasionally cause *pericardial rupture* with herniation of all or part of the heart; this has all the implications for entrapment of cardiac structures seen with congenital deficiencies of the pericardium (Chapter 6). *Pericardial laceration*, often with diaphragmatic rupture, is not rare with severe blunt (nonpenetrating) trauma, the laceration permitting cardiac displacement while diaphragmatic rupture permits intrapericardial and intrathoracic herniation of abdominal organs (page 365). Isolated uncomplicated pericardial laceration is rare and of significance only if sterile or infective inflammation ensues.

Complications

Pericardial injury only occasionally occurs in isolation. Concurrent disease or injury of other organs, particularly the heart (including iatrogenic heart injury), modify the clinical picture, the physiologic response to trauma, the electrocardiogram (ECG) and all imaging modalities. These complicate the diagnosis and treatment of pericardial lesions, especially when there is tamponade. These include injuries of the heart, the great vessels (especially the ascending aorta), the conducting system, the myocardium, the mediastinum and other chest and abdominal organs. Above all, *bleeding anywhere else can produce a picture of shock in which it may be difficult to separate the pericardial contribution.* Indeed, the accompanying *hypovolemia* facilitates the development of cardiac tamponade, including deceptive low-pressure tamponade (Chapter 11). Finally, ingested alcohol, even in small amounts, can seriously reduce cardiac mechanical performance in the presence of cardiopericardial injury.

Late Effects

Late pericardial and cardiac sequelae and complications are common after all types of pericardial injury *irrespective of initially successful management.* These include late pericardial effusion, hemopericardium and cardiac tamponade, post–cardiac injury syndrome (PCIS), false aneurysm, congestive failure, constrictive pericarditis and all combinations of these. They require monitoring and late follow-up, and any of them may require repeated surgical and medical therapy.

Pericardial Wounds

The pericardium can be injured by a wide variety of direct and indirect traumas of accidental, criminal or iatrogenic origin and cannot escape when the heart is traumatized during surgery or accidentally. Indeed, *single or multiple wounds of the heart, great vessels and other organs should be anticipated with all pericardial traumatic injuries.* Bullet wounds below nipple level also suggest diaphragmatic and abdominal involvement. All the diagnostic and therapeutic aspects of tamponade in general (Chapter 11) apply, and treatment is complicated extremely by damage to the heart and other organs, exsanguination and any urgency due to the patient's precarious condition. Any concomitant penetrating or blunt myocardial injury should be identified through appropriate enzyme studies and, in cases with skeletal muscle injury by the myocardium-specific troponin I (cTnI). Because cardiac tamponade, often atypical, is common in many forms of traumatic injury, the watchwords are "always expect the worst" and "always anticipate thoracotomy."

PENETRATING TRAUMA

With penetrating trauma, the most common causes of immediate death are exsanguination or cardiac tamponade and often both.

Traumatic Agents

Knives, needles, bullets and high-velocity projectiles (shrapnel) are the most common causes of accidental or criminal penetrating trauma, with death common in the prehospital phase. In general, bullets and shrapnel cause more damage than lacerating and puncturing instruments, the pathways of which may seal over. However, tamponade is much more common in cardiac stab wounds than bullet wounds when first seen. Any chamber may be involved, but the right ventricle is more common in anterior chest wounds. Right atrial, right ventricular and great vessel wounds are the most quickly tamponading and exsanguinating. The left atrium can be penetrated by posterior chest wounds and has been ruptured by external cardiac massage; because of the tight clasp of the pericardium over the left atrium (page 11), these wounds tend to bleed slower than do wounds of other chambers. They sometimes produce hemothorax rather than hemopericardium or pericardial hematoma localized to the overlying oblique sinus (which, however, may be hemodynamically significant.) Anterior esophageal penetration by instruments or swallowed foreign objects like bones, is rare and, like contaminated surgical instruments, likely to cause suppurative pericarditis.

Clinical and Management Considerations (See Also Chapter 11)

While some patients may have a rub signaling pericardial irritation, many do not, or rubs may appear with pericardial bleeding and effusion. Electrocardiograms are frequently not helpful in assessing pericardial damage but may show characteristic or atypical Stage I changes within or after 24 hr (Figure 21.1A and B). *"Surgical" cardiac tamponade* (page 153) due to hemopericardium or hemopneumopericardium, immediate or delayed, slow or sudden—*the principal cause of death*—is often difficult to diagnose because of blood loss, vasoconstriction and frequent hemothorax that are not characteristic of "medical" tamponade (page 154); yet the same diagnostic criteria apply to tamponade in almost any circumstances. However, with many wounds, *rapid intrapericardial bleeding can become critical before fluid can be transferred into the venous system, so that although jugular venous pulsations may be visible, venous distention is absent.* Pulsus paradoxus also may be absent or disappear with severe hypotension and shock (Chapter 13). There may be tachycardia commensurate with shock levels, but preterminal bradycardia often occurs via the vagal

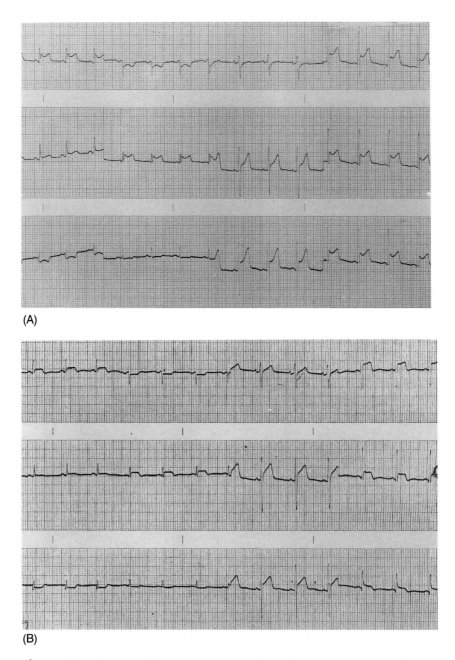

(A)

(B)

Figure 21.1 A.Pericardial stab wound. Stage I J (ST) elevations accompanying rub on day 2. Leads III and aVF make this atypical and may represent myocardial injury. B. Pericardial stab wound (same patient as Figure 21.1A). Day 4: Atypical evolution because of terminal T wave inversions in leads I, aVL, V4-V6 while J (ST) elevation remains.

effect of critical tamponade or abnormal rhythms due to concomitant cardiac injury or terminal electromechanical dissociation (EMD).

Tamponade and hemopericardium

Paradoxically, cardiac tamponade can be a correlate of survival. Patients with tamponade reaching the emergency rooms appear to survive better than non-tamponaded patients also arriving with detectable vital signs. The corollary of this is that *untimely release of tamponade without thoracotomy can cause rapid decompensation because clotting of the pericardial hematoma can be hemostatic for cardiac wounds* (as in many patients with dissecting aortic hematoma; page 356). Massive clotting can also produce an acute form of elastic pericardial constriction (page 254), precluding nonsurgical drainage. Thus, especially in unstable patients, thoracotomy in the emergency room or in the operating room (preferably via a left anterolateral approach) is optimal for repair of cardiac and pericardial wounds. This relegates pericardiocentesis to a desperation measure while simultaneously preparing surgery and administering treatment for shock (fluids, vasopressors, vasodilators). Indeed, patients in extremis not responding to volume infusion should be tapped without delay. However, a principal danger of all blind and restricted-vision procedures is relief of tamponade without control of bleeding sources.

In all cases, a central venous catheter should be advanced into the superior vena cava for delivery of fluids and medications and measurement of central venous pressure (CVP). A CVP of 15 cm H_2O or less suggests blood loss. In stable patients, *subxyphoid pericardial exploration* is feasible, with the option of extending to a full thoracotomy and, if necessary, laparotomy for any abdominal wounds, which can also reach the pericardium internally. *Appropriate sequencing—thoracotomy or laparotomy first?—must be individualized.* A transient or poor response to resuscitation in a severely hypotensive patient with a cardiopericardial wound mandates immediate anterolateral thoracotomy. Indeed, even favorable responses to "medical" resuscitation tend to be transient.

Both the patient's cardiac and total condition must be kept in mind with all injuries, and blood loss must be monitored. Chest and abdominal *x-rays* are essential. *Electrocardiograms* may or may not be helpful in evaluating the precise wounds but are necessary to monitor heart rate and rhythm. The *two-dimensional echocardiogram* is virtually indispensable to properly evaluate and monitor the heart and pericardium. In all cases initially negative results should not be accepted as final. *Transesophageal echocardiograms are optimal* but cannot be used with head, neck and esophageal trauma. *Transthoracic echocardiograms*, particularly the four-chamber view, are almost as useful, but any acoustic window may be precluded by wounds, bandages and drainage tubes. Some definitely stable patients may benefit from *computed tomography (CT)*, including helical CT, to demonstrate pericardial contents, including fluid, blood and air, as well as cardiac wounds and the integrity of the great vessels. Particularly after surgical trauma, CT may show increased density and thickening of the pericardium, especially in patients destined to develop the post-pericardiotomy syndrome (page 403).

Accidental iatrogenic pericardial wounds are produced by percutaneous transluminal coronary angioplasty (PTCA) instruments, pacing instruments (Figure 21.2), central venous and pulmonary flotation catheters and even insertion of needles and small catheters for pericardial drainage itself. Pericardial damage during PTCA can occur with coronary artery dissections, producing localized or generalized pericarditis with or without significant bleeding; the latter is accentuated by heparin therapy. PTCA balloon inflation and deployment of intracoronary stents may rupture an artery, especially if it is calcified.

Patients may have new pain or a rub or present with unanticipated tamponade; ECG registration of pericardial injury may be nonspecific or delayed 24 hr or more; with hemopericardium, T waves may become peaked, possibly due to potassium released by hemolysis. Pacing catheters and pulmonary artery flotation catheters may penetrate the right ventricle with (Figure 21.3) or without pericarditic signs or hemopericardium. Central venous catheters tend to penetrate the right atrium and rarely the superior vena cava; any fluids being administered through them may on their own provoke tamponade or exacerbate tamponade due to bleeding. Pericardiocentesis needles and catheters can lacerate the right atrium, the right ventricle or an epicardial vein, producing hemorrhage and causing or exacerbating tamponade. *Fetal tamponade* has been reported to complicate amniocentesis. Radiofrequency ablation of arrhythmia-associated structures has been attended by pericardial injury, as has epicardial pacing, particularly upon removal of the wires.

Unlike even densely hemorrhagic pericardial effusions of irritative or inflammatory origin, traumatic hemopericardium of any cause, particularly if

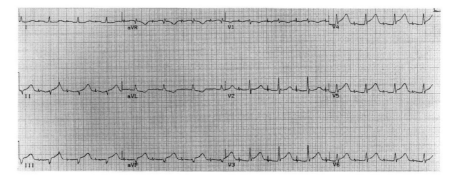

Figure 21.2 Acute pericarditis (stage I ECG) due to pacing wire. Atrial pacing spikes precede P waves. J (ST) elevation in most leads.

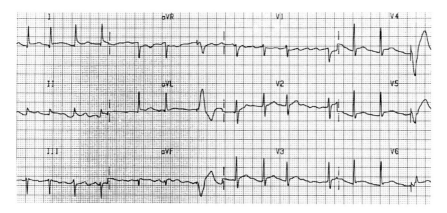

Figure 21.3   Acute pericarditis (stage I ECG) due to pacing wire. Ventricular pacing competes when responses to atrial flutter slow (leads R, L, F, V4, 5, 6).

rapid and voluminous, will tend to thrombose, so that *surgical evacuation remains the optimal method of management*. This includes rapid transfer to the operating room or thoracotomy in the emergency department. It is possible that pericardial catheterization or cannulation, particularly through the subxyphoid route, may permit thrombolysis of pericardial clots; this has been attempted with streptokinase and urokinase; before it can be a firm recommendation, however, further experience will be required, including sufficient follow-up to gauge its effect on recurrent and constrictive pericardial disease. Naturally, all wounds of the heart and great vessels must also be repaired.

　　Pneumopericardium, pneumohydropericardium and pyopneumopericardium (Table 21.2) should all be considered both early and late in patients with penetrating wounds involving gas-containing organs like the lungs or hollow abdominal viscera and even the esophagus. However, they can also follow blunt trauma (Figure 21.4) and thoracic surgery. *Pericardial infection* may appear at the initial presentation or may develop slowly, with pyopneumopericardium after repair of the pericardial and cardiac wounds; it must therefore be among the anticipated complications. Sometimes gas-producing organisms produce the picture of pneumopericardium. *Pneumopericardium and its variants* are usually demonstrated by any imaging technique, by precordial tympany and by the "mill-wheel sound" (page 38) on auscultation, but accurate examination may be difficult with multiple trauma. Moreover, these conditions may be deceptively "silent" (Table 21.3) until the onset of *tension pneumopericardium*, i.e., *pneumotamponade*. *Pneumomediastinum* may simulate this by roentgenography or other imaging, but with Hamman's sign (precordial crunch) on auscultation.

**Table 21.2   PATHOGENESIS OF PNEUMOPERICARDIUM AND ITS
VARIANTS Pneumohydropericardium, Pneumopyopericardium,
Pneumohemopericardium**

A. *Infection*
    1. Penetration of pericardium by disease of neighboring organs
        a. Pulmonary/pleural
        b. Mediastinal, *esp*. esophagus
        c. Subdiaphragmatic, *esp*. stomach
    2. Penetration by pericardial process into gas-containing organs
        a. Pericarditis, *esp*. suppurative
        b. Pericardial neoplasia
    3. Pericarditis due to gas-producing organisms

B. *Trauma*
    1. Penetrating ulcer of esophagus, stomach or colonic graft
        a. Benign
        b. Malignant
    2. Esophageal foreign body, *esp*. swallowed objects
    3. Chest trauma
        a. Blunt
        b. Penetrating
            1. Missiles
            2. Sharp objects
        c. Rib Fractures

C. *Iatrogenic*
    1. Positive-pressure ventilation
        a. Infants with immature pericardial sealing along vessels
        b. Adults with bronchopulmonary disease
    2. Closed chest cardiac resuscitation
    3. Pericardiotomy
    4. With pericardiocentesis (diagnostic, formerly also "therapeutic")
    5. Sclerotherapy of esophageal varices
    6. Dilation of esophageal structure

Catheter Injuries

While catheter penetration of the heart usually involves the right-sided chambers, misdirected catheters meant to enter the pulmonary artery, particularly for
arteriography, may penetrate or rupture the coronary sinus due to high-pressure injection of contrast material. Since a "right ventricular" pressure trace can
be obtained from the coronary sinus, this misdirection may not be appreciated.
The resulting hemorrhage can cause generalized tamponade or fill only the
pericardial oblique sinus (Figure 21.5) with localized compression of the left
atrium (Figure 21.4).

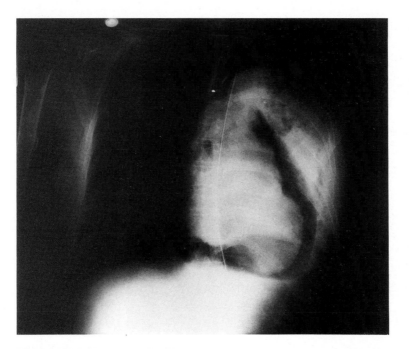

Figure 21.4   Pneumopericardium due to traumatic bronchopericardial fistula. Semi-oblique roentgenogram showing intrapericardial air as a broad black band outlining the heart.

Table 21.3   PHYSICAL EXAMINATION IN PNEUMOPERICARDIUM AND PNEUMOHYDROPERICARDIUM (Some, All or None Present)

A.   Precordial percussion
   1.   Precordial tympany (*esp.* supine)
   2.   Shifting precordial tympany
   3.   "Cracked pot" resonance
B.   Auscultation
   1.   "Mill-wheel sounds"
   2.   Loud splashing (sometimes heard without stethoscope)
   3.   Diminished to absent heart sounds, *esp.* supine
   4.   Pericardial rub
C.   Signs of cardiac tamponade (pneumotamponade)
D.   Chest wall signs
   1.   Subcutaneous emphysema/crepitus
   2.   Precordial systolic crunch (like Hamman's sign)

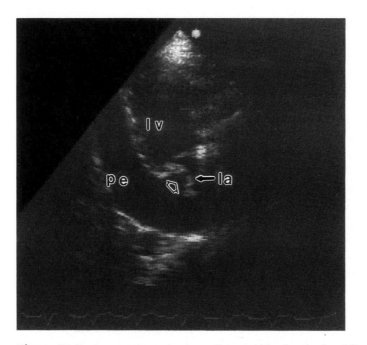

Figure 21.5   Low parasternal echocardiogram; bleeding in the oblique sinus of the pericardium (broad arrow) compressing the left atrium (narrow arrow). lv = left ventricle; la = left atrium; pe = pericardial effusion (pneumopericardium).

Malpositioned central venous catherers have a propensity to advance due to arm and neck motion and to perforate the right atrium or even the ventricle. When they are used to deliver parenteral fluids, tamponade ensues quickly. The catheter tip should lie in the superior vena cava proximal to the right atrium; this should put the tip above the pericardial reflection.

Catheter penetration of cardiac chambers may be clinically silent. The ECG is quite insensitive to any localized pericarditis so produced, although it is sensitive to generalized pericarditis (Figures 21.2 and 21.3). Moreover, even when recognized, the point of puncture may not be obvious. Some patients have precordial or dorsal pain, which can be severe, and some develop shock. Bleeding may be slow, but local or generalized compression by blood or clot, with or without contrast material, can occur very rapidly because of lack of time for pericardial "give" (page 181). For the same reason, x-rays may not show any significant change in the cardiopericardial silhouette. The slightest suspicion of such an event calls for emergency echocardiography, as well as attempts at drainage via the offending catheter; because of clotting, surgical drainage will often be necessary.

Pericarditis, with or without effusion, associated with catheter pacemaker penetration of the heart or an epicardial pacemaker is often associated with impaired sensing and reduced output voltage. Failure of timely recognition has resulted in effusion, hemopericardium and even constriction within weeks to months. Moreover, epicardial pacemaker implantation rarely produces brisk bleeding and has even resulted in simulation of constriction by a large clotted hematoma as well as the postpericardiotomy syndrome (page 403). Occasionally, infection of a pacemaker or defibrillator generator, usually one implanted in the abdominal left upper quadrant, can track to the pericardium, causing bacterial pericarditis with effusion.

Foreign-Body and Foreign-Substance Pericarditis (see also pages 427–428)

Smooth-edged foreign bodies less than 1 or 2 cm in diameter may be asymptomatic. Relatively large foreign bodies lying in or near the pericardium—usually metallic fragments, bullets or broken instruments, and needles—have been associated with recurrent pericarditis and effusion; they need not penetrate the heart (Figure 21.6). Implantable cardioverter-defibrillator patches may act similarly as foreign bodies. Silicone contaminating pacemaker insertion can provoke

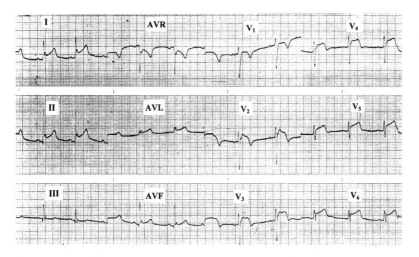

Figure 21.6 Foreign-body pericarditis in a 19-year-old man with precordial gunshot wound and bullet free in pericardium. The patient had pericardial rub and this atypical ECG. J-points elevated in most leads; terminal T-wave inversions in V1 to V4 may represent otherwise subclinical anterior myocardial injury. (Courtesy of Dr. Laurence M. Lesser.)

an exuberant pericardial foreign-body reaction, including giant cells. All these can progress to tamponade, adhesions or constriction. Definitive treatment is removal of the foreign material and any significant ahesions and fluid. Post-pericardiotomy syndrome (PPS; page 403) may follow with recurrent peri-carditis long after successful removal of the foreign body.

SURGICAL TRAUMA OF THE PERICARDIUM

Generalities

The pericardial effects of cardiopericardial surgical traumas resemble those of accidental trauma, although the wounds are under control and much less likely to be contaminated or complicated by damage and unchecked blood loss else-where. Following pericardiotomy, the pericardium is irregularly thickened, but usually regains a normal appearance in six months. Fortunately, there is a declining incidence of all of the many pericardial complications of surgery (Table 21.1B). Yet the critical *differential diagnosis* of postoperative pericar-dial inflammation, effusion, bleeding, and especially tamponade from other causes of low cardiac output, chest pain, fever and multiorgan failure is com-plicated by several factors:

1. The accompanying cardiac and chest wall wounds
2. The cardiac condition operated on
3. The often asymmetric, peculiar distribution of pericardial inflammation and adhesions, causing larger or smaller loculation of pericardial hema-tomas and effusions

Like trauma patients, postsurgical patients are not easily examined. They are supine, intubated or catheterized at various orifices, often unable to speak, and usually covered with surgical dressings; venous tone is abnormally in-creased, peripheral arterial constriction is common and there is a tendency for oliguria complicating clinical and physiologic evaluation.

Surgical Pericardial Inflammation and Effusion

Mild pericarditis and low-grade fever, usually with some bleeding and pericar-dial effusion, are common postoperatively and proportional to the amount of pericardial manipulation, which regularly causes loss of mesothelial cells and provokes fibrinous and leukocytic exudation; significant blood leukocytosis often indicates superimposed infection. The ECG tends to reflect this with minor nonspecific or local ST changes but often with generalized changes that usu-ally do not evolve beyond Stage I (Figure 21.7). A positive precordial gallium scan is common and nonspecific; an indium 111 scan may indicate super-infection.

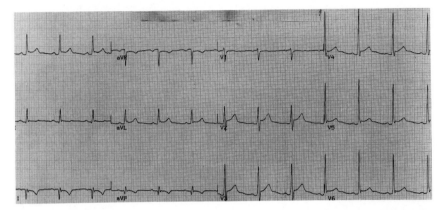

Figure 21.7 Surgical pericarditis following coronary bypass grafting: Stage I ECG changes with characteristic J (ST) and PR segment deviations. Leads III and aVF are "atypical" because of previous inferior myocardial infarction.

Detectable early pericardial effusions tend to appear by the fifth postoperative day and are common, usually small (under 1 cm echocardiographic depth), usually benign and frequently associated with a left pleural effusion. Moderate effusions (1 to 2 cm) are less common and large effusions (over 2 cm) relatively uncommon. These echo-free spaces due to effusion become more echo-dense as effusions decrease, while the posterior pericardium, initially flat, resumes its normal anterior systolic motion with the patient's improvement. Large, and especially increasing, early effusions, usually due to bleeding, are harbingers of tamponade (Figure 21.8). Late effusions (mainly 6 to 60 days postoperatively) may also be due to bleeding, especially in patients taking anticoagulants or with a coagulopathy, or due to the osmotic ("hydrophilic") effect of slow intrapericardial clot lysis or to immunopathic responses to cardiopericardial trauma. *Postoperative pneumopericardium* is relatively rare (Figure 21.9).

Owing to frequent pericardial adhesions, *postoperative pericardial effusions of any kind are more often loculated than circumferential*, particularly posteriorly, since most dense adhesions are anterior. Yet they can be localized over any cardiac chamber or combination of chambers (Figures 21.10 and 21.11). Intrapericardial thrombi and hematomas loculated over the right heart, especially the atrium, are relatively common after surgery and can cause a rapidly progressive low-output state. They are revealed by echocardiography, angiography or CT and cause flattening or even concavity of the right atrial or ventricular wall (Figure 21.12); occasionally, they extend to the superior vena cava. Tamponade of the *left* ventricle with diastolic collapse by echocardiography, with or without other chamber involvement, virtually occurs only after cardioperi-

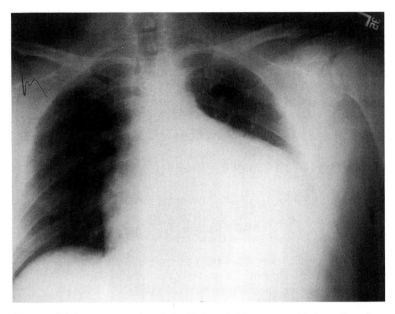

Figure 21.8 Large pericardial effusion (with tamponade) 2 weeks after coronary bypass. Left pleural effusion accompanies.

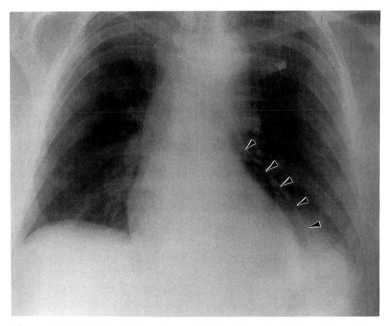

Figure 21.9 Postcardiotomy pneumopericardium. An air layer (arrows) separates the left cardiac border from the thin, normal-appearing pericardium. Left pleural effusion accompanies.

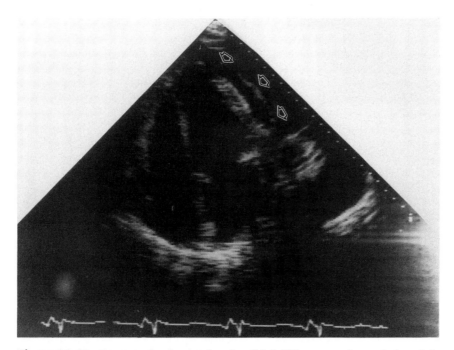

Figure 21.10   Postoperative loculated pericardial fluid/hematoma (arrows) along left ventricular border.

cardial surgery. It may also be recognized by *concavity of the LV posterior wall* and may cause the posterior pericardial space to decrease in systole and increase in early diastole. Loculated postoperative effusions with hemodynamic impairment are more likely than circumferential effusions to become significant late (10 days or more) after operation.

Early pericardial effusions appear to be slightly more common with coronary bypass surgery than with valve surgery and they are especially common following repair of atrial septal defects (which seem to have an unusual relation to pericardial disease). Early effusions do not correlate closely with pericardial rubs, chest pain, increasing sedimentation rate or arrhythmias. Their excess pericardial fluid, blood and clots may alter the cardiac contour by filling the pericardial oblique sinus (Figures 2.3 and 21.4) or any of the smaller pericardial sinuses and recesses (page 8), requiring CT or magnetic resonance imaging (MRI) for recognition.

Left or bilateral *pleural effusions* are common postoperatively (Figures 21.8 and 21.9) and can complicate recognition of pericardial effusions by echo as well as chest x-ray. Diagnosis may also be complicated because surgical severing of the sternopericardial ligaments allows the heart to sink posteriorly in

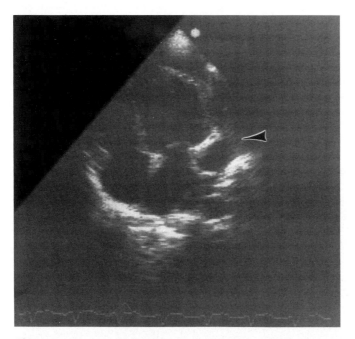

Figure 21.11 Postoperative loculated fluid/hematoma on the left A-V groove (arrowhead), indenting the left atrium.

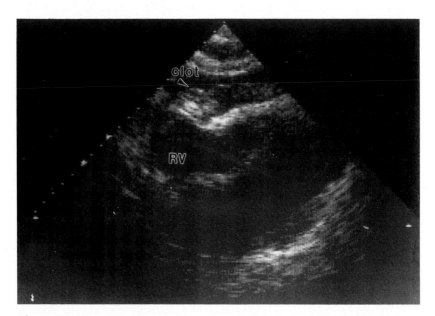

Figure 21.12 Postoperative thrombus (clot) indenting the right ventricular (RV) wall.

supine patients, a condition later to be "remedied" by the almost inevitable anterior adhesions that follow cardiac surgery.

Factors Associated with and Predisposing to Generalized or Loculated Postoperative Pericardial Adhesions, Hemopericardium and Cardiac Tamponade

While loculated effusions are more common than circumferential effusions, circumferential effusions are more frequent after valve surgery and loculated effusions are more frequent after coronary bypass. In general, larger effusions are more likely to cause tamponade (Figure 21.8). Certain conditions asociated with significant postoperative pericardial effusions and hemopericadium, include the following.

1. Drastic reduction of pericardial fibrinolytic activity from extensive manipulation, predisposing to adhesions and eventual constriction.
2. Copious mediastinal drainage, especially when it appears to stop rapidly.
3. Inadequate hemostatis with bleeding from suture lines, oozing vessels and coagulopathies. The latter include anticoagulant therapy, even with the prothrombin time at "therapeutic" levels. Patients with cyanotic congenital heart disease are especially likely to bleed.
4. Pleural effusion. Pericardial effusions are more common in patients with significant pleural effusions, especially on the left or bilaterally.
5. Epicardial fixation of permanent electrodes for defibrillation or pacing and electrodes for temporary pacing.

Leaving the pericardium open after surgery does not help to prevent tamponade. Indeed, most postoperative bleeding is extra-pericardial and *mediastinal bleeding and effusion can tamponade the heart*. Moreover, closing the pericardium tends to minimize both tamponade and significant adhesions, including those capable of bypass-graft occlusion; closure also facilitates localization of pericardial bleeding. Of course, in some patients increased postoperative heart size due to intravascular volume expansion or cardiac dilation does not permit pericardial closure.

Postoperative Cardiac Tamponade

Despite decreasing incidence, both circumferential and especially localized (individual chamber) tamponade remain challenging diagnostic and therapeutic problems. *Nearly all clinically significant effusions are present by the fifth postoperative day*. While anticoagulation is associated with tamponade at any time, its principal importance is in the first 3 to 5 days. During this period, hemopericardium is the most common cause, and most other tamponading effusions have at least blood-tinged fluid. *Late cardiac tamponade* is often associated with postpericardiotomy syndrome (page 403) and is probably of inflammatory or immunopathic pathogenesis.

While classic diagnostic signs of cardiac tamponade (Chapter 11) may be present postoperatively, *familiar clinical signs like pulsus paradoxus are often absent*. Similarly, echocardiographic and Doppler signs (Table 10.3) retain their specificity, but *their sensitivity is greatly reduced*, necessitating exceptional vigilance. Postoperative Stage 1 pericarditis ECG changes are common and of no help, while a swinging heart and electrical alternation are quite uncommon. Thus, *tamponade and its atypical presentation should be anticipated at any time postoperatively* by liberal monitoring of vital signs and catheterization data as well as diligent search by echocardiogram for diastolic chamber collapses and other evidence. Transesophageal echocardiography is better than transthoracic for both tamponade and pericardial thickening. Transvalvular Doppler flow may give further evidence of low cardiac output and, with exaggerated respiratory changes, functional cardiac tamponade (page 164).

Left ventricular tamponade is especially common postoperatively because of the tendency to posterior loculation of fluid. Indeed, left ventricular collapse is more reliable as a diagnostic sign than hypotension or pulsus paradoxus (Note: pulsus paradoxus is likely to be absent in any kind of localized or uneven cardiac compression and in patients with significantly decreased left or right ventricular compliance; Chapter 13). *Left atrial diastolic collapse* (LADC) can occur either with tamponading circumferential pericardial effusions or with fluid or bleeding confined to the adjacent oblique sinus amid the four pulmonary veins (Figures 21.5). It will decrease cardiac output with no increase in systemic venous pressure and no pulsus paradoxus. *Right atrial or ventricular collapse* also occurs with circumferential or localized fluid or hematoma. *Local* right atrial or right atrioventricular groove compression can occur with normal right ventricular end-diastolic pressures but is indicated by a tricuspid valve pressure gradient. Finally, *selective adhesive tethering of parts of chambers to the parietal pericardium can distort the images and restrict or prevent wall collapses.*

Diagnosing Postoperative Cardiac Tamponade

While dyspnea and chest pain are common after cardiac surgery, pericardial problems should be suspected in all patients doing poorly, even with nonspecific complaints, like lethargy and changing mental status. Although *respiratory alkalosis* is characteristic of uncomplicated tamponade, *metabolic acidosis* may accompany critical tamponade with severely depressed cardiac output, but it is nonspecific. Indeed, after surgery or any trauma, *typical* clinical and hemodynamic syndromes occur only with circumferential effusions and with generalized pericarditis. Definite pericardial effusion in any unstable patient strongly suggests cardiac tamponade.

Regional tamponade due to loculating adhesions is more common than circumferential tamponade. Dysphagia occasionally occurs due to esophageal encroachment by large posterior effusions and hematomas. In the common absence of indicative clinical findings (Chapter 11), critical information includes identifying and localizing pericardial fluid by imaging. Transesophageal echo-cardiography or CT, particularly, may be critical both to diagnosis and to guide catheter drainage and identify pericardial thickening and adhesions. It must be emphasized that chamber collapses and increased right heart–left heart respiratory reciprocation (page 181) may be lacking. Indeed, all conventional echocardiographic signs (Table 10.3) of tamponade have limited value postoperatively. *Any* chamber distortion and a *large* effusion are more sensitive and reliable. Indeed, clinical and hemodynamic deterioration in the presence of pericardial fluid, clots, or both should always raise the possibility or cardiac compression.

Cardiac catheterization is essential only if hemodynamic abnormalities will sort out a confusing picture, including cardiac output and right atrial, pulmonary artery and pulmonary capillary wedge pressures. For example, a right atrial pressure significantly above pulmonary capillary wedge pressure is consistent with localized right heart tamponade. Rarely, RA tamponade forces a right-to-left shunt across a patent foramen ovale. Gated technetium equilibrium radionuclide ventriculography can further evaluate both effusions and ventricular function.

Differential Diagnosis

Tamponade must be differentiated from *extrapericardial causes of low cardiac output*, including the following:

1. Ventricular hypokinesis with left, right or combined ventricular failure
2. Perioperative acute left or right ventricular myocardial infarction
3. Pulmonary embolism
4. Coronary insufficiency
5. Effects of prolonged aortic cross-clamping or inadequate coronary perfusion during cardiopulmonary bypass.
6. Severe pulmonary artery hypertension
7. Septic shock
8. Hepatitis (suggested by enzyme abnormalities), passive hepatic congestion or significant injury
9. Mediastinal hematoma or effusion causing extrapericardial cardiac compression

Apart from elastic constriction by clotted hemopericardium, constrictive pericarditis is not an early consideration; it can occur as soon as 2 to 7 weeks, but usually appears much later. Occasionally, acute cardiac dilatation within a repaired pericardium will have a comparable effect.

Management

Operative pericarditis usually responds quickly to brief therapy with a corticosteroid, but nonsteroidal agents are preferable if their effect is relatively prompt; noncompressing effusions often diminish with such medical treatment. Coagulation status and particularly prothrombin time and platelet levels should be monitored carefully.

Early postoperative tamponade is a surgical emergency, usually requiring thoracotomy; *later tamponade* may respond to drainage and observation. Either type may present as quite sudden clinical deterioration. Therefore, clinically and hemodynamically significant effusions of any size should be drained; urokinase or streptokinase can be instilled to aid drainage and inhibit adhesions if further bleeding is ruled out. While needle pericardiocentesis may be effective with large circumferential, easily reached effusions, surgical drainage is clearly optimal, particularly for complicated and loculated lesions. Moreover, coronary bypass grafts are endangered by any blind procedure. Options include the subxyphoid route (page 173) and drainage through the lower end of the chest incision, for which purpose easily removed interrupted sutures are useful. Reopening incisions, especially when there are anterior adhesion of parts of the heart or bypass grafts, is dangerous; *video-monitored thoracoscopy* (page XX), including right-sided approaches, may be safest, as determined by particular fluid locations. The pericardial oblique sinus must always be adequately evacuated.

Postoperative Pericardial Defects

Patients may have intended or unintended pericardial defects after pericardial resection for pericardial or mediastinal disease or to create, from pieces of pericardium, surgical patches, pledgets, or baffles. Unless closed by adhesions, these can permit part or all of the heart to herniate, much as with comparable congenital defects (Chapter 6). Moreover, cardiac herniation is not closely correlated with the size of the defect. Defects may be revealed by air entering the pericardium from a pneumothorax, for which CT or MRI are best for diagnosis.

Postoperative Pseudoaneurysms

Pseudoaneurysms occasionally follow cardiac surgery, especially when a chamber has been vented, requiring an opening in its wall. These resemble pseudoaneurysms following myocardial infarction (page 346; Figures 20.3 and 20.4). They are myocardial ruptures, with external leakage of blood contained by epicardium, epicardial fat and (especially with adhesions) parietal pericardium. They are recognized on imaging as a juxtacardiac zone into which blood flows in systole and reverses in diastole through a narrow neck that may only be visible on color-Doppler imaging (Figures 21.13A, B, and C). *They are prone to rupture and must be repaired urgently.*

Pericardial Involvement in Cardiac Transplantation

Broadly speaking, cardiac transplantation subjects the transplanted heart to many of the problems of any postsurgical heart, favorably modified by the usually normal new myocardium and valves and unfavorably by the possibility of varying degrees of rejection and antirejection treatment with corticosteroid and immunosuppressant therapy. Some epicardial inflammation and thickening is common in transplanted hearts. *Pericardial effusions*, usually of small to moderate size, are frequent after cardiac transplantation; they tend to develop in the first postoperative month and only rarely after 3 months. *Cyclosporine* treatment may be a key factor inducing these pericardial effusions. Most are small and localized posteriorly and laterally, owing to anterior adhesions to the recipient pericardium and sternum. Though uncommon, medium- to large-size effusions more often become tamponading. Decreasing ECG voltage generally indicates significant effusion. Constriction is quite uncommon and late.

Unlike other postsurgical effusions, which tend to be maximal by 10 days postoperatively, effusions in transplant patients increase and are increasingly frequent after the first postoperative week. Despite immunosuppression, postpericardiotomy syndrome can occur but is rare in adults. The precise association of transplant rejection with provocation of effusion is uncertain, disputed, and confounded by corticosteroid and immunosupressant treatment. However, pericardial effusion in transplant recipients is associated with more frequent and histologically more severe rejections. Rarely, *increasing* pericardial effusion is associated with (but not necessarily due to) late acute rejection.

There appears to be an association between preoperative diagnosis of idiopathic dilated cardiomyopathy and the appearance of transplant effusions. This may be related to a loose (and disputed) direct correlation between effusions and a recipient heart weight greater than donor heart weight. Moreover, since the absence of prior cardiopericardial surgery is also correlated with posttransplant effusion, dilated cardiomyopathy may be a surrogate for increased ventricular volume and representative of patients who would not have had prior cardiopericardial surgery. Thus, a preoperatively intact pericardium and a large *recipient-donor heart weight mismatch*, may favor the exudation of fluid into the pericardial space because the pericardium had enlarged to accommodate the recipient's original enlarged heart—a kind of effusion *"ex vacuo."*

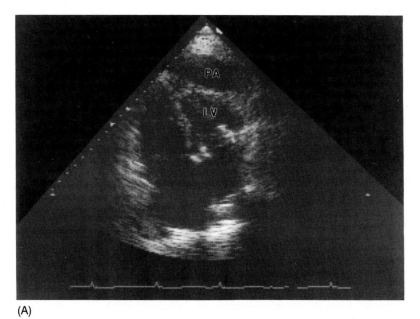

(A)

Figure 21.13   A. Left ventricular (LV) pseudoaneurysm (PA) following mitral valve replacement. Communication with left ventricle not visible. B. Same patient as in Figure 21.13A. Communication between pseudoaneurysm (PA) and left ventricle (LV) shown by Doppler flow during ventricular systole (jagged light streak from LV into PA). C. Same patient as in Figure 21.13A and B. Spectral Doppler flow recording showing higher-velocity flow into pseudoaneurysm (PA) and lower-velocity diastolic flow back into the left ventricle (LV).

Postoperative Chylopericardium (See Also Chapter 8)

Rarely, after any kind of cardiopericardial surgery, but more often in children and after extensive correction of congenital defects, a serious postoperative effusion is due to chylopericardium. The causes include injury to the thoracic duct or mediastinal lymphatic vessels, particularly when the superior or inferior vena cava is encircled by surgical occlusion tapes for extracorporeal circulation. Because of anatomic variations, the thoracic duct and various lymphatic channels, including those in the anterior mediastinum, may be unusually susceptible to operative trauma. Where posterior pericardial dissection causing direct trauma to lymphatic channels is unlikely, thrombosis of the thoracic duct or the left subclavian vein may be responsible. At reoperation to relieve the chylopericardium, the mechanism may or may not be apparent.

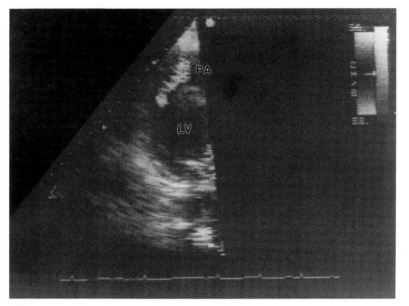

(B)

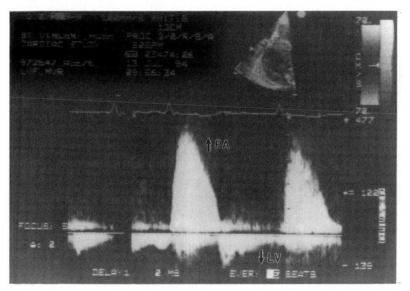

(C)

Chylopericardial effusions are large, ultimately tending to tamponade, and distinguished by a high triglyceride and total lipid level, producing a characteristically yellow, turbid, milky appearance. Cardiac tamponade, of course, forces immediate drainage. However, these large, relatively slowly developing effusions call for a stepwise therapeutic approach. After diagnostic or therapeutic pericardial drainage, a large subxyphoid pericardial drain should be left in with the patient on a low-fat diet. Persistent drainage may be poorly tolerated by children and debilitated patients and will necessitate reexploration to identify the source of the leak of chyle; this is not always identifiable but generally necessitates ligation of the thoracic duct above the diaphragm. A diet containing medium-chain triglycerides has frequently been successful, either as monotherapy or in addition to all the dirct measures for drainage and surgery. Failure necessitates pericardial resection or drainage through the pleural cavity via a pleuropericardial window.

Intrapericardial Pneumonectomy

Pneumonectomy, usually for malignancy but also for congenital and traumatic defects, is often aided by pericardial resection and intrapericardial ligation of the pulmonary vessels. A residual defect of any size may precipitate herniation of part or all of the heart, producing angulation and compression of the heart or great vessels. Right-sided resection is more likely to kink the atriocaval junctions and produce a right-sided cardiac volvulus; left-sided resection with escape of the ventricles into the left hemithorax is more likely to produce compression of the atrioventricular groove and portions of the ventricular myocardium, trapping of which may cause actual infarction. These herniations and torsions occur early, particularly within the first 24 hr postoperatively and before adhesions have formed. They may be precipitated by repositioning the patient, especially with the surgical side down, or during routine postoperative mechanical procedures. Symptoms are often sudden, including hypotension, shock, hypoxic signs and arrhythmias; superior vena cava syndrome may be accompanied by upper-body cyanosis. All are highly lethal events and call for rapid diagnosis and treatment. The situation is identified by physical signs of cardiac displacement, acute electrocardiographic changes, especially axis shifts, and—if there is enough time—appropriate imaging, including roentgenography and echocardiography. *Differential diagnosis* includes sudden hemorrhage, collapse of the remaining lung, airway obstruction, tamponade of other origin, and pulmonary embolus. *Definitive treatment is surgical correction*, which should be done as soon as diagnosis is made in the operating room or even in bed. First, the patient should be repositioned to favor gravitational return of the heart and mediastinum, usually by placing the patient in the lateral decubitus with the surgical side up. At the same time, airway pressure should be reduced if possible. Sometimes these simple measures relieve the acute situation, but the defect must be repaired.

Other Thoracotomy-Associated Traumas

Open-chest cardiac massage, an occasional necessity, necessarily traumatizes the epicardium, increasing the susceptibility to infection, pericardial effusion and tamponade, and ultimate constriction. *Removal of epicardial pacing wire*, routine after most cardiac operations, is usually effected without untoward event. Occasionally, however, an epicardial vein or other structure is traumatized and there is a hemopericardium. Tamponade must be anticipated in the early period after the wires are taken out.

PERICARDIAL FISTULATION

Fistulas to the pericardium producing either chemical injury or pneumopericardium result from pathologic communication between the pericardium and neighboring viscera. The most important of these is the esophagus (see also Chapters 7, 11 and 20) due to penetrating ulcers and malignancies as well as severe, particularly tuberculous, esophagitis. Replacement of resected esophagus with segments of colon may also result in penetration of the pericardium and heart by the same mechanisms, in each case sometimes precipitated by esophagoscopy. Deficiencies in the diaphragm—congenital, traumatic or iatrogenic—permit the stomach and the duodenum entry into the thorax where inflammatory, malignant and ulcer diseases have produced communications with the pericardium. Rarely, there may be a connection with herniated transverse colon with or without a subphrenic abscess. The results of these fistulations may be subtle, with vague complaints and only occasionally a pericardial rub; ultimately, however, they can progress to *pneumopericardium*. This may be appreciated by precordial tympany on percussion and roentgenography showing gas in the pericardial cavity, which does not rise above the level of the pericardial ensheathment of the ascending aorta (Figures 21.4 and 21.9). There are varying degress of toxicity, fever and systemic reaction; pericardial fluid may either be clear or grossly contaminated with a variety of organisms, including mixed bacterial and fungal infections. Although esophagoscopy and contrast media can demonstrate esophageal communications, the points of perforation are not always identifiable. Videotape recording improves the sensitivity of esophagography. Computed tomography may greatly improve the diagnostic yield for details of the process. *Pericardial fistulation is a surgical emergency calling for resection and repair.*

Chemical Injury

More or less sterile *chemical injury* of the pericardium may follow unusual communications with the biliary tract, the pancreas and the esophagus, particularly following sclerotherapy of esophageal varices. Pancreatitis itself is known to be accompanied by pericardial irritation and effusion even without chemical communication, and this is often ascribed to hematogenous and lymphogenous transportation of pancreatic enzymes to the pericardium.

ELECTRICAL TRAUMA

Electrical countershock during resuscitation or to electively convert arrhythmias applies high-voltage electricity to the pericardium, the results of which have not been conclusively investigated. However, following *lightning strikes*, with their well-known cardiac consequences, occasional survivors have had pericardial effusion with tamponade or recurrent pericarditis. The latter could represent a form of the post–cardiac injury syndrome.

RADIATION PERICARDIAL DISEASE

Radiation therapy for diseases in the vicinity of the pericardium—particularly mediastinal Hodgkin's disease and non-Hodgkin's and other lymphomas, and malignancies of the breast, lungs or thyroid—frequently involves the pericardium to a variable extent. This depends on the radiation dosage, the duration of treatment, the volume of the heart in the field and the source of the radiation. Because most significant pericardial involvement is delayed, often for many years, *all radiated patients remain indefinitely susceptible*. Accordingly, the incidence increases with increased follow-up time and survival from the radiated lesions. Recently, with improvements in radiation dosing, delivery and subcarinal shielding, there appear to be decreased pericardial involvement and longer latent periods from treatment to conditions like constrictive pericarditis. The peak incidence remains between 5 and 9 months after radiation. Fortunately, the prognosis is generally favorable for the pericardial lesions.

Pathogenesis

Of all cardiac structures, the pericardium is most susceptible to radiation injury, with pericardial syndromes sometimes complicated by injuries of the myocardium, coronary arteries or valves (radiation pancarditis). While direct radiation injury can be demonstrated, the majority of patients escape significant involvement and there is always a question of triggering of latent antigens or viral infections, particularly in the delayed forms. While some or all of the pericardium may be in the path of the radiation, all pericardial surfaces, internal and external, are affected simultaneously. Any effusion fluids may be serous, sanguineous or serosanguineous, with high concentrations of protein and lymphocytes, resembling malignant effusions. Late thickening is more conspicuous in the parietal pericardium, with or without occult or eventually obvious constrictive pericarditis (page 215). The endothelium of the lymphatics and capillaries is involved. Obstruction of these vessels produces pericardial effusion as well as microvascular ischemia—a factor that, along with collagenization of the fibrinous exudates, contributes to pericardial fibrosis.

Any radiation plan involving over 50% of the heart volume and delivering over 2500 rads or 40 Gy produces a definite risk, which increases sharply with increasing dose and volume of the heart radiated. (This also increases the risk of hypothyroidism.) Usually, if 100% of the pericardium is involved, especially in a mantle distribution, risk is as much as 20%. With effective subcarinal shielding, this can be reduced to almost 2%. Overall risk is higher with cobalt 60 or anterior weighting of the radiation dosage.

Clinical Aspects

Clinically, the range of involvement extends from immediate to variably delayed acute, subacute and chronic syndromes, the latter being much more common. Acute noneffusive ("clinically dry") and effusive pericarditis, with or without tamponade, are relatively uncommon. However, pericardial rubs may frequently be auscultated if diligently sought in otherwise silent cases during therapy or within weeks of its completion. Oddly, the acute syndromes do not correlate with late disease. Indeed, the infrequent typical acute pericarditis can be related to necrosis of larger adjacent tumor masses.

Echocardiography shows some degree of effusion in all patients with clinical evidence of pericardial involvement. Subacute disease may be demonstrated in a matter of months, including effusion, constriction and effusive-constrictive pericarditis. (Radiation-induced effusions most commonly occur 4-6 months after radiation.) More common is chronic effusion or constriction, even after many years of latency. Of course, after very long periods, other disease must be considered, either separately or as a precipitating factor, raising the question of whether radiation injury makes the pericardium more susceptible to infections. *Occult constrictive pericarditis* (page 294) is relatively common and is identified by catheter monitoring during an intravenous saline challenge. At all times, the condition must be differentiated from disease due to or combined with pericardial involvement by the primary disease for which radiation was given. Although radiation-induced pericardial effusions tend to be large, malignant effusions are more likely than radiation-induced effusions to be very large and have positive cytologic, chemical and enzymatic tests. Moreover, even treated malignancies can also cause pericarditis, tamponade and constriction. It is not certain whether chemotherapy affects pericardial susceptibility to radiation injury.

Diagnosis

Echocardiography usually defines the anatomic lesions. Although CT and MRI are more sensitive and specific, transesophageal echocardiography is excellent. Occult constriction may be overlooked in patients who have nonspecific complaints—like exertional dyspnea, edema and chest pains—which may be attributed to their primary illness. Involvement of the mediastinum by disease or fibrosis complicates anatomic and physiologic evaluations. However, *radiation therapy is the major cause of combined pericardial constriction and restrictive cardiomyopathy*, the latter being a notorious cause of a poor result from pericardiectomy. This makes myocardial biopsy desirable in any such case.

Treatment

Mild acute pericarditis and noncompressing effusion do not require specific therapy. Indeed, there is usually no reason to discontinue the radiation therapy. Prednisone may be needed for intractable pain but does not appear to be helpful in avoiding constriction. Occult constriction may not need resection, but definite constriction necessitates pericardiectomy, while always considering the patient's prognosis and quality of life. *Radiation constriction often presents a serious technical challenge to the surgeon.* Because of severe involvement of the pulmonary vessels and myocardium, it may be unsuccessful. Radiation-induced cardiac lesions—including myocardial fibrosis, conduction disturbances and valve dysfunction—also contribute to unsatisfactory surgical management.

INDIRECT (BLUNT/NONPENETRATING) PERICARDIAL TRAUMA

Many characteristics of penetrating pericardial trauma, including associated trauma to other organs, apply to nonpenetrating pericardial trauma, but indirect injuries to pericardium, heart and lung are often more complex. Blunt trauma to the chest and abdomen follows *nonpenetrating thoracic impacts* and *compression (crush), blast* and *traumatic deceleration.* These can produce an acute injury spectrum from contusion to rupture of the heart, the pericardium or both. Transportation injuries and falls are the common causes. Closed chest cardiac massage, even without rib fractures, can also traumatize the heart and pericardium. Any *cardiac* damage—including exacerbation of antecedent heart or pericardial disease—may complicate a range of *pericardial* injury, including *acute, "clinically dry" pericarditis* or *hemopericardium* with or without tamponade. Occasional patients develop *pneumopericardium*, early and late *constriction* and *recurrent pericarditis* (including the post–cardiac injury syndrome; PCIS). Cardiopericardial *pseudoaneurysms*, characteristically postinfarctional, are unusual sequelae of accidental and surgical trauma (Figure 21.13A, B, and C).

Nonpenetrating, indirect forces can displace numerous viscera as well as the heart. They may cause the heart and great vessels to acutely "trap" more blood than usual, with directional stresses capable of rupturing the pericardium as well as other structures. Common causes are *deceleration forces*, characteristic of transportation-associated accidents, acting in any plane or tangentially. Death usually follows cardiac rupture with acute hemopericardium or pericardial rupture and acute extrusion (herniation) of some or all of the heart. In general, the more serious the cardiac injury, the more serious the pericardial injury. (Note: Many such patients have no significant external marks of trauma.)

Range of Nonpenetrating Pericardial Injury

The sites and extent of pericardial injury depend on the direction and force of the chest trauma. Although frequently without clinical significance, at autopsy, *isolated parietal pericardial rupture*, with or without cardiac contusion from blunt injury, or after cardiac resuscitation, is not rare, although frequently without clinical significance. *Fibrinous pericarditis*, often with some hemorrhage, is common. As with penetrating injury, *septic pericarditis* follows bacteremia due to infected wounds or burns or contamination from gastrointestinal or respiratory organ damage, which are also sources of *pneumopericardium*. *Pericardial effusion* may be rapid or delayed, even for weeks, as may *cardiac tamponade* due to effusion or, more often, *hemopericardium*. Hemopericardium can also be an isolated lesion, but it is usually associated with contusion, laceration or rupture of the myocardium or great vessels. Subacute or late *constrictive pericarditis* may follow hemopericardium or purulent pericarditis from days to many years after injury.

Pericardial Laceration

Parietal pericardial tears are common, especially after falls and deceleration injuries. Lacerations are rarely isolated or clinically silent and characteristically accompany serious cardiac injury. The most serious consequence is *cardiac herniation*: extrusion of all or part of the heart in any direction, but usually into the left or less often the right pleural cavity, frequently with mediastinal and tracheal shift. *Herniation is nearly always a surgical emergency*. Moreover, such cardiac dislocations and other evidence of pericardial injury may occur either during the initial trauma or only after 48 to 72 hr, after which herniation tends to be restrained by adhesions. Even when delayed, cardiac herniation is characteristically sudden, most often when the patient changes position (page 394).

Rupture and laceration of the parietal pericardium occur mainly at two sites: its diaphragmatic or its pleural abutments (page 7) or both. *Pleuropericardial ruptures* are usually vertical and permit intrapleural cardiac displacements with a high immediate mortality due to either cardiac or vascular incarceration, producing myocardial injury or compression and angulation of cardiac chambers, the aortic root, coronary arteries and veins, the pulmonary trunk or the venae cavae. Ipsilateral lung damage can add atelectasis and pneumopericardium. In general, large pleuropericardial lacerations permit cardiac bleeding to produce hemothorax, so that tamponade may not result due to free drainage into the pleural space. *Diaphragmopericardial rupture* produces a communication between pericardial and abdominal cavities, resembling similar congenital deficiencies (page 68); cardiac herniation is unusual unless this is combined with pleuropericardial rupture. The associated diaphragmatic rupture permits upward herniation into the pericardial cavity of remarkable quantities and combinations of omentum, stomach, large and small bowel and even liver. Damage to the pericardiophrenic artery or other vessels can add acute hemorrhage.

Cardiac Rupture/Laceration

Any cardiac chamber, but usually the left ventricle, can be torn when "overstuffed" with blood by sudden nonpenetrating force, producing significant hemopericardium and often sudden death. Sometimes the hemopericardium is at least temporarily retarded by rapid clotting or, especially with left atrial bleeding, contained in the retroatrial oblique sinus. Although some patients survive longer, atrial injuries are less likely than left ventricular injuries to stop bleeding spontaneously.

Other Nonpenetrating Injury

Traumatic pneumopericardium with potential *pneumotamponade* (tension pneumopericardium) in the absence of direct communication with perforated viscera or gas-producing organisms can occur via three routes: (1) dissecting along perivascular sheaths of the pulmonary vessels or branches of the aorta, (2) downward along fascial planes of the neck or (3) upward from the peritoneal cavity along the esophagus or aorta. Intrapericardial air is demonstrated by chest X-ray film (Figure 21.4) and by streaky interruptions of the M-mode echocardiogram ("air-gap sign"). (Pneumopericardium is separately discussed in Chapter 7).

In addition to potential cardiopulmonary contusions and lacerations, *closed chest resuscitation* increases intrapericardial pressure, tending to decrease ventricular filling because of decreased transmural pressure (page 21). Diastolic blood pressure consistently falls, potentially compromising coronary flow.

Clinical Considerations

Symptoms following diverse blunt pericardial traumas can be nonspecific or multiple, with and without dyspnea or anterior chest or abdominal pain, and may be overshadowed by injuries elsewhere. *All significant or potentially significant chest injuries require careful monitoring with anticipation of progression or more or less sudden cardiocirculatory deterioration.* Although chest contusions, especially with rib and sternal fractures, should increase this anticipation, absence of significant external abnormalities is not rare. Many pericardial injuries are detected only at thoracotomy or autopsy. Indeed, *in hemorrhaging and other hypovolemic trauma patients, an initial favorable response to fluid administration may obscure and delay recognition and treatment of tamponade.* Moreover, because of many late sequelae, including delayed tamponade, the PCIS and constriction, posttraumatic patients must be followed indefinitely, the intensity of follow-up depending on the degree of abnormalities discovered by diligent clinical and laboratory searches. For example, acute intrapericardial abdominal organ herniation can induce vomiting, but may remain remarkably asymptomatic for long periods.

Cardiac enzyme rises may indicate myocardial injury, although excessive levels of total CPK generally reflect extracardiac trauma. Serious cardiac contusions may be identified by indium-111 antimyosin scintigraphy.

Nonpenetrating trauma can produce all of the cardiocirculatory physical findings of penetrating trauma and penetrating surgical injuries (page 373). A *pericardial rub*, easily missed because frequently transient, may be the only physical sign of pericardial involvement. *Hypotension* is the rule and *pulsus paradoxus* must be diligently sought but is often deceptively absent (page 198). With *pneumohydropericardium*, precordial tympany accompanies the typical "mill-wheel sound" of air and fluid that is sometimes audible without a stethoscope (page 38). It must be distinguished from a similar sound made by air embolism to the right heart. *Precordial tympany* with *precordial bowel sounds* can be detected after intrapericardial herniation of abdominal organs. Such herniated organs sometimes tamponade the heart with or without significant pericardial effusion or bleeding. On a *decubitus roentgenogram*, free air in the pericardium will rise to the uppermost part of the sac.

The ECG will confirm any *arrhythmias* and *conduction defects*; these depend on cardiac rather than pericardial injuries but may be delayed for 2 to 3 days. The ECG commonly shows only *ST-T wave changes*, which only occasionally suggest and only rarely are completely typical of acute pericarditis (Figure 21.14). With cardiac displacement, the *QRS axis* may or may not shift, although it occasionally becomes quite unusual and there may be altered precordial R-wave progression.

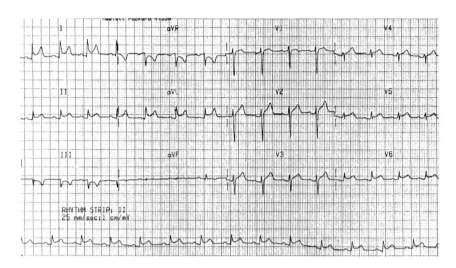

Figure 21.14 Blunt chest trauma: acute pericarditis. Stage I ECG in a patient with a pericardial rub 24 hr after steering-wheel injury. This tracing is a quasidiagnostic, typical variant (Chapter 5) because of the isoelectric J (ST) in lead aVF with QRS axis = 0°. The depressed J (ST) in lead III is equivalent to that in aVR with this axis. PR segment depressions accompany the nearly ubiquitous J (ST) elevations.

Imaging

Chest roentgenograms, optimally with the patient upright, may demonstrate rib and sternal fractures, any unusual gas collections, atelectasis, tracheal shift, and displacement of the herniated heart. Often the apex is elevated, moved laterally, and unusually clearly defined, sometimes with a "doubled" or "capped" appearance. The films may indicate intrapericardial migration of abdominal organs with unilateral (usually left) diaphragmatic elevation and unusual supradiaphragmatic densities, lucencies and organ shadows. Careful identification of herniated organs is especially valuable for anticipating both deterioration and bleeding. Rare patients tolerate this remarkably, not developing symptoms for months, years or ever.

Echocardiography, optimally transesophageal (TEE), is indispensable and so sensitive that if a high-quality study is negative, there is significantly decreased likelihood of complications and sequelae. It will disclose pericardial effusion and fibrinous exudate, right ventricular dilation and ventricular (especially right ventricular) thrombi, and traumatic true and false aneurysms. Finally, the physiologic effect of sufficient right ventricular contusion on the pericardium may simulate that of right ventricular infarction (see pages 349 and 339).

Computed tomography (or MRI if necessary and feasible) will disclose any other cardiac and vascular injuries, angulations and dilations, as well as acute hepatic lymphedema due to cardiac or inferior vena cava compression. These methods also discriminate hemopericardium by its density. In patients progressing satisfactorily, unexplained deterioration and hypotension indicate renewed imaging and, if necessary, *cardioangiography. Video-assisted thoracoscopy* is most specific and helps select the appropriate site and extent of thoracotomy incisions.

Following injury to the mediastinal vasculature, *mediastinal hemorrhage and thrombi* can compress the heart, like their intrapericardial counterparts; they may be distinguishable by not conforming to the pericardial contours. Sternal fractures and tracheal shift are common.

Management

Definitive treatment is surgical repair of wounds, especially those of the heart and vessels, and repositioning of displaced organs, including a herniated heart. The pericardium may have to be sutured, patched or resected and some pericardial lacerations may be temporarily enlarged to be able to replace the heart, especially if it is dilated. Later, if there is acute cardiac herniation due to patient movement, repositioning the patient may permit restitution of the heart's position before emergency thoracotomy. Relieving tamponade can be guided by the usual principles (pages 171–178); *surgical exploration and drainage is safest and permits better survival than paracentesis*, which can be reserved for immediate relief of life-threatening cardiac compression. Formation of ventricular (especially right ventricular) endocardial thrombi raises the question of anticoagulation therapy, which must be decided on an individual basis.

THE POST–CARDIAC INJURY SYNDROME; POSTPERICARDIOTOMY SYNDROME (PCIS/PPS)

The post–cardiac injury syndrome (PCIS) develops usually within days to months after cardiac, pericardial or cardiopericardial injury of all kinds, including cardiac perforations by catheters, left ventricular puncture, epicardial pacemaker and defibrillator fixation and even injury by lightning. The PCIS so strongly resembles the post–myocardial infarction syndrome (PMIS; pages 349–356) that they appear to be variants of a common process. Indeed, though not due to physical trauma, myocardial infarction implies cardiac and cardiopericardial injury. *The PCIS differs from the PMIS because it acutely provokes a much greater antiheart antibody (AHA; antiactin and antimyosin) response*, probably related to usually more extensive tissue trauma and more concentrated release of antigenic material. Moreover, because even surgery limited to the pericardium can cause the PCIS, it is commonly denoted the "postpericardiotomy syndrome" (PPS).

Pathogenesis

The leading hypothesis accounting for the PCIS/PPS considers it an immuno-pathy like the PMIS; myocardial injury releases cellular constituents that may be autoantigens, providing an autoimmune antibody reaction by AHAs; comple-ment is activated; C3 and C4 levels fall and leukocytes are mobilized. At least in the PPS, AHAs appear to be pathogenetic in the presence of a dormant or concurrent viral infection that "permits" them to act. Seasonal variability with peak incidence in April to July may be related. (Some trigger is necessary because it is questionable whether AHAs alone are pathogenetic.) A quantita-tive effect of AHAs is seen in the proportionality between occurrence of the PPS and the extent of surgery: correction of congenital defects and the Wolff-Parkinson-White syndrome have the highest relative incidences. Occurrences of the syndrome after strictly pericardial surgery ("pure PPS") partly challenges the immunopathic hypothesis, since no antipericardial antibodies have been iden-tified. It too may be related to frequent serologic evidence of community-ac-quired viral infection.

Evidence that the PCIS/PPS is likely to be an immunopathy may be sum-marized as follows:

1. Preceding latent period.
2. Frequent recurrences.
3. Prompt response to corticosteroid therapy.
4. Stimulation of antiheart antibodies and complement activation.
5. *Clinical characteristics*: fever, pulmonary infiltrates, frequent pleuritis (rarely the only clinical sign), and systemic inflammatory symptoms and signs.
6. The "complete" PCIS/PPs (page 405) correlates well with increased frequency of high titers of antiheart antibodies.
7. The PCIS/PPS is rare under 2 years of age, possibly due to carryover protection by the mother's immune defenses or hyporeactivity.
8. Incidence decreases at advanced ages, which may be related to an im-mune system that has had more extensive encounters with a variety of viruses and/or is senescent and therefore hyporeactive.
9. Extent of myocardial damage is not clearly correlated with provoca-tion of the PCIS/PPS.

Clinical Aspects

Like the postmyocardial infarction syndrome, which they resemble, the post-cardiac injury and postpericardiotomy syndromes have declined in incidence, making them recently somewhat less common among adult patients. The PCIS/ PPS differ from the usually self-limited postoperative or posttraumatic pericarditis in that more patients develop a form of PCIS than clinically significant postsurgical pericarditis. The characteristic postinjury latent period usually lasts a week to 6 months and the symptoms and signs are more severe, disabling, and prolonged (days to weeks per attack) than uncomplicated posttraumatic pericarditis. A few patients with the appropriate laboratory findings are asymptomatic and a very few develop tamponade or eventual constriction with high leukocyte counts with or without other clinical findings. Pericardial fluid tends to be serosanguineous. *Recurrences* are characteristic, occurring mainly within 6 months of the index attack, but they may continue indefinitely, especially in patients who are difficult to wean from corticosteroid therapy. Among patients without congenital heart disease, the PCIS/PPS appears to be more frequent in those with a past history of either pericarditis or of corticosteroid therapy (especially for rheumatoid arthritis), after aortic valve replacement and among those with B-negative blood type.

Most patients have tachycardia, malaise, pleuritic pain, new pericardial and sometimes pleural rub or both, and mild lymphocytosis or granulocytosis; *all patients have low-grade fever, which may simulate a continuation of postoperative or postinjury fever*. The pain of sternotomy may match the pain of the PCIS/PPS but should progressively decrease over several days; if not, PCIS/ PPS should be suspected. Most postsurgical pericardial rubs should likewise disappear in a day to a week. The PCIS/PPS is considered "complete" if fever, pericarditis and laboratory evidence of inflammation are present and "incomplete" if there are only two of these.

The Pleuropulmonary PCIS/PPS

Rarely, this syndrome will have strictly pericardial rather than pleural or pleuro-pericardial manifestations. Diagnosis of "pleuropulmonary PCIS" is one of exclusion, although more than half of the patients also have a pericardial effusion, a pericardial rub or both. (Indeed, thrombolytic therapy for pulmonary embolism has caused a hemopericardium.) Nearly all patients have signs of pleuritis—pleuritic chest pain which may be lateral rather than precordial—and pleural effusions, mostly left-sided or bilateral. The pleural fluid is serosanguineous or bloody with an early granulocytic exudate changing after 30 days to a late lymphocytosis. Pulmonary embolism may be difficult to differentiate, particularly in the rare patient with hemoptysis, so that a pulmonary arteriogram may be needed.

Diagnosis of the PCIS/PPS

In general, PCIS/PPS must be considered in patients who after 6 days post-surgery or posttrauma, develop fever above 37.8°C for over 8 hr with signifi-

cant pleuritic anterior chest pain and a pericardial rub or two of these, usually
with a sedimentation rate exceeding 40 mm/hr and leukocytosis exceeding
11,000 cells/mm³. The *echocardiogram* can be negative but usually shows a
small to moderate-sized pericardial effusion. *Chest roentgenography* shows left
or bilateral pleural effusion in most patients, a right pleural effusion in a few;
the cardiopericardial silhouette may be enlarged over previous films; a very few
patients have pulmonary infiltrates. With a strictly pleural rub and pleural effusion, PCIS/PPS can be suspected if these persist beyond the immediate postoperative period or occur along with increasing pericardial effusion or a new
pericardial rub. The *ECG* usually reflects myocardial abnormalities and very
rarely even suggests acute pericarditis.

The *principal differential diagnoses of the PCIS/PPS* include:

1. Other causes of postoperative fever, including infections and pneumonitis.
2. Pulmonary embolism, especially if there is only or mainly the pleuropulmonary variant.
3. Myocardial infarction; here the ECG may be helpful. Perhaps half the
   patients have changes consistent with acute pericarditis (Chapter 5). If
   the ECG shows new changes inconsistent with infarct or pericarditis,
   technetium-99 or gallium-67 scanning or comparable studies may be
   useful.

Fortunately, the cytomegalovirus (CMV)-provoked postperfusion syndrome
with hepatomegaly and atypical lymphocytes is now so rare as to be considered only remotely significant in differential diagnosis.

Management

The PCIS/PPS usually responds to aspirin or another non-steroidal anti-inflammatory drug (NSAID), usually within 48 hr, which should be maintained for
10 days. (Indomethacin should be avoided in patients with coronary disease.)
Corticosteroid therapy is effective but should be reserved for patients with severe symptoms who do not respond within 48 hr to a NSAID. The unusual tamponading effusion must be drained. Recurrences, which are often worse than
the index attack, should be managed similarly, adding colchicine as tolerated
if NSAIDs appear to be ineffective. If corticosteroid treatment can be avoided,
recurrences are less likely. Pericardiectomy is reserved for intractable effusions,
which may increase (despite even corticosteroid therapy), and, of course, for
constrictive or effusive-constrictive pericarditis. Pericardiectomy is not very
effective for recurrent pericardial pain.

COMPLICATIONS ASSOCIATED WITH CARDIOPERICARDIAL TRAUMA

Patients who have undergone surgical or other penetrating and nonpenetrating trauma involving the pericardium virtually always have important disease or injury of other organs and systems which complicate diagnosis and management beyond that of purely pericardial disease. These have been considered in the preceding pages but must be constantly kept in mind, even when they are not immediately manifest at the time the pericardial syndrome appears. They include *bleeding* anywhere outside the pericardium, which may be slow or rapid, as well as other *fluid loss* contributing to hypovolemia, which exacerbates cardiac tamponade and permits low-pressure tamponade (page 165). Surgical and accidental *trauma to neighboring organs* often accompanies pericardial wounds, permitting hernias and fistulas, which can become manifest simultaneously or later. These organs include lung, pleura and bronchi, which may be associated with pneumopericardium, pneumothorax and hemothorax; abdominal wounds involving the liver, other abdominal organs and the diaphragm (pages 364–365); and wounds of the esophagus, mediastinum and chest wall. *Flail chest* may seriously compromise both diagnosis and therapy. *Abnormalities of the heart* itself can be associated or unassociated with a traumatic condition, including iatrogenic (usually surgical) trauma. *These include* disease or damage to the myocardium; conduction system damage and arrhythmias; transection or occlusion of coronary vessels as well as coronary arteriovenous fistula; and cardiac thrombi, especially in the right ventricle. *Vascular injuries* include not only the coronary vessels but also tears and angulations of the aorta or one or both venae cavae, often with catastrophic consequences. Echocardiographers regularly encounter *paradoxic septal motion* after pericardiotomy. *Early and late infection* of the heart, pericardium or other structures is, of course, always possible, particularly after contaminated penetrating injuries and any kind of injury producing pathologic communications between the pericardium and abdominal or thoracic organs (page 395).

Pericardial Sequelae

Pericardial adhesions are generally proportional to the amount of epicardial and pericardial injury, bleeding which has not been drained, or any residual blood after drainage. They are to be expected and will be exacerbated by any new infection. *Loculated effusion or hemorrhage* may become manifest early or even many months postoperatively. In most cases, many adhesions disappear or remain quiescent indefinitely. In a few patients, continued inflammatory activity, also proportional to the degree of injury and bleeding, will result in *constrictive or effusive-constrictive pericarditis* (Chapter 15). These usually occur after weeks to months and even years but occasionally remarkably rapidly, even within 2 weeks. Some degree of *epicardial constriction* should be anticipated because, should pericardiectomy for constrictive or, particularly, effusive-constrictive disease be necessary, residual epicardial constriction may vitiate the operative results either immediately or after a latent period. Fortunately, postoperative forms of constrictive pericarditis are now quite uncommon because of improved management of tissues during surgery.

Recurrent pericarditis, probably of autoimmune origin, with or without effusion, may follow any pericardial injury including radiation pericarditis, and even following pericardial resection. *Pseudoaneurysm*, much like that which is the result of myocardial infarction with localized ventricular perforation (page 346), is a rare complication that must be resected because pseudoaneurysms rupture. Posttraumatic pseudoaneurysms of the left ventricle usually follow valve surgery; right ventricular pseudoaneurysms follow repair of congenital lesions like tetralogy of Fallot; atrial pseudoaneurysms are extremely rare. Finally, *pericardiolithiasis*, also extremely rare, has followed blunt chest trauma in a patient who developed cholesterol pericarditis (pages 85–86) with the formation of cholesterol stones, which have not been seen in cholesterol pericarditis of other etiology.

KEY POINTS

1. A very broad range of indirect and direct traumas, mainly involving the chest, the heart and adjacent organs, can produce all forms of acute, subacute and chronic pericardial disease. The most serious are acute and follow surgical and nonsurgical traumas, including hemopericardium, pyopericardium, pneumopericardium, cardiac tamponade (related to the preceding) and constrictive pericarditis. While penetrating trauma produces the most dramatic of these, blunt and indirect trauma can produce the same range of lesions.
2. Pericardial injuries may yield clinical and laboratory signs typical of nontraumatic pericardial disease (e.g., Stage I ECG changes after uncomplicated cardiac surgery). More often pericardial manifestations are masked by other lesions and their effects. Electrocardiograms are most often insensitive and nonspecific. Imaging, especially echocardiography (optimally TEE), is the most useful diagnostic modality.
3. Postoperative or other traumatic tamponade is a surgical emergency. Massive clotting may temporarily stabilize a traumatic hemopericardium but should not delay definitive surgery to evacuate the pericardium and treat the bleeding source. Traumatic, especially postoperative, pericardial bleeding may be deceptively loculated.
4. *Traumatic lesions elsewhere seriously complicate the diagnosis and management of pericardial wounds.*
5. A wide variety of instrumental procedures, including catheters and needles of all kinds, can injure the heart and pericardium, sometimes with deceptively delayed consequences.

6. Traumatic fistulation between the pericardium and injured viscera, especially the esophagus, can produce pneumopericardium and its variants, with a high susceptibility to microbial contamination and bleeding.
7. Pericardial laceration or rupture may permit an injured or intact heart to herniate, with critical entrapment of cardiac structures.
8. The postpericardiotomy syndrome (PPS)/post–cardiac injury syndrome (PCIS) is probably immunopathic and may last indefinitely, necessitating repeated therapy of pericarditic recurrences with or without effusion. As in the related postmyocardial infarction syndrome (PMIS), systemic symptoms accompany chest symptoms.

BIBLIOGRAPHY

Adams JE III, Davila-Roman VG, Bessey PQ, Blake DP, Ladenson JH, Jaffe AS. Improved detection of cardiac contusion with cardiac troponin I. Am Heart J 1996; 131:308–312.

Borrie, J., Lichter, I. Pericardial rupture from blunt chest trauma. Thorax 1974; 29:329–337.

Cabalka, A.K., Rosenblatt, H.M., Towbin, J.A., et al. Postpericardiotomy syndrome in pediatric heart transplant recipients—Immunologic characteristics. Texas Heart Inst. J. 1995; 22:170–176.

Chuttani, K., Tischler, M.D., Pandian, N.G., et al. Diagnosis of cardiac tamponade after cardiac surgery: Relative value of clinical, echocardiographic, and hemodynamic signs. Am. Heart J. 1994; 127:913–918.

Cimino, J.J., Kogan, A.D. Constrictive pericarditis after cardiac surgery: Report of three cases and review of the literature. Am. Heart J. 1989; 118:1292–1301.

Cross, J.H., DeGiovanni, J.V., Silove, E.D. Use of streptokinase to aid in drainage of postoperative pericardial effusion. Br. Heart J. 1989; 62:217–219.

Hastillo, A., Thompson, J.A., Lower, R.R., et al. Cyclosporine-induced pericardial effusion after cardiac transplantation. Am. J. Cardiol. 1987; 59:1220–1222.

Hauptman, P.J., Couper, G.S., Aranki, S.F., et al. Pericardial effusions after cardiac transplantation. J. Am. Coll. Cardiol. 1994; 23:1625–1629.

Hollerman, J.J., Fackler, M.L., Coldwell, D.M., Ben-Menachem, Y. Gunshot wounds: 1. Bullets, ballistics, and mechanisms of injury. A.J.R. 1990; 155:685–690.

Keogh, B.E., Oakley, C.M., Taylor, K.M. Chronic constrictive pericarditis caused by self-mutilation with sewing needles: A case report and review of published reports. Br. Heart J. 1988; 59:77–80.

Kim S, Sahn SA. Postcardiac injury syndrome. An immunologic pleural fluid analysis. Chest 1996; 109; 570–572.

Kronzon, I., Cohen, M.L., Winer, H.E. Cardiac tamponade by loculated pericardial hematoma: Limitations of M-mode echocardiography. J. Am. Coll. Cardiol. 1983; 3:913–915.

Nagy, K.K., Lohmann, C., Kim, D.O., Barrett, J. Role of echocardiography in the diagnosis of occult penetrating cardiac injury. J. Trauma Injury Infect. Crit. Care 1995; 38:859–862.

Ni, Y., von Segesser, L.K., Turina, M. Futility of pericardiectomy for postirradiation constrictive pericarditis? Ann. Thorac. Surg. 1990; 49:445–448.

Schrank, J.H., Jr., Dooley, D.P. Purulent pericarditis caused by Candida species: Case report and review. Clin. Infect. Dis. 1995; 21:182–187.

Slack, J.D., Pinkerton, C.A. The electrocardiogram often fails to identify pericarditis after percutaneous transluminal coronary angioplasty. J. Electrocardiol. 1986; 19:399–402.

Spodick, D.H. Critical care of pericardial disease. In: Rippe, J.M., Irwin, R.S., Alpert, J.S., Fink, M.P. Intensive Care Medicine, 2d ed. Boston: Little, Brown, 1991, pp. 282–295.

Symbas, P.N. Cardiothoracic trauma. Curr. Probl. Surg. 1991; 28:745–797.

Thomas, P., Saux, P., Lonjon, T., et al. Diagnosis by video-assisted thoracoscopy of traumatic pericardial rupture with delayed luxation of the heart: Case report. J. Trauma Injury Infect. Crit. Care 1995; 38:967–970.

Van Gelderen, W.F.C. Stab wounds of the heart: Two new signs of pneumopericardium. Br. J. Radiol. 1993; 66:794–796.

22

Drug- and Toxin-Related Pericardial Disease

GENERAL CONSIDERATIONS; DIAGNOSTIC IMPORTANCE

Certain oral and parenteral medications and toxic substances and some irritants contacting the pericardium can induce *acute or subacute pericarditis and effusion, and, depending on the abnormal substance, tamponade, adhesions, fibrosis or constriction*. Anticoagulants and thrombolytic agents may cause pericardial bleeding in an already inflamed sac, even leading to adhesions and constriction, but this is not a specific "pericardiotoxic" effect. Most drug and toxin responses are either acute pericarditis of some form, inflammatory pericardial effusion, or, less commonly, hydropericardium. A wide variety of agents (Table 22.1) and mechanisms are responsible, some poorly understood.

The importance of this class of relatively uncommon "pericardiopathies" lies in diagnostic recognition and in its corollary: excluding other causes of pericardial disease. Most of the agents in Table 22.1 are used to treat specific diseases, many of which themselves can cause pericarditis or effusions, making the distinction particularly important. In general, the acute reactions to these agents resolve when exposure to the agent ceases. However, those that can go on to constriction and even recurrent pericarditis pose continuing threats to the patient. The disorders for which many of these are given include malignancies, infections and renal failure, each of which can itself cause pericarditis, and arrhythmias. Moreover, distinguishing drug or toxin-induced pericarditis from idiopathic pericarditis is crucial, so that *exposure to a pericarditis-inducing agent*

Table 22.1 DRUG- AND TOXIN-RELATED PERICARDIAL DISEASE

A. Drug-induced lupus erythematosus
    Procainamide
    Tocainide
    Hydralazine
    Methyldopa
    Mesalazine
    Reserpine
    Isoniazid
    Hydantoins (diphenylhydantoin, dantrolene)
    ? Quinidine
B. Hypersensitivity reaction (often with eosinophilia)
    Penicillins (ampicillin, procaine penicillin)
    Cromolyn sodium
    ? Praziquantel
C. "Idiosyncratic" or hypersensitivity

Methysergide	Para-aminosalicylic acid (PAS)	
Minoxidil (? also lupus)	Thiazides	5-Fluorouracil
Practolol	Streptomycin	Vaccines
Bromocriptine	Thiouracils	Smallpox
Psicofuranine	Sulfa drugs	Yellow fever
Polymer fume inhalation	Cyclophosphamide	GMCSF (granulocyte-
Cytosine arabinoside	Cyclosporine	macrophage colony
Phenylbutazone	Amiodarone	stimulating factor).
Amiodarone	Mesalazine (Rowasa)	
Streptokinase		

D. Anthracycline derivatives
    Doxorubicin
    Daunorubicin
E. Serum sickness
    Foreign antisera (e.g., antitetanus)
    Blood products
F. Venenation
    Scorpion fish sting
G. Foreign-substance reactions (direct pericardial application)
    Talc (magnesium silicate)
    Silicones
    Tetracycline and other sclerosants
    Asbestos
H. Secondary pericardial bleeding/hemopericardium
    Anticoagulants
    Thrombolytic agents

must be considered in the differential diagnosis of idiopathic pericarditis (Chapter 23). Indeed, in every new case of pericarditis, the customary thorough history obtained from the patient must include use of any drug and any exposure to noxious agents.

LUPUS REACTIONS

Drug-induced lupus erythematosus must lead the list for iatrogenic pericarditis, because the most commonly responsible drugs are procainamide and hydralazine, which nearly always induce a form of lupus complete with the appropriate antinuclear antibodies. Procainamide, in particular, is known to provoke classic acute pericarditis, pericardial effusions, cardiac tamponade and quite rapid constrictive pericarditis (acute and subacute constriction; page 217). Tamponade due to hydralazine has been a component of the presenting syndrome of hydralazine toxicity. Lupus pericarditis associated with methyldopa, reserpine, isoniazid and the hydantoins is much less common.

IDIOSYNCRASY

A large number of drugs appear to induce *idiosyncratic pericardial responses*, although hypersensitivity (without eosinophilia) is always possible (Table 21.1C). Among these, psicofuranine, an antineoplastic drug, is uniquely characteristic because its only known tissue toxicity is confined to pericarditis in both human beings and animals. Methysergide, which induces widespread fibrosis, is responsible for constrictive pericarditis both due to aggressive mediastinal fibrosis and as a sequela of fibrinous pericarditis. Minoxidil presents problems in that, while it has appeared to provoke a lupus syndrome and can cause isolated pericarditis, it is not clear that minoxidil-associated hydropericardium in many patients was not due to the hypertensive disease for which the drug was prescribed. This is equally true of amiodarone. Drug-induced acute cardiomyopathy may be responsible for cyclophosphamide-associated hydropericardium. Cyclosporine seems strongly associated with pericardial effusion in cardiac transplant patients. Phenylbutazone, which can be used to treat acute pericarditis, can also cause it. Finally, recombinant human granulocyte-macrophage stimulating factor (GM-CSF) has caused pericardial effusion, polyserositis and constrictive pericarditis.

OTHER PERICARDIOPATHIC RESPONSES

Serum sickness, due mainly to antisera and parenterally delivered blood products, occasionally includes an element of pericarditis. Pericarditis following *poisoning* by the sting of a scorpion fish appears to be unique. On the other hand, *foreign-substance reactions* due to direct pericardial application are quite understandable. Magnesium silicate (talc), used to produce pericardial adhesions in unsuccessful attempts to revascularize the heart, produces relatively mild pericarditis with adhesions. On the other hand, tetracycline and other sclerosants, introduced intrapericardially to prevent stubbornly recurrent, malignant effusions, evokes a painful acute reaction. Silicones, inadvertently deposited in the pericardium during surgical implantation of defibrillation patches, and on epicardial pacemaker leads, have provoked pericarditis foreign body reactions and adhesions. Asbestos, possibly by lymphatic spread, has acted comparably.

HYPERSENSITIVITY AND IMMUNOPATHY

Hypersensitivity by whatever mechanism, "idiosyncratic," "allergic" or via lupus is clearly the most common cause of pericardial drug and toxin reactions. Patients reacting to a single dose of an agent may be considered to be unduly sensitive to that agent. With multiple doses, this may also be true or may represent toxicity. Where there is strong evidence for the pathogenic role of circulating immune complexes, some drugs act as a hapten, binding to plasma proteins, with this complex evoking an immune response, particularly during serum sickness–type reactions. On the other hand, antinuclear antibodies may be induced without necessarily being pathogenic. *Allergic-type hypersensitivity reactions*, often with eosinophilia, occur with a variety of medications, but various penicillins and cromolyn sodium have definitely been incriminated in producing pericarditis. Praziquantel, a mixture of isomers with pyrazinoquinoline ring structures, has produced pericarditis as a part of a polyserositis, but it is not clear whether this was due to the sudden release of antigens from dead schistosomas. "Hypersensitive" patients with pericarditis may have fever, rashes, arthralgias, lymphadenopathy, albuminuria, vasculitis, arthritis and sometimes eosinophilia.

ALTERNATE CATEGORIZATION BY TARGET DISORDER

Regrouping most pericarditogenic pharmaceutical agents by the kind of disease at which they have been aimed should heighten awareness of the possibility of drug-induced pericardial reactions. The following may be included:

    Antiarrhythmic: procainamide, practolol, amiodarone, diphenylhydantoin, and possibly quinidine

    Antineoplastic: daunorubicin, doxorubicin (Adriamycin), psicofuranine

    Anti-infectious: isoniazid, streptomycin, sulfa drugs; possibly praziquantel

    Antihypertensive: hydralazine, methyldopa, reserpine, minoxidil, practolol, thiazides, reserpine

MYOPERICARDITIS AND CARDIOMYOPATHY

Some of the pericarditis-inducing agents, like the anthracycline derivatives, tend to induce *myopericarditis* (Chapter 9), particularly during early reactions. With cumulative toxicity, they produce a cardiomyopathy, which may be accompanied by hydropericardium due to congestive failure.

KEY POINTS

1. A wide variety of medications and toxins, including immunity-inducing agents, can cause the gamut of structural and functional pericardial disease, making indispensable a careful history of ingestants, injectants, known allergies and insect venenation.
2. Agents inducing "pericardiopathies" include antiarrhythmics, antineoplastics, antimicrobials and antihypertensives.
3. Several chemically unrelated drugs can cause systemic lupus erythematosus with acute pericarditis and sometimes relatively rapid constriction.
4. Idiosyncrasy and hypersensitivity (including "allergy") to inducing agents may cause pericarditis with eosinophilia.

BIBLIOGRAPHY

Alarcon-Segovia, D. Drug-induced lupus syndromes. Mayo Clin. Proc. 1969; 44:664–669.

Browning, C.A., Bishop, R.S., Heilpern, R.J., et al. Accelerated constrictive pericarditis in procainamide-induced systemic lupus erythematosus. Am. J. Cardiol. 1984; 53: 376–377.

Harbin, A.D., Gerson, M.C., O'Connell, J.B. Simulation of acute myopericarditis by constrictive pericardial disease with endomyocardial fibrosis to methysergide therapy. J. Am. Coll. Cardiol. 1984; 4:196–198.

Harrington, T.M., Davis, D.E. Systemic lupus-like syndrome induced by methyldopa therapy. Chest 1981; 79:696–698.

Haugtomt, H., Haerem, J. Pulmonary edema and pericarditis after inhalation of Teflon fumes. Tidsskr. Nor. Laegeforen 1989; 109:584–587.

Krehlik, J.M., Hindson, D.A., Crowley, J.J. Jr., Knight, L.L. Minoxidil-associated pericarditis and fatal cardiac tamponade. West. J. Med. 1985; 143:527–529.

Lipworth, B.J., Oakley, D.G. Surgical treatment of constrictive pericarditis due to practolol: A case report. J. Cardiovasc. Surg. 1988; 29:408–412.

Martin, W.B., Spodick, D.H., Zins, G.R. Pericardial disorders occurring during open-label study of 1,869 severely hypertensive patients treated with Minoxidil. J. Cardiovasc. Pharmacol. 1980; 2:(suppl. 2):S217–S227.

Miller, D.H., Haas, L.F. Pneumonitis, pleural effusion and pericarditis following treatment with dantrolene. J. Neurol. Neurosurg. Psychiatry. 1984; 47:553–556.

Ratliff, N.B., McMahon, J.T., Shirey, E.K., Groves, L.K. Silicone pericarditis. Cleve. Clin. Q. 1984; 51:185–187.

Schoenwetter, A.H., Silber, E.N. Penicillin hypersensitivity, acute pericarditis and eosinophilia. JAMA 1965; 136:191–193.

Slater, E.E. Cardiac tamponade and peripheral eosinophilia in a patient receiving cromolyn sodium. Chest 1978; 73:878–880.

Spodick, D.H. Pericarditis in systemic diseases. Cardiol. Clin. 1990; 8:709–716.

Spodick, D.H. Diseases of the pericardium. In: Chatterjee, K.C., Korliav, J., Rapaort, E., et al. (eds.). Cardiology: An Illustrated Text/Reference. Vol. 2. New York and London: Gower, 1991, Chap. 10, pp. 38–64.

Yates, R.C., Olson, K.B. Drug-induced pericarditis: Report of three cases due to 6-amino-9-D-psicofuranosylpurine. N. Engl. J. Med. 1961; 265:274–277.

23

Idiopathic Pericarditis; Pericarditis of Unknown Origin (Nonspecific Pericarditis; "Acute Benign Pericarditis")

TERMINOLOGY

Oxford English Dictionary (new Shorter Ed.)

Idio - own, personal, private, distinct.

Idiopathic - of a disease: not consequent on or symptomatic of another disease; having no known cause.

Webster's 3d Ed.

Idio - one's own; personal; self-produced; arising within.

Idiopathic - peculiar to the individual. Innate. Arising spontaneously or from an obscure or unknown cause. Primary.

Stedman's 26th Ed.

Idio - (G. *Idios*, one's own). Combining form meaning private, distinctive peculiar to.

Idiopathic - (idio - + G. *pathos*, suffering).

1. Agnogenic; denoting a disease of unknown cause.
2. Denoting a primary disease.

Idiopathic pericarditis or "acute benign pericarditis" was named in the 19th century at a time when searches for pathogenetic agents, particularly identification of viruses and many bacteria, were impossible or impractical. We now recognize that "idiopathic" pericarditis refers to either the general meaning of idiopathic (i.e., by any dictionary definition) or to a particular syndrome indistinguishable from viral pericarditis (pages 260–265). In the broader sense that diagnostic testing is often unrewarding, it will be seen that *pericarditis of unknown cause* is the result of a variety of *causes that are not demonstrable at the time pericarditis appears*; most of these are probable viral infections. Others are immunopathic processes associated with some tendency to recur. For example, post–myocardial infarction syndrome (PMIS) after clinically silent infarcts may appear to be "idiopathic pericarditis."

No disease processes are sui generis—i.e., truly "idiopathic"; their actual causes only remain to be discovered. Moreover, while the majority of cases of "idiopathic pericarditis" do fall into the *"acute benign"* category, *no form of acute pericarditis deserves this traditional label*, since many patients develop pericardial effusions, cardiac tamponade and constrictive pericarditis. Moreover, as in viral pericarditis, careful follow-up (e.g., by echo-Doppler study approximately every 2 to 4 weeks and careful observation of neck veins) will show that many patients who recover clinically go through a transient constrictive phase that is nearly always asymptomatic (page 254).

Idiopathic pericarditis, in the sense of either probable viral origin or any attack that resolves without specific diagnosis, is the commonest form of acute pericarditis in clinical practice. Yet because it is not truly one disease, it will receive only brief discussion here. Moreover, *many diseases occasionally present first as a pericardial disorder* and may not be diagnosed until well after pericardial illness appears. Examples include the *vasculitis-connective tissue disease group*, in which a pericarditic initial presentation is not rare, particularly in systemic lupus erythematosus (page 321); *unrecognized myocardial infarction*, which may first become symptomatic as infarct pericarditis or even the post–myocardial infarction syndrome (PMIS; page 349); *dissecting hematoma of the aorta* (page 356); *primary and metastatic malignancies* of the pericardium (Chapter 18); some forms of *acute tuberculous pericarditis* (page 269); *brucellosis with pericarditis as the presenting or major manifestation; Lyme disease* (page 286); *traumatic pericarditis* appearing relatively late after trauma (PCIS, pages 403), the *seronegative spondyloarthropathies* and *intestinal inflammatory diseases* (page 326); *acute pancreatitis* first presenting as a pericardial effusion; some patients with *cholesterol pericarditis* may have had preceding idiopathic pericarditis with cholesterol-free effusion (page 85); finally, rare diseases—for example, *"yellow-nail syndrome"*. The physician encountering undiagnosed acute pericarditis with or without effusion may often safely attribute it to viral infection, especially in cases that truly prove to be "benign," but must always keep in mind the occasional to rare initial presentation of more serious illness as pericarditis.

Some cases go on to overt constrictive pericarditis; a few develop pericardial adhesions and even calcification with or without a clinical counterpart. *Recurrent (relapsing) "idiopathic" pericarditis* tends to follow a pattern seen in patients with viral pericarditis, including precipitation by exposure to antigenic stimuli, including microorganisms that do not necessarily involve the pericardium. Indeed, many patients with "idiopathic" pericarditis that is stubbornly recurrent have a personal or family history of allergic disorders. In those with a missed nonviral pathogenesis the disease process ultimately surfaces after the index pericarditis or during a recurrence. Rare causes, exemplifying the extreme etiologic range, include *celiac disease* and *dermatitis herpetiformis* with recurrent pericarditis responsive to a gluten-free diet. Pericarditis in *eosinophilic fasciitis* may precede eosinophilia.

In all large prospective studies of patients with acute pericarditis, the largest single group, often the majority, is "idiopathic," mainly because there have not been comprehensive searches for evidence of viral infection or systemic disease like lupus. While certain viruses like enteroviruses, particularly the Coxsackie group, are especially "pericardiotropic," community prevalence of viruses varies from year to year; therefore, even with a determined search, certain etiologies will be missed. In areas of endemic disease—for example, those with certain parasitoses—pericardial involvement may be considered idiopathic unless there are telltale signs like unusual eosinophilia or positive skin or antibody tests. Indeed, *a travel history may be important in any new case of pericarditis*. However, positive antibody and skin tests may be "red herrings," which are common in individuals without pericarditis (for example, in areas of high prevalence of tuberculosis, where many patients with positive skin tests will not have tuberculous pericarditis). (Note: Some patients with aggressive tuberculous pericarditis have negative skin tests.)

When "idiopathic" pericardial disease first presents as a pericardial effusion, the question of differential diagnosis often becomes more urgent. However, there are conditions like *hypertension with pericardial effusion of unknown origin* that may be related to the vascular disease itself or to intercurrent disease. All the foregoing considerations make *"pericarditis of unknown origin" preferable to the classic "idiopathic pericarditis."*

Because they are probably due to viral pericarditis, most cases of "idiopathic" pericarditis syndrome are the clinical epitome of acute pericarditis. Thus, most such patients tend to have easily recognizable acute pericardial disease with frequent rubs and Stage I ECG changes, often preceded by upper respiratory infection. Any fluid is usually serous or serosanguineous but, by definition, yields no specific diagnostic material. As with demonstrably viral and other infective pericarditis, pleuritis is common with or without pneumonitis. The white blood cell count may or may not be elevated, with varying differential counts. A *high lymphocyte proportion, for example, is compatible with tuberculosis or lymphoma as well as viral infection*. The acute illness lasts days to several weeks, but sporadic cases may endure for much longer. As with viral pericarditis, "idiopathic" pericarditis syndrome is often self-limited, but one or many recurrences are not rare. Unless they are due to a specific illness, recurrences are generally negative for diagnostic material and are likely to be due to an immune mechanism, often termed "autoreactive," in which investigation may demonstrate antibodies, e.g., antimyolemmal antibodies of IgG and IgA isotypes. Culturable or otherwise identifiable microorganisms are long gone.

Treatment is as usual for acute, clinically dry pericarditis (pages 107–108) and for effusion and tamponade (pages 172–178) as needed. Eventual identification of any specific pathogenesis requires adequate follow-up followed by specific treatment.

KEY POINTS

1. Acute "idiopathic" pericarditis usually resembles and most often probably is typical acute viral pericarditis. It is typically but by no means always benign and must be followed up indefinitely for sequelae, including recurrences and constrictive pericarditis.
2. So many of the large etiologic variety of pericardial diseases can present as idiopathic pericarditis that many cases must initially be investigated and later followed up for the possibility of serious systemic disease, including neoplasia, infections, the vasculitis-connective tissue group (especially SLE), post–myocardial infarction syndrome (PMIS) following silent infarction, and many exotic disorders. A travel history may be helpful, especially in patients with eosinophilia and patients exposed to zones of endemicity for particular communicable diseases.

BIBLIOGRAPHY

Anger, R.C., Gallis, H.A. Pericarditis—Differential diagnostic considerations. Arch. Intern. Med. 1979; 139:407–412.

Farley, J.D., Thomson, A.B.R., Dasgupta, M.K. Pericarditis and ulcerative colitis. J. Clin. Gastroeneterol. 1986; 8:567–568.

Johnson, A.G., Stokes, J.F. Allergic pericarditis. Br. Med. J. 1964; 1:481–482.

Ling LH, Oh JK, Seward JB, Danielson GK, Tajik AJ. Clinical profile of constrictive pericarditis in the modern era: A survey of 135 cases. J Am Coll Cardiol 1996; 27:32A-33A.

Maisch, B., Drude, L. Pericardioscopy—A new diagnostic tool in inflammatory disease of the pericardium. Eur. Heart J. 1991; 12(suppl. D): 2–6.

Millaire, A., Goullard, L., deGroote, P., Ducloux, G.: Use of colchicine in acute or recurrent pericarditis. Eur. Heart J. 1990; 11:(suppl.):409.

Mocchegiani, R., Capestro, F., Grancesconi, M., et al. Idiopathic acute pericarditis: A 10 year follow-up. Eur. Heart J. 1990; 11(suppl.):404.

Permanyer-Miralda, G., Sagrista-Sauleda, J., Soler-Soler, J. Primary acute pericardial disease: A prospective series of 231 consecutive patients. Am. J. Cardiol. 1985; 56:623–630.

Sagrista-Sauleda, J., Permanyer-Miralda, G., Candell-Riera, J., et al. Transient cardiac constriction: An unrecognized pattern of evolution in effusive acute idiopathic pericarditis. Am. J. Cardiol. 1987; 59:961–966.

Sagrista-Sauleda, J., Permanyer-Miralda, G., Soler-Solder, J. Tuberculous pericarditis: Ten year experience with a prospective protocol for diagnosis and treatment. J. Am. Coll. Cardiol. 1988; 11:724–728.

Saner, H.E., Gobel, F.L., Nicoloff, D.M., Edwards, J.E. Aortic dissection presenting as pericarditis. Chest 1987; 91:71–75.

Spodick, D.H. Infective pericarditis: Etiologic and clinical spectra. In: Reddy P.S. (ed.). Pericardial Disease. New York: Raven Press, 1982, pp. 307–312.

Spodick, D.H. Pitfalls in the recognition of pericarditis. In: Hurst, J.W. (ed.). Clinical essays on the heart. New York: McGraw-Hill, 1985, pp. 95–111.

Spodick, D.H. Pericarditis in systemic disease. Cardiol. Clin. 1990; 8:709–716.

Variyam, E.P., Shah, A. Pericardial effusion and left ventricular function in patients with acute alcoholic pancreatitis. Arch. Intern. Med. 1987; 147:923–925.

Wakasa, M., Imaizumi, T., Suyama, A., et al. Yellow nail syndrome associated with chronic pericardial effusion. Chest 1987; 92:366–367.

Zayas, R., Anguita, M., Torres, F., et al. Incidence of specific etiology and role of methods for specific etiologic diagnosis of primary acute pericarditis. Am. J. Cardiol. 1995; 75:378–382.

24

Recurrent and Incessant Pericarditis

DEFINITIONS AND PATHOGENETIC CONSIDERATIONS

Perhaps 15 to 20% of patients do not recover permanently following an initial attack of acute pericarditis of a variety of etiologies. Table 24.1 presents an etiologic-pathogenetic ("etiopathic") summary of the origins of recurrent pericarditis, with the disorders grouped for clinical convenience. While the exact incidences and natural histories are uncertain, *the vast majority of patients have had acute idiopathic, presumably viral or manifestly viral pericarditis*; in them, *recurrent pericarditis* or continuously active *incessant pericarditis*—frequently recurrent or incessant provocation of pericardial pain—appear to be immunopathic processes. "Incessant" designates pericarditis (or identical pain) in patients who continue to need treatment for unremitting symptoms or are symptom-free for periods of less than 6 weeks. The 6 week figure is selected arbitrarily because of the overwhelming failure of pericardiectomy to end these syndromes after they become chronic: postoperatively, nearly all patients have a brief, unexplained symptom-free period of between 1 and 6 weeks. A few patients either appear to be cured completely or for months to years before symptoms return. It is possible that meticulous removal of nearly all the pericardium (pedestals must be left for the phrenic nerves) may yield improved results, but very long-term follow-up will be needed for such patients. Anecdotal evidence suggests better results in patients with recurrent pain who also have recurrent pericardial effusions.

Incessant pericarditis involves continuous activity that surfaces whenever anti-inflammatory, usually corticosteroid, therapy is reduced or discontinued.

Table 24.1   **Etiopathogenesis of Recurrent and Incessant Pericarditis**

A. Idiopathic pericarditis
B. Infective/reinfective pericarditis
    1. Viral
    2. Bacterial, *esp.* tuberculosis, streptococcus, meningococcus
    3. Other (e.g., histoplasmosis; rickettsiosis)
C. Hemopericardium-initiated
D. Post–myocardial and pericardial injury syndromes
    1. Post–myocardial infarction syndrome (PMIS)
    2. Post-traumatic pericarditis
       a. Surgical: postpericardiotomy syndrome (PPS)
       b. Other traumata
    3. Foreign-body pericarditis
    4. Epicardial instrumentation: defibrillator, pacemaker
    5. Electric injury (lightning strike; ? other)
E. Systemic disorders involving the pericardium
    1. Vasculitis–connective tissue disease group
    2. Thalassemia major
    3. Dermatitis herpetiformis
    4. Inflammatory bowel disease
    5. Familial Mediterranean fever (periodic polyserositis)
F. Metabolic (*esp.* uremia)
G. Hypersensitivity/"allergy"
    1. Ingestants
       a. Drug: with and without drug-induced lupus
       b. Food (e.g., gluten: celiac disease; ? related to E3)
    2. Injectants
       a. Immunization
       b. Immunotherapy; allergic "desensitization"
       c. Serum sickness
H. Malignancy
I. Hypothetical pathogenetic factors. (no conclusive evidence)
    1. Inadequate anti-inflammatory treatment of the index or subsequent attacks
    2. Corticosteroid treatment too early (during active viral multiplication)
    3. Uneradicated "septic foci"

The majority of such patients may be said to be "steroid hooked"—a term of art, more dramatic than "steroid dependant" reflecting their desperation. Naturally, in a relatively small minority of patients, repeated or chronic exposure to the inciting agent or process is clearly responsible for recurrences. Examples include viral and bacterial reinfection (or reactivation of dormant organisms) and, more commonly, systemic disorders, notably the vasculitis–connective tissue disease group and especially exacerbations of lupus erythematosus.

Certain pathogenetic possibilities may apply to recurrent and incessant pericarditis, a heterogenous grouping, although without definitive proof:

1. Inadequate anti-inflammatory treatment of the index or subsequent attacks. This is difficult to judge because, as with most kinds of pericarditis, there are no controlled clinical trials to indicate how much treatment, over what period and with what agents is "adequate."
2. Corticosteroid treatment given early during active viral multiplication is known to promote and prolong viral infection.
3. French authors have incriminated "septic foci," mentioning dental, tonsillar, ear, nose, throat and appendiceal infections, following eradication of which pericarditic recurrences ceased. However, this was not adequately documented.
4. Poorly understood cyclic immune or autoimmune responses to specific or nonspecific agents and processes, like respiratory infections or fatigue as mechanisms for recurrences and both precipitating and perpetuating the syndrome.
5. The capability of viral RNA sequences in pericardial tissue to serve as constant sources of antigen, although not themselves capable of replication.

RECURRENT IDIOPATHIC PERICARDITIS: THE PROTOTYPE OF RECURRENT AND INCESSANT PERICARDITIS

"Idiopathic pericarditis" is usually of viral origin (Chapter 23); its recurrences and also recurrences after demonstrably viral pericarditis are virtually the same syndrome. Moreover, following the index attack, evidence of concurrent infection cannot be demonstrated. Recurrent idiopathic pericarditis is perhaps the greatest therapeutic challenge among the disorders of the pericardium and encompasses both the *intermittent type* with widely varying symptom-free intervals without therapy and the *incessant type* in which discontinuation, or even attempts to wean patients from anti-inflammatory, especially corticosteroid, therapy nearly always ensures a relapse. Indeed, it is characteristic for many patients to have a *threshold level* of prednisone therapy, below which relapse is certain. If weaning is too fast, a patient who has been on 60 mg prednisone daily may find the threshold between 30 and 40 mg. With slower, more judicious weaning, the threshold is commonly between 10 and 20 mg, frequently close to 15 mg. Particularly remarkable in these cases is the virtual absence of tamponade. Although effusion and tamponade may occur in the index attack, effusions are uncommon and tamponade is rare during recurrences, even over many years. Constrictive pericarditis appears not to occur in the great majority—those cases considered to be idiopathic. Indeed, specimens of pericardial tissue obtained by biopsy or at pericardiectomy typically show only nonspecific changes: light fibrosis, sometimes with adhesions, rare fibrinous exudates, or variably increased pericardial vascularity; tissue obtained during more active disease may show pericardial thickening and edema. Some of this nonspecificity may be due to suppression of inflammation and fibrosis by corticosteroids or nonsteroidal agents. In any case, recurrent idiopathic pericarditis and sterile recurrences following viral pericarditis practically do not occur without a background of initial or continuing corticosteroid treatment, usually with prednisone. Yet the majority of patients, despite corticosteroid therapy, escape recurrences, notably those given a brief course following cardiopericardial surgery. Thus, most recurrent pericarditis seems to represent individual pericardial reactivity to a variety of poorly understood pathogenetic agents and processes and their corticosteroid suppression.

PERICARDIAL IMMUNOPATHY

Strong evidence that most recurrences of pericarditis, including the most common—recurrent idiopathic and postviral pericarditides—are of immunopathic origin includes the following:

1. The latent period after the index attack, lasting days to years, but usually months.
2. Antiheart antibodies in some cases, probably those with significant myopericarditis (Chapter 9) in the index attack.
3. (Related to #2): Similarity to illnesses like the post–myocardial infarction and postpericardiotomy syndromes (Chapters 20,21). These have in common similar symptoms and frequent recurrences.
4. Frequent allergic personal and/or family history.
5. Rapid response to corticosteroid therapy and relapses with decreasing doses or discontinuance. (Corticosteroids have immunosuppressive effects on T cells, B cells and phagocytes, blunting immune and inflammatory responses.)
6. Acute recurrent pericarditis during allergic disorders, such as reactions to drugs and to foods like gluten in patients with celiac disease and dermatitis herpetiformis.
7. Acute recurrent pericarditis in classic serum sickness, including reactions to immunizations (e.g., smallpox; yellow fever).
8. Recurrence of relapsing pericarditis in patients with diseases of demonstrably autoimmune pathogenesis, like systemic lupus erythematosus.
9. Occasional occurrence of other kinds of serositis, mainly pleuritis and rarely peritonitis.

10. Frequent arthralgias, especially in the post–myocardial injury and postmyocardial infarction syndromes (as well as arthritis in the vasculitis–connective tissue disease group).
11. Occasional eosinophilia.

Recurrences vary from one to dozens over periods of weeks to decades. In no individual case is the pattern of recurrences precisely predictable except during corticosteroid weaning with an established threshold level for recurrences. Some patients can predict a relapse to follow fatigue or various kinds of premonitory malaise.

CLINICAL ASPECTS

Symptoms during recurrences are quite similar among patients and usually stereotyped for each patient. The constant feature is *pain*, which resembles the pain of the index attack, often but not exclusively with strong pleuritic components. In most cases, it is best described as "annoying" and "disabling," nearly always making life extremely unpleasant. *Objective manifestations* are much less uniform and, while frequently detectable in the first recurrence, rapidly become less and less common. Thus, with chronicity (though even with the first recurrence), most patients lose their original fever, pericardial rub, electrocardiographic (ECG) changes, elevated sedimentation rate and any dyspnea. If significant pericardial effusion does not accompany the first recurrence, it is less likely in subsequent recurrences, irrespective of any degree of effusion in the index attack. This is equally true of tamponade, which is rare in recurrent pericarditis. Exceptional patients may experience increasing severity in recurrences, during which tamponade may first appear. It is worth reiterating that *recurrent idiopathic pericarditis does not appear to cause constriction.* Any significant arrhythmias are the result of myocardial irritation or independent cardiac disease (page 56). Finally, the male predominance for most forms of pericarditis is much less apparent in the recurrent forms.

RECURRENT IDIOPATHIC PERICARDITIS

Recurrent "idiopathic" pericarditis is frequently of remote viral origin (Chapter 23). Enterovirus-specific IgM responses have been found in many patients with chronically relapsing pericarditis, whereas comparable patients after acute enterovirus—mainly Coxsackie B—infections elsewhere have had only transient evidence of such viral infection. Indeed, among patient with acute pericarditis, the level of IgM antibody was significantly higher in those who later relapsed. The influence of host genetic factors is suggested in such individuals by significantly higher levels of HLA A2 haplotypes in those who were IgM positive (although extracardiac sites of viral persistence could not be excluded).

Thus, many patients with recurrent pericarditis may experience persistent viral antigenic stimulation. Recurrences frequently follow new exposure to or infection by viral illnesses. It is not clear why constrictive pericarditis can follow a single attack of viral pericarditis, while recurrent pericarditis follows apparently comparable attacks but appears not to constrict.

NONIDIOPATHIC RECURRENT PERICARDITIS

Although rare, it is axiomatic that reexposure of susceptible patients to *bacterial, particularly tuberculous, and other infections* can result in recurrent pericarditis, i.e., *reinfection pericarditis*. This may be the case also with insufficient suppressive treatment during the index attack. For example, bacteriostatic agents may not be as effective as bactericidal agents given over a sufficiently long period. Finally, tamponade and constriction may follow severe recurrent infection.

Hemopericardium of any cause, particularly with injury to the pericardium, may be associated with recurrent pericarditis. Most patients with a frank, clinically detected hemopericardium have had tamponade and usually pain and fever in the index attack. Unlike recurrent idiopathic pericarditis, these cases, like cases of recurrent bacterial pericarditis, may eventually constrict. Indeed, some degree of hemopericardium may be another prerequisite for those cases of viral pericarditis that constrict after a single episode rather than resolve or become recurrent, since many such cases have a serosanguineous effusion in the index attack.

The *postmyocardial and pericardial injury syndromes* (post—cardiac injury syndromes; PCIS, pages 349; 403) are especially prone to recurrence. Although almost certainly on an immunopathic basis, these syndromes are subject not only to recurrence but also, less commonly, to constrictive pericarditis. The relationship to hemopericardium in the index attack is also evident in many patients, who will also have had early tamponade more frequently than with other kinds of acute pericarditis. Unusual cases of pericardial injury result from lightning and perhaps other electrical trauma or epicardial instrumentation, like epicardial pacemaker or defibrillator implantation.

Foreign-body pericarditis (page 381) has been observed with projectiles retained in the thorax following industrial accidents, explosions and, notably, bullets and shrapnel. Such objects lie either within or adjacent to the pericardium. Pericarditis may occur at the time of injury and recur days to weeks later and over a period of years, with susceptibility to recurrent effusions as well as recurrent pain. (Variability results from interim movement and migration of the foreign body.) These may respond to corticosteroid therapy, with the usual penalties of side effects and potential steroid dependence. Surgical removal of the foreign body may be advisable for treatment of recurrent or constrictive pericarditis, to prevent embolism of the foreign material or associated thrombi, and because of the danger of infection and myocardial damage.

Systemic disorders involving the pericardium are outlined in Tables 7.1 and 8.1. The most important of these are in the vasculitis–connective tissue disease group (pages 314–333), especially disseminated lupus erythematosus. An unusual cause among these is the hypocomplementemic urticarial vasculitis syndrome that involves the skin and pericardium (page 328), characterized by recurrences related to immune complex disposition in the pericardium. In young patients with thalassemia major, the frequency of recurrent pericarditis remains unexplained, although it is somewhat more common in those having had splenectomy. Recurrent pericarditis with inflammatory bowel disease (page 326) is on a fairly firm immunopathic basis, as is that accompanying dermatitis herpetiformis. Dermatitis herpetiformis may be related to celiac disease in that there may be both malabsorption and deposition of IgA, IgG and complement in the pericardium—that is, immune complex deposition as the common basis of recurrent pericarditis. Rarely, patients with inflammatory bowel disease have pericarditis as the first manifestation, in advance of gastrointestinal symptoms, and only later relapse. Here, an immunopathic basis is suggested also by accompanying migratory large-joint arthritis. However, recurrent pericarditis in such patients can occur with and without symptoms, asymptomatic recurrences being revealed by pericardial rubs and occasional effusions. The recurrent polyserositis of familial Mediterranean fever only rarely involves the pericardium and does not appear to predispose to constriction.

Further examples of the probable immunopathic basis of many pericarditic recurrences is the group involving *hypersensitivity* and manifest *"allergy,"* particularly with repeated exposures to ingestants, inhalants and injectants. Pericarditic responses to *drugs* occur with and without drug-induced lupus and include agents including phenylbutazone, quinidine, procainamide and hydralazine (Table 22.1). Food allergies include pericarditis in response to gluten ingestion, specifically with celiac disease. In any case, celiac disease rarely may first present as a recurrent pericarditis that responds to a gluten-free diet. Injectants include immunizations for various illnesses and for immunotherapy or allergic "desensitization," which has provoked recurrent pericarditis, as has the serum-sickness syndrome following parenterally administered agents, including blood products.

Malignancies involving the pericardium (Chapter 18) are obvious causes of pericardial relapses, although these usually occur within a brief time period and are due either to inadequate eradication of malignant tissue in the initial attack or to new metastases. Patients with pericardial malignancies, either primary or metastatic, have a prognosis for life of at best only a few months, curtailing any propensity to recurrence or chronicity.

MANAGEMENT

With a confirmed etiology, there may be specific management. For the majority of patients suffering mainly from recurrent idiopathic pericarditis—irrespective of whether the index attack was demonstrably viral—treatment has been extremely difficult. This is because a corticosteroid agent (nearly always prednisone) has either been used injudiciously or when other anti-inflammatory agents have failed to suppress this extremely uncomfortable syndrome. The patient is thus maintained in a steroid-dependent state, producing *incessant pericarditis*, which, by definition, is due to inability to discontinue corticosteroid therapy without relapses. Patients with the *intermittent recurrent form* are much luckier, since they require treatment only for relapses and generally avoid the many corticosteroid side effects that appear sooner or later in most patients receiving chronic corticosteroid treatment. (A single uncontrolled trial of high dose prednisone with aspirin requires confirmation by appropriately designed studies.) Consequently, the most important consideration to prevent recurrent and incessant pericarditis is to avoid corticosteroid therapy if at all possible and to reduce corticosteroid dosage to zero by weaning patients judiciously, relying on aspirin or one of the newer nonsteroidal anti-inflammatory drugs (NSAIDs), particularly ibuprofen. (Other agents, specifically immunosuppressant and cytotoxic drugs often used in oncology and in organ transplantation, have not proved to be dependably effective for recurrent pericarditis. A prospective, well-designed clinical trial may determine their value.) In patients in the "coronary" ages, indomethacin, which reduces coronary flow, should be avoided. Side effects of NSAIDs are summarized in Table 8.5.

Any effective NSAID may be tried at the lowest adequate dose; all NSAIDs attack the gastrointestinal mucosa. Overall, ibuprofen is the safest, and it has the widest dose range. Observation is required for possible gastrointestinal and other side effects, including renal damage, and particularly in older patients. The largest challenge, requiring high doses of ibuprofen, is to wean patients who are "steroid hooked." It must be emphasized that there are *no appropriately designed controlled prospective studies*; in their absence, *absolute recommendations cannot be given.* One can only offer "experience" as a potentially useful tenth-rate alternative to an appropriately controlled trial. In my experience, escalating doses of ibuprofen, while slowly reducing prednisone, appear to have given good results. *There are no fixed rules.* This must be a trial of "permutations and combinations," fine-tuned for the individual patient by the physician. Prednisone may be reduced from whatever level keeps the patient symptom-free in decrements of as little as 1 mg. Doses can be reduced at intervals of between 1 week and 2 months, while introducing colchicine (see below) and ibuprofen beginning with 800 mg every 8 hr to a maximum of 1200 mg every 6 hr, if the patient can tolerate this, under careful observation.

Chapter 24

Colchicine appears to be an extremely promising adjunct to treatment (perhaps ultimately a principal treatment). Indeed, it should probably be used for the index attack of viral or idiopathic pericarditis in patients who can tolerate it (in my experience, most patients), because it clearly appears to reduce recurrences. It is also useful during weaning from prednisone, can accompany NSAID therapy and has been effective as monotherapy. The dose is 0.5 to 1 mg per day (1 mg probably being better); it is uncertain whether a loading dose of 2 to 3 mg is needed at the beginning of treatment. Colchicine is amazingly well tolerated, even by patients who develop diarrhea or nausea and even mild leukopenia; it requires especially careful observation for these usually dose-dependent effects and a variety of rare but important complications usually accompanying long-term use. Since successful NSAID treatment itself should be carefully weaned over a period of weeks to months, colchicine therapy may be maintained for 4 to 6 months after apparent success. Colchicine is also useful in postpericardiotomy and post–myocardial infarction syndromes and has been used in systemic lupus erythematosus.

Colchicine is a remarkable drug with many actions. It is traditionally known as an effective agent for gout and for inhibiting mitoses in the cell nucleus; it binds to tubulin; it inhibits various polymorphonuclear leukocyte functions; it interferes with transcellular movement of collagen. In these roles, it may help to reduce or block immunologic triggering mechanisms when given early enough and probably has immunosuppressant and antifibroplastic properties when used early or late. As with NSAIDs and even corticosteroids, the precise place of colchicine therapy awaits large, well-controlled clinical trials.

Recurrent pericardial effusions are rarely a problem under the foregoing conditions. If they are large or there is any degree of tamponade, they should be drained; if they quickly refill, there should be catheter drainage for several days, while drug therapy is maintained. Failure mandates pericardiectomy. Malignancies, of course, often require sclerosing agents that may be needed to "dry" the pericardium by causing adhesions, or a pericardiopleural fenestration (window) or pericardioperitoneal shunt (pages 309–310).

Rare patients with *chronic hemopericardium* have had fluctuating symptoms that might be grouped under recurrent pericarditis. Among these, some are tuberculous, though most are idiopathic. Drainage of some of these effusions seems to provoke rapid constriction (like that in some cases of cholesterol pericarditis; pages 85–86). Such patients are probably better treated with pericardial resection following a diligent search for specific "treatable" diagnoses.

EXERCISE RESTRICTION

As with most other treatment of recurrent pericarditis, the absence of appropriately designed controlled trials limits the objectivity of exercise restriction.

Personal experience over more than 20 years strongly suggests that exercise contributes to exacerbations and recurrences of pericarditis and that restriction of exercise can be a decisive component of treatment in these always very difficult cases. It is uncertain exactly when to seriously restrict exercise. However, when a patient being weaned from prednisone or other corticosteroid has relapses during the process or approaches a previously known threshold dose for relapses, it appears important not only to restrict deliberate exercise but also most exertion involved in daily living beyond what is necessary to perform essential domestic tasks and do sedentary work. The psychologic effects of any unaccustomed illness must be considered. The exact amount of restriction, of course, cannot be known without clinical trials. Yet it appears that the quieter a patient's life-style can be physically, the less difficult it is to eventually reduce anti-inflammatory treatment to zero. The appropriate compromise for each patient must be reached between patient and physician by trial and error. Recent evidence suggesting that exercise affects T lymphocytes in a significant way may be related to this factor in dealing with such self-cycling immunopathies as most recurrent pericarditides appear to be.

KEY POINTS

1. Almost any kind of acute pericarditis can recur indefinitely. Most cases are "idiopathic," presumably originally viral. Others are typically recurrent syndromes like the post–cardiac injury syndrome (PCIS), including the postpericardiotomy syndrome (PPS), and the post–myocardial infarction syndrome (PMIS). Direct and indirect evidence ascribes such recurrences to probable immunopathic mechanisms that are well demonstrated among members of the vasculitis–connective tissue disease group.
2. A few infections, particularly by chronically aggressive and incompletely suppressed organisms, can cause limited pericarditic recurrences.
3. *Incessant pericarditis* denotes mainly "idiopathic" pericarditis that flares upon reduction or cessation of anti-inflammatory treatment, nearly always a corticosteroid. The main symptom is disabling chest pain, usually without objective signs of inflammation. Medical treatment is difficult, requiring individualized, carefully tailored reduction of steroid intake and introduction of a nonsteroidal anti-inflammatory drug and colchicine, as tolerated, while reducing physical activity at critical dosage thresholds for symptom breakthrough. Surgical therapy nearly always fails if the patient had been corticosteroid-dependent.

BIBLIOGRAPHY

Adler, Y., Zandman-Goddard, G., Ravid, M., et al. Usefulness of colchicine in preventing recurrences of pericarditis. Am. J. Cardiol. 1994; 73:916–917.

Clementy, J., Jambert, H., Dallacchio, M. Les pericardites aigues recidivantes: 20 observations. Arch. Mal Coeur 1979; 72:857–864.

Fowler, N.O., Harbin, A.D. III. Recurrent acute pericarditis: Follow-up study of 31 patients. J. Am. Coll. Cardiol. 1986; 7:300–310.

Kopecky, S.L., Callahan, J.A., Tajik, A.J., Seward, J.B. Percutaneous pericardial catheter drainage: Report of 42 consecutive cases. Am. J. Cardiol. 1986; 58:633–635.

Laine, L.A., Holt, K.M. Recurrent pericarditis and celiac disease. JAMA 1984; 252:3168–3170.

Millaire, A., DeGroote, P., Decoulx, E., et al. Treatment of recurrent pericarditis with colchicine. Eur. Heart J. 1994; 15:120–124.

Molnar, T.F., Jeyasingham, K. Pericardioperitoneal shunt for persistent pericardial effusions: A new drainage procedure. Ann. Thorac. Surg. 1992; 54:569–570.

Muir, P., Nicholson, F., Tilzey, A.J., et al. Chronic relapsing pericarditis and dilated cardiomyopathy: Serological evidence of persistent enterovirus infection. Lancet 1989; 1:804–807.

Permanyer, M.G., Sagrista-Sauleda, J., Shabetai, R., et al. Pericarditis aaguda: Algunos aspectos del diagnostico etiologico del tratamiento. In: Soler-Soler, J., Premanyer-Miralda, G., Sagrista-Sauleda, J. (eds.). Enfermedades del Pericardio. Barcelona: Ediciones Doyma, 1988, pp. 5–22.

Spodick, D.H. Infective pericarditis: Etiologic and clinical spectra. In: Reddy, P.S. (ed.). Pericardial Disease. New York: Raven Press, 1982, pp. 307–312.

Spodick, D.H. Pericarditis in systemic diseases. Cardiol. Clin. 1990; 8:706–716.

Spodick, D.H., Southern, J.F. A 55-year-old man with recurrent pericarditis and pleural effusions after aortic valve replacement: Case Records of the Massachusetts General Hospital, case 23-1992. N. Engl. J. Med. 1992; 326:1550–1557.

Spodick, D.H. Diseases of the pericardium. In: Chatterjee, K.C., Karliner, J., Rapaport, E., et al. (eds.). Cardiology: An Illustrated Text/Reference. Vol. 2. New York and London: Gower, 1991, chap. 10, pp. 38–64.

Spodick, D.H. Postmyocardial infarction syndrome (Dressler's syndrome). ACC Curr. J. Rev. 1995; 4:35–37.

25

Chronic Pericardial Effusion and Chronic Cardiac Tamponade

Definition and General Perspective

Chronic pericardial effusion represents excessive pericardial fluid remaining, arbitrarily for at least 3 months, in association with disorders of diverse etiology and pathogenesis. The vast majority of cases are idiopathic, presumably following viral or other burnt out infectious effusions, and are large to massive—a good example of pericardial adaptation over time. Table 25.1 outlines recognized etiologies, including inflammations of the pericardium and the heart and noninflammatory conditions predisposing to local and generalized fluid accumulation. Untreated chronic effusions present for months to many years can measure as much as 3 or 4 L, particularly those of inflammatory origin. They tend to be larger than acute effusions because chronicity with slow fluid formation permits greater relaxation of the parietal pericardium. Problems may be confined to the pericardium or may include cardiac and systemic diseases. Relatively few patients give a reliable history of acute pericarditis and the time of onset usually cannot be estimated. Yet some chronic effusions of known etiology behave exactly like chronic idiopathic cases, because of the slow tempo of the process. An interesting difference from idiopathic and other acute pericarditis is that there appears to be a female predominance in this group not only, as expected, in the large vasculitis–connective tissue disease group but also in chronic idiopathic effusion.

Chapter 25

Table 25.1 Etiopathogenesis of Chronic Pericardial Effusion and Chronic Tamponade

A. Idiopathic
B. Others
    I. Congestive heart failure (any etiology, mainly hydropericardium)
        a. Cardiomyopathies (dilated, restrictive, obstructive)
        b. Congenital heart disease (*esp.* atrial septal defect (ASD): hyrdo-pericardium or fibrinous)
        c. Other
    II. Heart disease without failure
        a. Cor pulmonale
        b. Chronic rheumatic
        c. Endomyocardial fibrosis
        d. Other
    III. Infections—active or remote
        a. Virus/idiopathic pericarditis syndrome
        b. Tuberculosis/pericardial cold abscess
        c. Fungi (*esp. Histoplasma, Actinomyces*)
        d. Parasites (e.g. *Toxoplasma, Echinococcus*, amebas)
        e. AIDS: multiple organisms; ? HIV
        f. Other
    IV. Vasculitis–connective tissue disease
        a. Rheumatoid arthritis
        b. Systemic lupus erythematosus
        c. Scleroderma
        d. Polyarteritis
        e. Grand cell arteritis
    V. Trauma
        a. Radiation
        b. Chest trauma
        c. Cardiopericardial surgery
        d. Other
    VI. Immunopathies
        a. Post–myocardial/pericardial injury
            1. Post–myocardial infarction syndrome (PMIS)
            2. Postpericardiotomy syndrome (PPS), *esp.*
                a. Congenital defect repair (e.g. ASD; endocardial cushion defect)
                b. Transplantation: cyclosporine a major factor
                c. Others
        b. ANA-positive patients without lupus
        c. Hypothyroidism, *esp.* myxedema following primary atrophic thyroiditis
        d. Postmyocarditis/myopericarditis
        e. Other

Table 25.1   Continued

   VII.   Metabolic disorders
         a. Renal
            1. Uremia
            2. Nephrotic syndrome
         b. Myxedema (tamponade rare)
         c. ? Acromegaly
         d. ? Alcoholism (? cardiomyopathy)
         e. Hypoalbuminemia
         f. Scurvy
         g. Other
  VIII. Cholesterol pericarditis:
         Idiopathic, myxedema, rheumatoid arthritis, tuberculosis
    IX.   Chylopericardium: primary, secondary
         Note: If not following inflammation, possibly inducing secondary inflammation
         due to chylous irritation
     X.   Lymphopericardium (pericardial lymphangiectasis)
    XI.   Neoplasia: benign or malignant (slow-growing)
         a. Atrial myxoma
         b. Angiosarcoma
         c. Mesothelioma
         d. Kaposi's sarcoma (primary; AIDS)
         e. Thymoma; thymic cyst
         f. Metastases
             1. Solid (e.g., lung, breast, pheochromocytoma)
            2. Leukemia, lymphoma
            3. Pericardial lymphangioma, lymphangiectasis
            4. Other
   XII. Hematologic disorders
         a. Severe anemias (*esp.* congenital)
            1. Thalassemia
            2. Pernicious anemia
            3. Other
         b. Polycythemias
         c. Clotting disorders
         d. Bleeding disorders (including scurvy)
         e. Heterotopic myelopoiesis in pericardium
  XIII. Drug-induced, *esp.* procainamide, hydralazine, cyclosporine, methyldopa
  XIV. Pregnancy
   XV. Massive pulmonary embolism
  XVI. Idiopathic polyserositis

Importance of Chronic Pericardial Effusions

Chronic pericardial effusions may cause problems stemming solely from their own manifestations or from effects on the signs, symptoms, diagnosis and management of other conditions, particularly intrinsic heart disease. These problems include:

1. Chronic cardiac tamponade
2. Symptoms and signs owing to local effects of persistent inflammatory activity
3. Combination with or progression to constrictive pericarditis, including effusive-constrictive and localized constrictive pericarditis
4. Production of inflammatory pericardial cysts and diverticula
5. Distortion of clinical, pathophysiologic and graphic signs of associated or coexistent heart disease

Incidence

Except in some recognized forms like myxedema (page 296) the incident of chronic pericardial effusions is uncertain. *Large postinflammatory chronic effusions* appear only sporadically and are the source of most of the clinical problems. Various kinds of *noninflammatory hydropericardium* (pages 130–131) are common, particularly those recognized at autopsy, but these are likely to be relatively small and clinically silent, while most patients with effusion-related chest symptoms are diagnosed during life.

Classification and Etiology

While the association of pericardial effusion with a systemic or even a cardiac disorder is not of itself proof of an etiologic connection, diseases typically causing acute pericardial effusion are potential sources of chronic effusion and tamponade; noninflammatory disorders are more likely to produce chronic noncompressing hydropericardium. Pathogenetic classification by etiology is indicated in Table 25.1. A working *clinical classification* is as follows:

A. Anatomic
    1. Without significant pericardial changes
    2. With pericardial thickening
    3. With pericardial adhesions, including loculations
B. Functional
    1. Noncompressing, with or without symptoms
    2. Causing chronic cardiac tamponade
    3. Associated with some form of constrictive pericarditis

General Comments on Etiologic Forms

Idiopathic effusions of inflammatory origin may represent viral infection or "burnt out" bacterial, fungal or connective tissue disease. *Pyogenic bacteria* tend to cause acute effusions but have been found in chronic pericardial exudates and may be an unexpected postmortem finding. *Tuberculosis* can cause chronic pericardial effusions including larger or smaller pericardial cold abscesses (pages 269–274). The same is true of actinomycosis and other *fungi*. While *pericardial trauma* of any origin (page 369) can cause critical acute tamponade or constriction, trauma may be followed by *chronic hemopericardium*, which is also occasionally seen with some neoplasms, including *primary pericardial sarcoma* and *Kaposi's sarcoma*, and various *hemorrhagic diseases*. The main *connective tissue and related disorders* associated with chronic effusions include *lupus erythematosus, rheumatic heart disease, scleroderma, polyarteritis*, and especially *rheumatoid arthritis*. *Lympho-pericardium* is uncommon and follows lymphatic obstruction, lymphangioma, or rarely, communication of the thoracic duct with the pericardium (usually after cardiothoracic surgery). Chronic effusive *cholesterol pericarditis* has multiple causes (pages 85–86). *Endomyocardial fibrosis* may be accompanied by and can present as a large pericardial effusion. *Congenital heart lesions*, especially *atrial septal defect*, and *atrial thrombi* rarely are associated with massive chronic pericardial effusions. *Supervoltage irradiation* for thoracic and cervical tumors occasionally produces large, slowly absorbed or nonabsorbed effusions. *Metabolic causes* include *myxedema* and *uremia*. Chronic pericardial effusion in patients who seem to have only hypertension is probably not a direct result of the hypertension, as was once believed. *Hematologic disorders* associated with chronic pericardial effusion include polycythemia and severe, mainly "congenital" anemias—notably *thalassemia* and *pernicious anemia*; rarely, *heterotopic myelopoiesis* in the pericardium provokes a large effusion. *Scurvy* produces both acute and chronic hemopericardium.

PATHOLOGIC CHARACTERISTICS

Generalities

Structural pericardial abnormalities and the characteristics of the pericardial fluid in chronic effusion largely depend on the causative disorders. The fluid, especially in idiopathic chronic effusion, is usually clear and straw-colored with mainly exudative characteristics: specific gravity exceeding 1.014 and protein levels 4 to 5 g/dL. However, *transudate and exudate borderlines may be indistinct* and a transudate, which is characteristic of heart failure–induced effusions, can occur even with inflammatory changes in pericardial tissue. Pericardial tissue usually shows no acute changes and may be strictly fibrotic, with variable adhesions and loculations, sometimes with cyst formation, with or without chronic cardiac tamponade. Indeed, specific histologic changes are uncommon even in cases related to a known disease process. Yet subacute inflammation and a fibrinous pericarditis is occasionally superimposed on chronic changes. Sometimes blood pigment is deposited in the pericardium, following hemopericardium of any origin and in patients with severe congenital anemias.

In general, when the effusion is not inflammatory, the pericardium may be normal or only slightly thickened and without adhesions and the fluid tends to be a transudate. In contrast, inflammation causes one or both pericardial layers to be thickened and fibrosed with internal adhesions, including loculations containing exudative fluids, blood or pus. Inflammatory fluids are more often under pressure, producing chronic tamponade with or without associated constriction. Occasional *pericardial calcification* is usually confined to the visceral pericardium.

Relation to Congestive Heart Failure

Unless complicated by uremic or other pericarditis, non-compressing hydropericardium (pages 130–131) accompanying congestive failure usually results from the abnormal cardiocirculatory physiology, particularly venous hypertension and the general tendency to retain fluid. Such effusions tend to be small, even in rheumatic heart disease, unless there is rheumatic activity.

Association with Constrictive Pericarditis

Constriction is not a rare concomitant or sequela of chronic pericardial effusions of inflammatory origin, probably due to incomplete absorption of fluid and blood after acute or subacute pericarditis. Indeed, residual fluid is one cause of apparent cardiomegaly in constrictive pericarditis (page 230). Such effusions may or may not contribute independently to cardiac compression, which depends on the state of a parietal pericardium that is sometimes sufficiently scarred to limit yielding, thereby permitting cardiac compression by even slowly accumulating pericardial fluid. However, *constrictive epicarditis* (page 253) is the principal cause of constriction accompanying chronic effusion, i.e., *chronic effusive-constrictive pericarditis*. Occasionally, both pericardial layers are separated by fluid, but independently cicatrized without adhesions, or there may be local constriction. Distortion by scarring may involve one or both venae cavae. *Amebic pericarditis* (page 284) usually causes effusive-constrictive pericarditis only after an interval of acute or chronic effusion if the patient survives the initial pericardial invasion and the culprit organism.

Many large, chronic effusions, even when accompanied by pericardial calcification, do not develop significant cardiac compression, either by constriction or tamponade. Yet *constriction sometimes develops rapidly after drainage of a long-standing effusion*, possibly by exciting previously low-grade inflammatory activity.

Pathogenesis

Chronic pericardial effusions can be produced by serosal injury in experimental subjects surviving the phase of acute pericarditis. The pathogenesis of clinical disease—symptoms and signs—is probably that of acute effusions (pages 126–128), accentuated by pericardial thickening and prolonged obstruction of lymphatics and veins. This can be seen, for example, in patients with a history of acute rheumatic fever with or without rheumatic heart disease. *Idiopathic effusions* may increase osmotically due to high protein levels, since large molecules are poorly transported, even by the normal pericardium. In *chronic hemopericardium*, osmotic attraction may additionally occur from fragmentation of blood constituents, resembling the mode of fluid accretion in pleural and subdural hematomas; it is accentuated by any generalized fluid retention, resistance to normal fluid removal (venous hypertension; lymphatic blockade) and decreased plasma oncotic pressure (e.g. hypoalbuminemia), some or all of which may complicate chronic effusions, especially those leading to chronic cardiac tamponade.

PATHOPHYSIOLOGY

Chronic pericardial effusions give rise to four functional situations:

1. Slow production of small amounts of fluid undetected during life
2. Clinically demonstrable effusion without apparent symptoms or signs of cardiac compression
3. Smaller or larger effusion at a rate appropriate to compress the heart but eventually balanced by compensatory mechanisms to stabilize at some level of compression
4. Recurrent or progressive chronic cardiac tamponade

As in acute effusions, these functional states depend on the capacity of the pericardial fibrosa to stretch; any scarring limits this. Significant degrees of cardiac compression evoke compensatory responses that may or may not succeed in maintaining the circulation in the face of increasing intrapericardial pressure (page 187). Thus, the physiologic borderline between a stabilized though compressing effusion and progressive tamponade is indistinct; *tam-*

ponade, acute or chronic, is not "all or none" (page 181). There is persistent danger of destabilization and decompensation by hemorrhage or increased exudation due to renewed inflammatory activity. Yet, many chronic effusions remain indefinitely at relatively low or modestly increased pressure (see low-pressure tamponade; pages 165–167).

In some patients with congestive failure and a hydropericardium, pericardial pressure decreases with drainage, along with decreased cardiac pressures, indicating mild cardiac compression. Alternately, pericardial pressure may be somewhat elevated, well on the positive side of zero, but less than right atrial pressure; drainage reduces the pericardial pressure without significant effect on the cardiac pressure. In either case, mean atrial pressures and ventricular diastolic pressures are significantly different from pericardial pressure; this is not expected with overt cardiac tamponade.

Physical Effects

The mere presence of significantly increasing pericardial fluid resembles the effect with acute effusions. *Insulation of the heart* may diminish heart sound integrity. Electrocardiographic (ECG) changes include modestly decreased voltage (sparing the P waves, which generally remain normal) except in myxedema, where true QRS-T microvoltage tends to occur; T waves may be inverted, probably an effect of inflammation if there is no heart disease. Drainage usually improves QRS- and T-wave voltage. Clinically, the most important physical effect of large effusions is *encroachment on contiguous structures*, causing restrictive pulmonary impairment with dyspnea on exertion, hoarseness, hiccough and dysphagia. Large, chronic effusions are most likely to cause a Bamberger-Pins-Ewart sign (page 131).

CHRONIC CARDIAC TAMPONADE; COMPENSATION, STABILIZATION, DECOMPENSATION

Chronic tamponade resembles chronic constrictive pericarditis. Diminution in cardiac output is comparable, resembling that in both constriction and acute tamponade. In chronic tamponade, if there is no scarring of the epicardium, ventricular filling halts less abruptly than in constriction. While compensatory mechanisms are similar, the circulating blood volume is likely to be more expanded than in acute tamponade. Within limits, tachycardia maintains minute cardiac output in the presence of a relatively fixed stroke volume. Many patients tolerate even very large stable chronic effusions amazingly well with minimal or no symptoms and signs, at least at rest. Others reach a stage of relentlessly increasing cardiac compression—or one of prolonged debility with serious complications owing to chronically diminished cardiac output and congested viscera.

CLINICAL MANIFESTATIONS

General Considerations

Most symptoms and signs of chronic effusions are directly referable to the burgeoning pericardial mass, any degree of chronic cardiac compression, and residual pericardial inflammation, modified by any cardiac disease. Noninflammatory effusions rarely cause significant tamponade and their clinical setting is dominated by the underlying disease. Chronicity makes symptoms "late" or nil, and such quiet chronic effusions, particularly in idiopathic cases, are often accidentally discovered. This can be by chest films showing a discrepancy between the "enlarged heart" and the clear lung fields. Others first present as systemic congestion with signs of increased blood volume and reduced renal function due to chronic tamponade, or chronic effusive-constrictive pericarditis. Unless precipitated or complicated by recent intercurrent illness or residual inflammation, there are no abnormal acute phase reactants, like elevated white cell counts, sedimentation rates and C-reactive protein. Patients with *noninflammatory effusions* usually have had clear-cut signs and symptoms of the responsible disease, particularly by the time the effusion is large. Symptomatic patients with *inflammatory infusions* occasionally have had one or more recognized attacks of acute or recurrent pericarditis with a well-defined transition to the chronic stage in some, but this history is remote in the majority. A few have had pleurisy or vague chest pains; others give a history consistent with some provoking disorder, such as trauma (Chapter 21). Usually, however, there is no recognizable acute phase and illness begins more or less insidiously with progressive pericardial enlargement that may stabilize or progressively compress the heart.

Symptoms and Signs

In general, manifestations can resemble those of acute effusions (pages 130–131) or tamponade (pages 154–158). However, many patients have only vague chest discomforts or aches and chronic fatigue. Indeed, systemic complaints like fatigue, anorexia and weight loss may dominate the picture. Some have exercise-induced tachycardia and palpitations. Yet in the absence of anemia, others have relatively good exercise tolerance. Blood pressure tends to be low but occasional patients are hypertensive, even with some degree of cardiac compression. There is no abnormal third heart sound unless due to effusive-constrictive pericarditis or to accompanying heart disease.

Course

The course varies according to pathogenetic factors: bland versus actively inflammatory effusion; pure chronic tamponade; or effusive-constrictive pericarditis. With any degree of tamponade, resemblance to chronic constriction includes a *tendency to develop atrial fibrillation* as well as *myocardial atrophy* with chronicity; *liver congestion*, which can ultimately induce "cardiac cirrhosis"; *the nephrotic syndrome*; and *protein-losing enteropathy*. Chronic tamponade can also exist as a form of low-pressure tamponade (page 165) with pericardial and right atrial pressures only 4 to 8 mm Hg; after drainage, the pericardial pressure becomes negative. Drainage, however, frequently results in refilling; in some cases drainage appears to provoke rapid constrictive or effusive-constrictive pericarditis. These complications may also be precipitated by systemic or respiratory infections following long periods of stability. When constrictive epicarditis supervenes in an untapped effusion, signs of increasing circulatory impairment appear with little or no change in the enlarged cardio-pericardial silhouette; more typical pericardial constriction follows drainage when such signs are accompanied by a shrinking silhouette. In any case, the possibilities of increasing tamponade or eventual constriction make indefinitely prolonged observation mandatory in all patients in whom pericardiectomy has not been performed.

DIAGNOSIS: CLINICAL AND GRAPHIC

General Considerations

Clinical findings can help suggest the diagnosis of chronic pericardial effusion with or without tamponade but are of limited value. A definite history of antecedent pericarditis and the occasional presence of a chronic rub give added weight to probable inflammatory etiology. However, these are the exceptions; identifying pericardial fluid and tamponade by clinical and graphic methods is the same as for acute effusion and tamponade. Readily available *imaging methods, especially echocardiography*, easily demonstrate the fluid and any accompanying heart disease, related or not to the pericardial disorder. Evidence of pericardial calcification is characteristic of a chronic postinflammatory state. *The ECG* is of little value, low voltage of the QRS-T being common and quite nonspecific as are any T-wave abnormalities (Figure 25.1). Low voltage is probably related to myocardial atrophy, fluid retention and any pleural effusions as well as the pericardial effusion. *Noninflammatory effusions* produce little or no ECG evidence other than that of any underlying heart disease.

Effusions with an inflammatory background may have any or all the ECG abnormalities of constrictive pericarditis—i.e., those associated with chronic subepicardial myocarditis and chronic cardiac compression. These include persistence of the widespread Stage III T-wave inversions of acute pericarditis (page 41) and frequently wide, bifid P waves due to interatrial block, which predisposes to *atrial arrhythmias*, notably fibrillation and occasionally flutter.

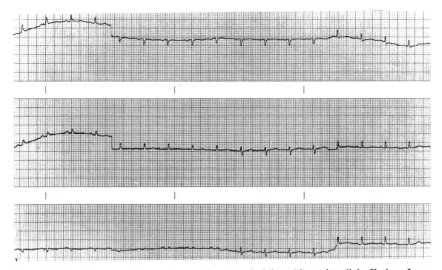

Figure 25.1 Electrocardiogram in massive chronic idiopathic pericardial effusion. Low voltage of QRS-T and nonspecific T-waves abnormalities (all T waves disproportionately low). P waves normal.

"Regional" ECG effects of any unequal epicardial constriction (page 253) may also affect the ECG because, unlike generalized cardiac compression, individual cardiac chambers and structures are differentially compressed; thus, for example, compression of the left atrium or A-V groove can give ECG as well as clinical and physiologic signs suggesting mitral stenosis. Complications like myocardial atrophy and atrial thrombosis may also contribute.

Etiologic diagnosis depends on conclusive demonstration of causative disorders—usually not possible in the vast majority of idiopathic cases and those following "burned out" infectious pericarditis. Pericardial fluid and tissue obtained surgically, by biopsy or necropsy may yield evidence from appropriate bacteriologic, immunologic and histologic techniques. Indeed, histologically "nonspecific" tissue may yield evidence of prior infection, like traces of tuberculous or viral RNA sequences.

MANAGEMENT OF CHRONIC PERICARDIAL EFFUSION

Treatment of patients with chronic pericardial effusion must be individualized, considering presence *or absence* of (1) cardiac compression, (2) a detectable causative disorder, (3) inflammatory manifestations, and (4) symptoms due to encroachment on adjacent structures. In general, *inflammatory effusions* tend to require surgical intervention sooner or later, particularly if they cause chronic tamponade; *noninflammatory effusions* usually respond to treatment of associated disease. Ancillary procedures like *aspiration of pleural effusions and ascites* often contribute greatly to symptomatic relief as well as preoperative management.

Although frequently not rewarded, *search for a cause is mandatory*, particularly for curable etiologies like tuberculosis, toxoplasmosis or myxedema, since these give specific therapeutic targets. Management in general is the same as for acute pericardial effusion and tamponade—diagnosis from fluid and biopsy; drainage for relief. However, drainage without resection is seldom adequate, particularly in the idiopathic cases where refilling is common. In contrast, myxedematous effusions respond readily to thyroid therapy, nearly always without drainage. Specific etiologies like tuberculosis require specific therapy. Signs of persistent inflammation call for anti-inflammatory therapy, particularly nonsteroidal agents. Because of potential dependency, corticosteroids should be used only if absolutely necessary—often the case in lupus; nonabsorbable agents may be given intrapericardially. In patients for whom complete pericardial resection is not contemplated, chronic systemic congestion calls for sodium restriction and diuretics.

Decompression by nonsurgical drainage—pericardicentesis—should be relatively slow to avoid cardiac overloading in patients with poor myocardial function; the expanded blood volume and any myocardial atrophy make this more likely than in acute tamponade. After paracentesis, incomplete or tardy improvement in the absence of refilling may be due to myocardial impairment; total failure to improve may signify constrictive epicarditis. After paracentesis, rubs may first appear; preexisting rubs (usually exopericardial; page 27) either disappear or persist. However, *pericardiectomy remains the procedure of choice for chronic inflammatory effusions with or without tamponade*. It may be postponed in the occasional patient who has sustained relief from paracentesis or restricted surgical drainage and appropriate medical measures. However, the tendency of inflammatory chronic effusions to eventually constrict and the morbidity from recurrences strongly favor pericardiectomy. Pleuropericardial fenestration ("window"; page 173) is feasible in patients in whom full thoracotomy or thoracoscopic resection are considered unwarranted. Balloon pericardiostomy (page 143) has been a very successful method. However, fenestration has important disadvantages, including (1) frequent resealing of the stoma,, (2) impossibility of complete dependent drainage, (3) potential constrictive scarring due to irritant action of the procedure, (4) inadequate inspection of the epicardium and (5) incomplete removal of adhesive or inflamed and infected tissue.

INDIVIDUAL FORMS OF CHRONIC PERICARDIAL EFFUSION (TABLE 25.1)

Chronic Idiopathic Effusions

This is *the most common form of chronic pericardial effusion*, with many aspects, other than chronicity, in common with idiopathic acute effusions (page 80), but characterized by *absence of specific findings in pericardial tissue or fluid*, irrespective of whether the fluid is exudative, transudative, clear or hemorrhagic, or whether the patient has cardiac compression. Of course, "idiopathic"—absence of specific findings—is qualified by the extent of investigation in any given case, so that "idiopathic" is a descriptive catch-all. Indeed, the idiopathic group is obviously heterogeneous in origin, although acute viral pericarditis may have been the most common progenitor.

Chronic Infectious Effusions

The etiology, pathology, diagnosis and treatment of tuberculous and other *granulomatous infections* are discussed on pages 269–274. *Tuberculosis* may be the most important of this group. It can be quiescent or indolent for many years and is sometimes loculated ("cold abscess"). More than other identifiable pathogenetic forms, it produces chronic tamponade with or without constrictive epicarditis. The frequency of tuberculous adhesions, particularly at the base of the heart, may distort x-ray and echographic findings, necessitating computed tomography or magnetic resonance imaging. Chronic tuberculous pericarditis is one cause of *cholesterol pericarditis* (page 85), which also produces copious effusions. *Histoplasmosis* and *actinomycosis* can produce pericardial effusions that behave very much like chronic tuberculous effusions. *Pyogenic bacteria*, usually causing acute pericarditis, occasionally appear responsible for chronic effusions. *Viruses* may be an increasingly recognizable underlying cause; newer means of identifying viral evidence should reduce the number of idiopathic effusions.

Chronic Hemopericardium

Hemopericardium is an important result of trauma, bleeding disorders and vascular anomalies, although in chronic hemopericardium the pathogenesis may be untraceable. The pericardial fluid is frankly sanguineous or serosanguineous, particularly in neoplasia, tuberculosis and vasculitis–connective tissue disease. A pericardial fluid hematocrit approaching the blood hematocrit suggests active bleeding.

Rarely, even following wounds of the heart (pages 372–377), tamponade may be sufficiently delayed to qualify as chronic, possibly because of a sealing thrombus or fibrinous adhesions. There is a potential for constriction from intrapericardial bleeding and precipitation of rapid constriction following non-surgical drainage. The pericardium usually contains large quantities of old, chocolatey blood, which may be loculated, often with some evidence of more recent hemorrhage. Bloody sludge and clots rich in fibrin tend to cover the inner parietal pericardium and the epicardium; organization of these is the usual cause of constriction in hemopericardium and may be well advanced at the time of surgical intervention. Pericardial tissue itself usually shows chronic inflammatory changes, evidence of old and recent hemorrhage, blood pigment deposition and occasionally calcification.

Vasculitis–Connective Tissue Disease Group

Small amounts of pericardial fluid are present chronically in many if not most patients with *rheumatoid arthritis* and may or may not reflect activity. Chronic tamponade, like acute tamponade, is rare in this group, always necessitating consideration of other etiologies. *Rheumatic heart disease* appears to have caused many cases of chronic hydropericardium associated with congestive heart failure. Other vasculitides are included in Table 25.1, notably *scleroderma*, in which pericarditis is not rare and diagnostic problems arise from complications like cor pulmonale and congestive heart failure. In scleroderma, pericardial fluid can be unrevealing—an exudate with an electrophoretic pattern like blood plasma. Skin biopsy may indirectly aid the diagnosis.

Neoplastic Effusions

Primary pericardial tumors (page 306), including mesothelioma, hemangioma and lymphangiomatous hamartoma are common neoplastic causes of chronic effusion. The *benign tumors* (page 308) may cause relatively quiescent chronic effusions. *Metastatic and primary malignancies* of the pericardium tend to cause acute effusion and tamponade (Chapter 18). However, even malignant effusions can last for many months if the patient does not die of complications; they may even be noncompressing, although always with a danger of acute tamponade provoked by hemorrhage, rapid increase in exudation, or by irradiation or drug therapy. Rarely, there is deceptive spontaneous regression without treatment. Neoplasia, especially malignancy, should always be considered in effusions of unknown origin, and especially of unknown duration.

Irradiation Pericarditis

Radiation therapy may cause acute pericarditis, with or without effusion and tamponade, or pericardial scarring, including constriction (page 215). Occasionally, irradiation of a thoracic, mediastinal or cervical lesion appears to initiate a chronic pericardial effusion. In some cases, radiation of mediastinal lesions provokes pericardial fibrosis and calcification or superior vena cava obstruction which may complicate differential diagnosis.

Chronic Pericardial Effusions of Metabolic Origin

These have much in common with all metabolic forms of effusive pericarditis (Chapter 17). In the *nephrotic syndrome*, anasarca may be accompanied by excessive pericardial fluid. *Chronic uremia* apparently can produce effusions of fairly long duration, especially with resistance to renal dialysis (page 295). The principal danger in these cases is precipitation of acute tamponade by hemorrhage into an already filled sac. In *myxedema*, pericardial effusion is virtually constant in both experimental and human forms and may precede other manifestations of the disease. There are virtually never any signs of pericardial inflammation, but myxedematous effusions frequently contain many leukocytes, predominantly lymphocytic or even polymorphonuclear. Hemorrhagic effusions are uncommon although pericardial hemorrhage is one mechanism for the rare occurrence of frank tamponade in chronic myxedematous effusions. The fluid is characterized by (1) high cholesterol content, though usually well below the serum cholesterol level; (2) total protein concentrations approaching that of serum proteins but with less globulin; (3) specific gravity well within the "exudate" range. Accompanying myxedematous ascites or anasarca may falsely suggest the picture of chronic cardiac compression. This disorder is nearly always completely reversible by thyroid therapy.

Chronic Effusions Associated with Hematologic Disorders

Chronic effusions, usually hydropericardia of uncertain origin, occur in *thalassemia major* and *pernicious anemia* as well as other severe anemias. In patients with malignancies and bone marrow suppression, *heterotopic myelopoiesis* in the pericardium itself can provoke a small to moderate-sized effusion.

Hydropericardium Associated with Heart Disease

Most patients with congestive heart failure who have not had pericardial disease have minor effusions, which may be chronic and accompanied by general fluid and electrolyte retention. In patients like those who have had acute rheumatic fever, where the pericardium has been scarred, or hydropericardium due to antecedent acute pericarditis, fluid accumulation appears to be larger, without causing tamponade or constriction. Cardiomyopathies, notably dilated cardiomyopathy, and amyloid myocardial disease often have considerable hydropericardium. Isolated *pericardial amyloidosis* can also produce an effusion. Chronic hydropericardium frequently accompanies congenital heart abnormalities, ventricular aneurysms and, notably, *endomyocardial fibrosis* which is associated with large effusions. Although these are noncompressive hydropericardium, an erroneous diagnosis of tamponade is suggested by the markedly restrictive physiology of endomyocardial fibrosis and most amyloid heart muscle disease.

CHYLOPERICARDIUM (SEE ALSO PAGES 84–85)

Chronic chylopericardium with or without tamponade characteristically refills rapidly after drainage; even during thoracotomy, reaccumulation of fluid may be visible. Some communication with the thoracic duct is indicated by the presence of chyle in the pericardium and the intrapericardial appearance of ingested lipophilic dyes, as well as successful treatment by ligation of the thoracic duct. Unlike acute forms, chronic cases have not followed surgical and other trauma or erosive malignancy and are often referred to as *primary chronic chylopericardium*. While chylous pleural and peritoneal effusions usually cause no adhesions, chylopericardium is associated with pericardial inflammation, scarring, and, rarely, constriction. Because chyle is bactericidal, these are likely to be due to the chyle and not to contaminating infections. In any case, the tendency to very large progressive effusion favors chronic tamponade. Definitive treatment is ligation of the thoracic duct low in the right side of the chest, plus resection of any tumor tissue in cases due to neoplasm. Resection of the pericardium should always be considered.

CHOLESTEROL PERICARDITIS
("GOLD-PAINT PERICARDITIS," "LIPID PERICARDITIS")

Chronic Cholesterol Pericarditis (See Also Pages 85–86)

Chronic cholesterol pericarditis is characterized by (1) high pericardial fluid cholesterol and cholesterol crystals, cholesterol deposition, and cholesterol clefts in pericardial tissue, singly or in combination; (2) copious effusions of long duration; (3) apparent multiplicity of etiology and (4) frequently normal serum cholesterol level except in patients with hypothyroidism. Although occasionally clear, the fluid often has a striking variety of colors—white, golden brown, red, greenish or egg yolk; it is usually turbid and can be brightly scintillating (hence, "gold-paint pericarditis"). Moreover, the *cholesterol concentration can vary from high to absent in successive drainages*. The *average cholesterol* in series of cholesterol pericarditis has been approximately 250 mg/dL; *total lipids* may reach almost 3000 mg/dL. After centrifuging, cholesterol concentration in the supernatant usually is considerably less than the total and may even be lower than the approximately 70 mg/dL "normal" threshold (page 449). Most patients have crystals in the fluid most of the time, visible under polarizing light as Maltese crosses; over half of the pericardial biopsies show cholesterol deposits with or without cholesterol clefts.

Grossly, the pericardium is thickened by scarring, frequently with variable amounts of fibrin, yellowish nodules, plaques and papillomatous masses of cholesterol lining its interior. The epicardium may be visibly inflamed and constrictive epicarditis is not uncommon. *Microscopically,* there is variable fibrosis with hyaline changes, infiltrations by lymphocytes, plasma cells, many mononuclear cells and frequently many cholesterol clefts, cholesterol crystals and other lipid crystals in plates, needles and rhomboids; phagocytes, macrophages and giant cells often contain crystals or blood-derived iron pigment. Both intracellular and extracellular lipid can be identified as birefringent particles and by staining with lipophilic dyes. Cholesterol crystals themselves are often surrounded by elements of chronic granulomatous inflammation as well as foreign body giant cells. (In contrast, *hypothyroid cholesterol pericarditis is nearly always the exception* because the pericardial tissue is frequently normal despite high fluid cholesterol. Inflammatory responses and crystallization are extremely rare and when present suggest a pathogenetic role of unrelated pericarditis or pericardial trauma).

Etiology and Pathogenesis

Since approximately half of all patients have no identifiable disease, they qualify as having *idiopathic cholesterol pericarditis.* Many other cholesterol-laden effusions are associated with a wide variety of diseases that cause pericarditis, many of them granulomatous. Rarely, they may accompany conditions like atrial septal defect, mitral stenosis and metastatic malignancy and have been discovered following myocardial infarction. Such associated conditions may be incidental.

Only occasional patients have a history suggesting acute pericarditis or chest trauma. Granulomatous diseases, like rheumatoid arthritis and tuberculosis, seem to be directly implicated, since chronic granulomas are rich in cholesterol. Although it is exceptional to find evidence of active tuberculosis, many patients have positive tuberculin reactions. Pericardial fluids obtained at operations for heart disease suggest that 70 mg/dL cholesterol is the threshold for abnormality. (There is some evidence that acute pericarditis per se can be associated with temporarily increased pericardial cholesterol, because cholesterol is poorly reabsorbed by diseased pericardium.) Moreover, there is slow equilibration of labeled cholesterol between pericardial fluid and serum, suggesting an abnormality of cholesterol transport. This is reinforced by finding chronic pericardial inflammation in almost all biopsies. Three hypotheses have been proposed:

1. Inflammation-induced necrosis of pericardial cells liberates cholesterol, which is then poorly reabsorbed.
2. Chronic hemopericardium, with precipitation of lipids from dissolved red blood cells and inflammatory reactions to lipid fractions perpetuating low-grade pericarditis, sometimes leading to constriction. Indeed, pericardial bleeding can occur at some stage in most forms of pericarditis and is unavoidable during cardiopericardial surgery. However, significant tissue injury is probably needed, as well as chronicity of the hemopericardium, since blood disappears relatively rapidly from the intact pericardium. (However, after most trauma, notably cardiopericardial surgery, even with copious pericardial bleeding and hemolysis, cholesterol pericarditis remains rare.)
3. Inflammatory changes damage lymphatics, decreasing cholesterol absorption, the cholesterol mainly being held in solution as lipoprotein complexes, which have a solubilizing effect. Loss of solubility leads to precipitation of cholesterol crystals. Indeed, mere aging of serous effusions is a significant factor in losing their initially high tendency to keep cholesterol in solution. Thus, *blood is certainly the main source of increased pericardial cholesterol*, and any long-standing effusion could be responsible for cholesterol pericarditis, particularly in the presence of a rich source like hemorrhage. Bacterial modification of cholesterol solubility and subepicardial fat necrosis could be subsidiary mechanisms. Regardless of how cholesterol becomes trapped and precipitates within the pericardium, foreign-body giant cells from granulomatous and other reactions to crystals appear to initiate or perpetuate pericardial inflammation and presumably further effusion. Thus, pericardial disease can cause cholesterol precipitation, which in turn exacerbates pericardial disease.

Hypothyroid patients are fundamentally different. Pericardial inflammation is not necessary and cholesterol is derived from an increased serum cholesterol, which is well transported into and out of the pericardium in the absence of pericardial damage. Unimpeded reabsorption is also part of the excellent response to thyroid hormone therapy if given early enough. Only rarely does long persistence or delayed thyroid therapy become associated with cholesterol pericarditis of a more serious nature. In such cases, inflammatory pericardial responses always pose a question of unassociated pericarditis, hemopericardium or trauma.

Clinical Considerations

Cholesterol effusions tend to be very large, up to 4000 mL, and have been documented for up to 20 years. Chest pain and fever may occur. A few patients develop severe cardiac tamponade. Drainage may give some relief, but the rule is swift refilling. Drainage also occasionally provokes acute epicardial constriction or unremitting tamponade, making pericardiectomy the treatment of choice.

KEY POINTS

1. Most chronic inflammatory pericardial effusions are of unknown etiology ("idiopathic"). Those of clinical significance are large to massive. Noninflammatory hydropericardium is rarely very large and is related to cardiac failure and fluid-retentive systemic diseases; although sometimes complicating diagnosis, it is rarely a therapeutic problem.
2. The wide etiologic spectrum of chronic pericardial effusion necessitates a detailed search for treatable pericardial, cardiac and systemic disorders.
3. Chronicity itself implies that most chronic effusions can be "silent" for long periods. The largest effusions have physical effects on neighboring structures that can be a source of symptoms. The degree and distribution of pericardial scarring determines whether a chronic effusion will progress to chronic tamponade or to constriction or effusive-constrictive pericarditis, which may be precipitated by paracentesis.
4. Although a hydropericardium may have modest compressive effects, chronic cardiac tamponade is nearly always of remote, or reignited, inflammatory origin and resembles both chronic constrictive pericarditis and acute tamponade.
5. Large postinflammatory effusions tend to require surgical intervention. Noninflammatory effusions usually respond to successful management of associated diseases. It *is essential to identify all associated or unassociated cardiac and systemic disorders for differential diagnosis and appropriate management.*
6. Chronic chylopericardium and chronic cholesterol pericarditis are primarily diagnosed from pericardial fluid composition, although biopsy may be necessary for the latter. Each can cause chronic tamponade and constrictive pericarditis. Each refills rapidly after simple drainage. Optimal management is pericardiectomy.
7. Cholesterol pericarditis is usually idiopathic and probably depends on crystal formation following hemopericardium or infective and noninfective granulomatous diseases, like rheumatoid arthritis and tuberculosis. In myxedema, cholesterol-laden effusions are not associated with crystallization or inflammation.

BIBLIOGRAPHY

Brown, A.K. Chronic idiopathic pericardial effusion. Br. Heart J. 1966; 28:609–614.

Cathcart, E., Spodick, D.H. Rheumatoid heart disease: A study of the incidence and nature of cardiac lesions in rheumatoid arthritis. N. Engl. J. Med. 1962; 266:959–964.

Connolly, D.C., Dry, T.J., Good, C.A., et al. Chronic idiopathic pericardial effusion without tamponade. Circulation 1959; 6:1095–1105.

Doherty, J.E., Jenkins, B.J. Radiocarbon cholesterol turnover in cholesterol pericarditis. Am. J. Med. 1966; 41:322–330.

Hastillo, A., Thompson, J.A., Lower, R.R., et al. M.L. Cyclosporine-induced pericardial effusion after cardiac transplantation. Am. J. Cardiol. 1987; 59:1220–1222.

Kane, G.C., Figueroa, W.G. Encroachment upon the lungs of large chronic pericardial effusion—Pulmonary tamponade? Chest 1988; 93:434–436.

Kelly, J.K., Butt, J.C. Fatal myxedema pericarditis in a Christian Scientist. A.J.C.P. 1985; 86:113–116.

Maisch, B. Myocarditis and pericarditis—Old questions and new answers. Herz 1992; 17:65–70.

McCabe, J.C., Engle, M.A., Ebert, P.A. Chronic pericardial effusion requiring pericardiectomy in the postpericardiotomy syndrome. J. Thorac. Cardiol. Vasc. Surg. 1974; 67:814–817.

Pietras, R.J., Lam, W. Large pericardial effusions associated with congenital heart disease: Five-and-eight year follow-up. Am. Heart J. 1988; 115:1334–1336.

Sagrista-Sauleda, J., Permanyer-Miralda, G., Juste-Sanchez, C., et al. Huge chronic pericardial effusion caused by Toxoplasma gondii—Case reports. Circulation 1982; 66:895–897.

Soloff, L.A., Bello, C.T. Pericardial effusion mistaken for cardiac enlargement in severe anemia—Report of two cases. Circulation 1950; 2:298–303.

Spodick, D.H. Chronic pericardial effusion. In: Spodick, D.H. Chronic and constrictive pericarditis. New York: Grune & Stratton, 1964; chap. 25, pp. 279–321.

Spodick, D.H. Clinical manifestations of chronic pericardial effusions. Mod. Med. 1965; 32:289–301.

Spodick, D.H.: "Low voltage ECG" and pericardial effusion. Chest 1979; 75:113–114.

Index

Abnormal breathing, 102
Absence of pulsus paradoxus, 198
Acquired heart lesions, murmurs due to, 38
Actinomyces, 278
Acute benign pericarditis. *See* Idiopathic pericarditis
Acute ischemia, pain in acute pericarditis vs. pain in, 101
Acute myocarditis, 15
Acute pericarditis, 27, 41-56
    atypical ECG variants, 50-55
    early repolarization as mimic of, 59-60
    electrocardiographic variants, 50
    electrogenesis of ECG abnormalities, 45-50
    etiologies of, 98-100
    rate and rhythm abnormalities, 56
    See also Clinically "dry" (noneffective) acute pericarditis
Acute renal failure, uremic pericarditis in, 292, 295
Acute rheumatic fever, 315, 319-320
Adrenal failure, 298
AIDS (and related complex):
    hydropericardium and, 80
    pericardial disease in, 279-282

[AIDS (and related complex)]
    clinical aspects, 281-282
    neoplasia in AIDS, 281
    nonmalignant pericardial disease in AIDS, 280-281
    pericardial effusion in, 5-6
Amebiasis, 284
Amiodarone, 413
Aneurysm, ventricular
    pseudoaneurysm vs., 348
    See also Dissecting aneurysm
Anisotropy, pericardial, 15-16
Anticoagulants, 78
Antiinflammatory agents, 124
Aorta, intramural hemorrhage of, 356-359
Arrhythmias in constrictive pericarditis, 61
Asymptomatic pericardial effusions, 126-128
Atropine, 172
Atypical ECG variants, 50-55
Atypical forms of cardiac tamponade, 188-189
Auscultatory phenomena, 27-39
    ausculatory characteristics, 30-31
    clicks, 28, 37
    effects of pneumohydropericardium, 28, 38

453